a CORE Curriculum for Diabetes Education
Fifth Edition

Diabetes Management Therapies

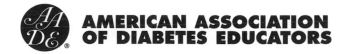

AMERICAN ASSOCIATION OF DIABETES EDUCATORS

a CORE
Curriculum
for Diabetes
Education
Fifth Edition

Diabetes Management Therapies

Editor
Marion J. Franz, MS, RD, LD, CDE

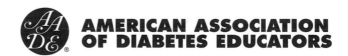

AMERICAN ASSOCIATION OF DIABETES EDUCATORS

a CORE Curriculum for Diabetes Education, 5th Edition
Diabetes Management Therapies
Published by the American Association of Diabetes Educators

©2003, American Association of Diabetes Educators, Chicago, Illinois.
ISBN 1-881876-12-8 (Volume Two)
ISBN 1-881876-15-2 (Four-Volume Set)

Library of Congress Control Number: 2003108781

Printed and bound in the United States of America.

a CORE Curriculum for Diabetes Education

Diabetes Management Therapies

In this Volume:

Table of Contents

Introduction/Acknowledgements vii

Editors ix

Authors x

Reviewers xi

Diabetes Management Therapies

1 Medical Nutrition Therapy for Diabetes 3

2 Physical Activity/Exercise 61

3 Pharmacologic Therapies for Glucose Management 95

4 Pharmacologic Therapies for Hypertension and Dyslipidemia 157

5 Monitoring 189

6 Pattern Management of Blood Glucose 215

7 Insulin Pump Therapy and Carbohydrate Counting for Pump Therapy:

Insulin-to-Carbohydrate Ratios 249

8 Hypoglycemia 279

9 Illness and Surgery 313

Index 337

Other Volumes in CORE Curriculum, 5th Edition:

Diabetes and Complications

1 Pathophysiology of the Diabetes Disease State

2 Hyperglycemia

3 Chronic Complications of Diabetes: An Overview

4 Diabetic Foot Care and Education

5 Skin and Dental Care

6 Macrovascular Disease

7 Eye Disease and Adaptive Diabetes Education for Visually Impaired Persons

8 Nephropathy

9 Diabetic Neuropathy

Diabetes Education and Program Management

1 Applied Principles of Teaching and Learning

2 Psychosocial Assessment

3 Behavior Change

4 Cultural Competence in Diabetes Education and Care

5 Teaching Persons With Low Literacy Skills

6 Psychological Disorders

7 Management Diabetes Education Programs

8 Payment for Diabetes Education

Diabetes in the Life Cycle and Research

1 Lifestyle for Diabetes Prevention

2 Type 1 Diabetes in Youth

3 Type 2 Diabetes in Youth

4 Pregnancy With Preexisting Diabetes

5 Gestational Diabetes

6 Diabetes in Older Adults

7 Biological Complementary Therapies in Diabetes

8 The Importance of Research

Introduction/Acknowledgements

It is an exciting and challenging time for diabetes education. Exciting because of the many advances that help people better manage their diabetes—new medications, technologies, research that makes lifestyle recommendations easier to understand and apply, the empowerment approach to education, to name just a few. The challenges and frustrations are the difficulties of sharing this information with individuals with diabetes, the lack of opportunities to individualize care, and the lack of time to assist in facilitating behavior changes. Resources—personnel, payment for services, maintaining education centers—are other challenges. The CORE Curriculum cannot solve all the challenges, but it can update healthcare providers' knowledge and skills and provide suggestions for facilitating behavior changes in persons with diabetes.

The CORE Curriculum was originally planned to help educators prepare for the Certified Diabetes Educator (CDE) exam. This has continued to be a goal for subsequent editions; however, the use and the scope of the CORE Curriculum has expanded. It is a key reference for the Advanced Diabetes Management credential exam. The CORE Curriculum has also evolved into being an authoritative source of information for diabetes education, training, and management. Just as all medicine is moving toward evidence-based practice, this must also be a goal for education. Chapters must have appropriate and adequate references, and as a reader you have the right to question statements in the CORE Curriculum that do not have adequate documentation. Continuing this focus will result in the CORE Curriculum becoming more evidence-based. Another goal is to have the CORE Curriculum reflect a team approach to education and management. It is exciting to see the number of management chapters written by a team of healthcare providers.

As with all projects of this size, there are many individuals to whom we are indebted. It begins with the chapter authors, who are willing to share their expertise and provide up-to-date information and management skills for the reader. It continues to the chapter reviewers, who provide suggestions to make the chapters stronger. The authors and reviewers are listed in each volume of the CORE Curriculum. When you see these individuals, please extend your thanks to them for the valuable service they provide. The Editorial Board—Janine Freeman, Barbara McCloskey, Charlotte Nath, and William Polonsky—provide suggestions to improve the CORE Curriculum and valuable reviewer assistance. Dr. Lois Book, RN, Director of Professional Relations, at the AADE National Office provides valuable suggestions for CORE content and support for the process of writing and editing of the CORE Curriculum. We are fortunate to work with very competent editorial and publishing professionals. Mary Beach at Stenson Bauer Communications keeps the process moving efficiently. Nancy Williams uses her copyreader and editing skills to make sure small details and mistakes are not missed. Karen Lloyd provides editorial assistance for the new chapters, and Michele Montour at Montronics makes sure text is accurately typeset. To all these important professionals, the AADE owes a great deal of gratitude.

The CORE Curriculum would not be possible without the contributions of previous editors—Diana Guthrie, Julie Meyer, Kathryn Godley, Virginia Peragallo-Dittko, and Martha Funnell. Each edition moved the professionalism of the CORE Curriculum forward, and those who worked on this edition sincerely hope to have continued that tradition. As authors, reviewers, and editors, we have done our best to make this edition a valuable resource for all diabetes educators and healthcare providers. We welcome suggestions from you as you read and use the CORE Curriculum as to how it can become a better and more useful resource. Please use the CORE Curriculum to improve the education and care that you provide for people with diabetes. That ultimately is the final goal, to enrich the lives of persons with diabetes who have been, for all of us, our best educators!

Marion J. Franz, MS, RD, LD, CDE
Editor, CORE Curriculum, 5th Edition

Editor

Marion J. Franz, MS, RD, LD, CDE
Nutrition Concepts by Franz, Inc.
Minneapolis, Minnesota

Editorial Board

Janine Freeman, RD, LD, CDE
Diabetes Nutrition Specialist
Atlanta, Georgia

Barbara A. McCloskey, PharmD, BCPS, CDE
Diabetes Services
Baylor Medical Center
Irving, Texas

Charlotte R. Nath, MSN, RN, EdD, CDE
West Virginia University Department of Family Medicine
Robert C. Byrd Health Sciences Center
Morgantown, West Virginia

William H. Polonsky, PhD, CDE
Department of Psychiatry
University of California
San Diego, California

Authors

Ann Marie Brooks,
MSN, RN, BC-ADM, CDE
St. Marks Hospital
Diabetes Center
Salt Lake City, Utah

R. Keith Campbell,
RPh, MBA, CDE
Washington State University
Pullman, Washington

Karen Hanson Chalmers,
MS, RD, CDE
Joslin Clinic
Boston, Massachusetts

Belinda P. Childs,
MN, ARNP, CDE
Mid-America Diabetes
Associates
Wichita, Kansas

Marion J. Franz,
MS, RD, LD, CDE
Nutrition Concepts
by Franz, Inc.
Minneapolis, Minnesota

Judy Friesen,
RD, LD, FADA, CDE
Via Christi Regional
Medical Center
Wichita, Kansas

Linda A. Gonder-
Frederick, PhD
University of Virginia
Behavioral Medicine Center
Charlottesville, Virginia

Diana W. Guthrie,
PhD, ARNP, FAAN,
BC-ADM, CDE
Professor Emeritus
University of Kansas
School of Medicine
Wichita, Kansas

Richard A. Guthrie,
MD, CDE, FAACE
Mid-America Diabetes
Associates
Via Christi Regional
Medical Center
University of Kansas
School of Medicine
Wichita, Kansas

Deborah Hinnen,
MN, ARNP, BC-ADM, CDE
Via Christi Regional
Medical Center
Wichita, Kansas

Tommy Johnson,
PharmD, CDE
University of Georgia
College of Pharmacy
Athens, Georgia

Elaine Boswell King,
MSN, RN, CS, CDE
Vanderbilt Diabetes Research
and Training Center
Nashville, Tennessee

Karmeen Kulkarni,
MS, RD, BC-ADM, CDE
St. Marks Hospital
Diabetes Center
Salt Lake City, Utah

Janie Lipps,
MSN, RN, CS, CDE
Vanderbilt Diabetes Research
and Training Center
Nashville, Tennessee

Catherine A. Mullooly,
MS, RCEP$_{SM}$, CDE
Joslin Clinic
Boston, Massachusetts

Virginia Peragallo-Dittko,
APRN, BC-ADM, MA, CDE
Diabetes Education Center
Winthrop-University Hospital
Mineola, New York

Diana Speelman Rhiley,
EdS, LCMFT, CDE
Via Christi Regional
Medical Center
Wichita, Kansas

John V. St. Peter,
Pharm D, BCPS
Hennepin Center for
Diabetes and Endocrinology
College of Pharmacy,
University of Minnesota
Minneapolis, Minnesota

John R. White, Jr.,
RPh, PharmD, PA-C
Washington State University
Spokane, Washington

John Zrebiec, MSW
Harvard University
Joslin Diabetes Center
Boston, Massachusetts

Reviewers

Patricia K. Andronica,
RN, MS, CDE
Suffolk County Department
of Health Services
Hauppauge, New York

Gary M. Arsham, MD, PhD
Arsham Consultants, Inc.
San Francisco, California

Roger R. Austin,
MS, RPh, CDE
Henry Ford Health System
Detroit, Michigan

Belinda Childs,
RN, MN, ARNP, CDE
Mid-America Diabetes
Associates
Wichita, Kansas

Anne Daly,
MS, RD, LD, BC-ADM, CDE
Springfield Diabetes and
Endocrine Center
Springfield, Illinois

Janet Davidson,
BSN, RN, CDE
International Diabetes Center
Minneapolis, Minnesota

Janine Freeman,
RD, LD, CDE
Diabetes Nutrition Specialist
Atlanta, Georgia

Sandra J. Gillespie,
MMSc, RD, LD, CDE
Diabetes Resource Center
Piedmont Hospital
Atlanta, Georgia

David M. Kendall, MD
International Diabetes Center
Minneapolis, Minnesota

Barbara A. McCloskey,
PharmD, BCPS, CDE
Diabetes Services
Baylor Medical Center
Irving, Texas

Charlotte R. Nath,
MSN, RN, EdD, CDE
West Virginia University
Department of Family
Medicine
Robert C. Byrd Health
Sciences Center
Morgantown, West Virginia

Diane M. Reader, RD, CDE
International Diabetes Center
Minneapolis, Minnesota

Pamela Scarborough,
PT, MS, CDE, CWS
Education 2000 Plus
Dallas, Texas

Jane W. Schultz,
RN, MSN, CDE
Consultant/Diabetes Educator
Spotsylvania, Virginia

Hope S. Warshaw,
MMSc, RD, CDE
Hope Warshaw Associates
Alexandria, Virginia

Donald K. Zettervall,
RPh, CDE, CDM
The Diabetes Center
Old Saybrook, Connecticut

A Core Curriculum for Diabetes Education
Diabetes Management Therapies

Medical Nutrition Therapy for Diabetes 1

Marion J. Franz, MS, RD, LD, CDE
Nutrition Concepts by Franz, Inc.
Minneapolis, Minnesota

Introduction

1 Diabetes is a chronic progressive disease that usually requires lifestyle changes, especially in the areas of nutrition and physical activity. The goal of medical nutrition therapy (MNT) is to assist persons with diabetes in making self-directed behavior changes that will improve their overall health and the management of their diabetes.

2 Achieving optimal nutrition through healthy food choices is the underlying principle of the American Diabetes Association (ADA) nutrition recommendations for people with diabetes.[1] However, in addition to concerns related to improved health through healthy food choices and physical activity, MNT for diabetes focuses on goals and strategies for the treatment and prevention of diabetes and on achieving optimal metabolic outcomes related to glycemia, lipid profiles, and blood pressure levels.[1-3]

   A The ADA nutrition recommendations for health are similar to the nutrition recommendations for the prevention of chronic diseases from other major health organizations (eg, US Department of Agriculture and US Department of Health and Human Services,[4] American Heart Association,[5] American Institute for Cancer Research[6]).

   B Although many studies have focused on the role of single nutrients, foods, or food groups in disease prevention or promotion, emerging research suggests health benefits from certain food patterns that include a mixture of foods containing multiple nutrients and nonnutrients.[4,7-12]

     • A healthy diet consists of multiple servings of fruits and vegetables, whole grains, low-fat dairy products, fish, lean meats, and poultry.

3 Persons with diabetes report that making changes in their lifestyle is one of the greatest challenges they face in managing their diabetes.[13] Therefore, it is essential that recommendations take into account lifestyle changes the individual with diabetes is willing and able to make and maintain. This requires the person with diabetes to be involved in the decision-making process. Cultural and ethnic preferences also must be taken into consideration.

4 MNT is an essential component of successful diabetes management.[14-18]

5 Medical nutrition therapy (or nutrition therapy) is the preferred term and replaces other terms such as diet, diet therapy, and dietary management. MNT involves the use of specific nutrition services to treat an illness or condition and incorporates the process or system for providing individualized nutrition care and specific lifestyle recommendations for that care. The process of providing care includes assessment, intervention/education, goal setting, and evaluation of outcomes. Lifestyle recommendations include food/nutrition and physical activity strategies.

6 Every individual with diabetes needs a comprehensive treatment approach, which includes

   A An assessment of the individual's knowledge, skills, attitudes, behaviors, cultural and ethnic concerns and what the individual desires to gain from the nutrition sessions.

B An intervention that includes an individualized food/meal plan appropriate for his/her lifestyle and diabetes management goals and education related to diabetes and nutrition therapy and food/meal planning.

C Mutually agreed-upon short-term and long-term goals for lifestyle changes.

D Evaluation of lifestyle change outcomes with appropriate recommendation for changes in lifestyle and/or medication.

E Ongoing education and nutrition care, with regular review and modification, as necessary, of the food/meal plan, management goals, and self-management education.

7 For persons requiring insulin therapy, the goal of MNT is to provide a food/meal plan that integrates an insulin regimen into usual eating and activity patterns.[1,2] For persons with type 2 diabetes, the goal of MNT is to normalize metabolic outcomes. Strategies that can be implemented to achieve this goal are the following: improving eating habits; restricting energy intake; achieving moderate weight loss; having consistent carbohydrate intake at meals and for snacks; decreasing fat intake, especially saturated and trans fats and cholesterol; increasing physical activity levels; and/or adopting new behaviors and attitudes.[1,2]

Objectives

Upon completion of this chapter, the learner will be able to

1 Identify medical nutrition therapy goals for diabetes management.

2 State the primary strategy for achieving the goals of MNT for persons with type 1 diabetes.

3 List 5 nutrition-related strategies for achieving the goals of MNT for persons with type 2 diabetes.

4 Describe the role of carbohydrate in food/meal planning for persons with diabetes.

5 State guidelines for the use of sucrose and fiber.

6 Explain how the term acceptable daily intake (ADI) relates to the use of nonnutritive sweeteners.

7 State guidelines for the role of protein in food/meal planning for persons with diabetes.

8 List nutrition recommendations for the amount and type of fat appropriate in the food/meal plan for persons with diabetes.

9 State general principles related to the role of certain vitamins and minerals in diabetes management.

10 List guidelines for the use of alcoholic beverages.

11 Describe how assessment, implementation/education, goal setting, and evaluation apply to nutrition care for diabetes.

12 Individualize a food/meal plan.

13 Describe the rationale for carbohydrate counting and how to implement this method for food and meal planning.

14 Explain the concept of exchange lists including the nutritive values for each list and their use in assessing eating habits.

15 Describe nutritional concerns for persons with diabetes and celiac disease and for persons with cystic fibrosis–related diabetes.

16 Implement nutrition recommendations at acute-care and long-term healthcare facilities.

Goals of Medical Nutrition Therapy for Persons With Diabetes

1 The primary goal of MNT is to assist in attaining and maintaining optimal metabolic outcomes, including

A Blood glucose levels in the normal range, to the greatest extent possible. This is achieved by balancing food intake, physical activity, and diabetes medications (when needed) and is necessary to prevent the complications of diabetes.[19,20] Blood glucose recommendations for adults with diabetes are listed in Table 1.1.

B Lipid and lipoprotein profiles that are associated with a decreased risk for cardiovascular disease. Recommended values are shown in Table 1.2[23] and Table 1.3.[24]

C Blood pressure levels that are associated with a decreased risk for vascular disease. Optimal blood pressure for adults with respect to cardiovascular risk is <130/80 mm Hg.[23]

Table 1.1. Glucose Recommendations for Adults with Diabetes Mellitus

A1C	<7.0%*
Preprandial plasma glucose	90–130 mg/dL (5.0–7.2 mmol/L)
Peak postprandial plasma glucose	<180 mg/dL (<10.0 mmol/L)

*Referenced to a nondiabetic range of 4.0–6.0%.
Source: Reprinted with permission from the American Diabetes Association.[21]
Note: The American Association of Clinical Endocrinologists (ACE) consensus statement recommends the following goals: A1C of 6.5% or less; preprandial glucose of 110 mg/dL or less; and a postprandial glucose of 140 mg/dL or less.[22]

Table 1.2. Risk for Macrovascular Disease Based on Lipoprotein Values in Adults With Diabetes

Risk	LDL Cholesterol Levels	HDL Cholesterol* Levels	Triglyceride Levels
High	≥130 mg/dL (3.4 mmol/L)	<40 mg/dL (1.1 mmol/L)	≥400 mg/dL (4.4 mmol/L)
Borderline	100–129 mg/dL (2.6–3.3 mmol/L)	40–59 mg/dL (1.1–1.7 mmol/L)	150–399 mg/dL (1.7–4.4 mmol/L)
Low	<100 mg/dL (2.6 mmol/L)	≥60 mg/dL (1.7 mmol/L)	<150 mg/dL (1.7 mmol/L)

*For women, the HDL cholesterol values should be increased by 10 mg/dL.
Source: Reprinted with permission from the American Diabetes Association.[23]

Table 1.3. Recommended Lipoprotein Values for Children and Adolescents

	Cholesterol Levels	LDL Cholesterol Levels	Triglyceride Levels
High	≥200 mg/dL (5.2 mmol/L)	≥130 mg/dL (3.4 mmol/L)	
Borderline	170–199 mg/dL (4.4–5.2 mmol/L)	110–129 mg/dL (2.9–3.3 mmol/L)	
Desirable	<170 mg/dL (4.4 mmol/L)	<110 mg/dL (1.1 mmol/L)	<100 mg/dL (2.9 mmol/L)

Source: Adapted with permission from the American Academy of Pediatrics.[24]

2 Improve health through healthy food choices and physical activity. Nutrition guidelines and nutrient needs are outlined and illustrated in Dietary Guidelines for Americans[4] and the diabetes version of the food pyramid from the American Diabetes and the American Dietetic Association, The First Step in Diabetes Meal Planning.[25]

3 Individualize nutrition care to achieve health-related goals with attention to personal preferences, cultural appropriateness, and the need/willingness to change lifestyle habits.

Goals of Diabetes Medical Nutrition Therapy for Specific Populations and Conditions

1 For youth with type 1 diabetes, provide adequate calories to ensure normal growth and development. The meal plan is not a restriction of calories but is intended to ensure reasonably consistent food intake and a nutritionally balanced eating pattern. Insulin needs to be adjusted to cover the amount of food consumed.

2 For youth with type 2 diabetes, recommend changes in lifestyle to decrease the risks associated with diabetes. Achieving and maintaining a healthy weight through healthy eating habits and exercise can delay the progression of diabetes. Changes in eating and exercise habits are important for the entire family.[26]

3 For pregnant and lactating women, provide adequate energy and nutrients. By monitoring glucose levels, ketones, appetite, and weight gain, appropriate nutrient and energy adjustments can be made.

4 For older adults, provide for the nutritional and psychosocial needs of an aging individual.

5 For individuals treated with insulin or insulin secretagogues, provide appropriate nutrition guidelines to prevent and/or treat acute complications of diabetes (eg, hypoglycemia, acute and catabolic illnesses, exercise-related blood glucose problems).

6 For all persons with diabetes, provide appropriate nutrition guidelines to prevent and treat chronic complications associated with diabetes (eg, nephropathy, hypertension, cardiovascular disease, gastropathies, obesity).

7 For individuals at risk for diabetes, recommend ways to decrease the risk by improving lifestyle factors. Becoming physically active and maintaining activity[27-29] or sustained weight loss[30,31] can prevent or delay the onset of type 2 diabetes.[32,33]

Nutrition-Related Strategies for Achieving Metabolic Goals for Type 1 Diabetes

1 The food/meal plan is based on the individual's appetite, preferred foods, and usual schedule of food intake and activities. The insulin regimen can then be integrated into usual eating habits.[1,2]

2 Individuals using flexible or intensive insulin regimens consisting of basal (background) insulin and bolus (mealtime) insulin doses or insulin pumps have more flexibility in timing and frequency of meals, amount of carbohydrate eaten at meals, and timing of physical activity[34] (see Chapter 6, Pattern Management of Blood Glucose, and Chapter 7, Insulin Pump Therapy and Carbohydrate Counting for Pump Therapy, in Diabetes Management Therapies).

 A The total carbohydrate content of meals (and snacks, if desired), not the source, is the first priority. The amount is based on the individual's preference.

 B The amount of carbohydrate in the meal determines the mealtime doses of rapid-acting insulin (lispro or aspart) or short-acting (regular) insulin and is adjusted accordingly.[34-36]

 C In people with type 1 diabetes, a skills training program, Dose Adjustment for Normal Eating (DAFNE), which promotes dietary freedom with appropriate insulin adjustments, improved quality of life and glycemic control without worsening of hypoglycemia or cardiovascular risk.[34]

3 Individuals taking fixed doses of insulin, which often consists of injections of rapid-acting or short-acting insulin and NPH insulin before breakfast and the evening meal, need to eat similar amounts of carbohydrate at consistent times that are synchronized with the time actions of their insulin(s). Consistency in the amount of day-to-day carbohydrate intake is associated with improved blood glucose control.[37]

4 Improved glycemic control with intensive insulin therapy is often associated with increased body weight. Although it is important to try to prevent weight gain, the benefits of improved blood glucose control outweigh concerns about added pounds.[38] However, because of the potential for weight increases to adversely affect lipids and blood pressure, it is desirable to prevent weight gain.[39,40]

 A To prevent weight gain and hypoglycemia, insulin therapy should be integrated into usual eating and exercise habits, and insulin doses should be adjusted accordingly.

 B Overtreatment of hypoglycemia should be avoided. In general, treatment for glucose levels <80 mg/dL (4.4 mmol/L) consists of consuming 15 g of carbohydrate. Individuals should retest glucose levels in 15 minutes and in 1 hour after consuming carbohydrate to see if additional carbohydrate is needed (see Chapter 8, Hypoglycemia, in Diabetes Management Therapies).

C Adjustments in insulin and possibly carbohydrate intake should be made for physical activity. In general, it may be more helpful to decrease the dose of rapid-acting or short-acting insulin during the time of the activity. If additional carbohydrate is needed, 15 g to 30 g can be ingested (depending on the intensity of the physical activity), either before or after an hour of exercise[41] (see Chapter 2, Physical Activity, in Diabetes Management Therapies).

D Although the carbohydrate content of the meal determines the mealtime insulin dose, meat/meat substitutes and fat servings cannot be ignored. To prevent weight gain, attention also needs to be given to the total number of calories ingested.

Nutrition-Related Strategies for Achieving Metabolic Goals for Type 2 Diabetes

1 MNT for persons with type 2 diabetes focuses on lifestyle strategies that can assist in improving and maintaining normal/optimal metabolic parameters: optimal glucose control, improved lipid profiles, and control of blood pressure.[1,2]

2 Several strategies are available to assist individuals in accomplishing these goals. MNT must be individualized, and goals must be based on what the individual with diabetes chooses to focus on.

A As research continues to clarify why weight loss,[42,43] particularly maintenance of weight loss,[44] is difficult for many persons to achieve, the emphasis for persons with type 2 diabetes needs to shift from weight loss to achieving and maintaining metabolic goals. Both energy restriction and moderate weight loss decrease insulin resistance[45] and are especially helpful early in the course of the disease.[16] Energy restriction, independent of weight loss, is associated with increased insulin sensitivity; significant improvements in glycemia generally occur before much weight is lost.[46,47]

- Energy restriction is, therefore, an independent factor for improved glycemic control. Glycemic control improves within 24 hours of caloric restriction and before any weight loss occurs.

- One of the major lessons learned from the United Kingdom Prospective Diabetes Study (UKPDS) is that type 2 diabetes is a progressive disorder and therapy needs to be intensified over time.[20] Early in the course of the disease, when insulin resistance is most prominent, MNT alone may maintain adequate metabolic control. As the disease progresses and the pancreatic beta cells fail, insulin deficiency becomes more of a factor. Oral medication(s) and, for many individuals, insulin eventually need to be combined with MNT to maintain adequate metabolic control.

- In the UKPDS study, the greatest reduction in A1C was approximately 2% during the first 3 months with intensive diet and 5% weight loss. The initial glucose response was related more to the decrease in energy intake than to weight loss; the decrease in body weight was a secondary response.[16] Fasting plasma glucose levels (FPG) of 110 mg/dL (6.11 mmol/L) were only maintained in patients who continued a restricted caloric intake. In patients who increased their caloric intake, FPG levels increased even if the weight loss was maintained.

B Moderate weight loss of 10 to 20 lb (5 to 9 kg), irrespective of starting weight, has been shown to improve hyperglycemia, dyslipidemia, and hypertension in some,[47-49] but not all patients with type 2 diabetes.[50] If glycemia has not improved after a weight loss of approximately 10 lb (5 kg), oral glucose-lowering agents or insulin (alone or in combination) are generally needed.

- *Body mass index* (BMI, in kg/m^2) defines overweight and obesity and is based on weight/height squared.[51] To determine BMI, a chart such as Figure 1.1 can be used. In adults, a BMI >25 but <29.9 is defined as an overweight state, a BMI >30 but <39.9 is classified as obesity, and a BMI ≥40 is considered extreme obesity. In children and adolescents, a BMI between the 85th and 95th percentiles of weight indicates an increased risk for overweight and a BMI >95th percentile is used to define overweight. As body adiposity increases so does insulin resistance.

- In the US in 2001, the prevalence of obesity (BMI >30) was 20.9% compared to 12% in 1991, an increase of 74%.[52] In 2001, the prevalence of a BMI >40 was 2.3% compared to 0.9% in 1991.

- In 2001, the prevalence of diabetes increased to 7.9% compared to 4.9% in 1990, an increase of 61%.[52] Overweight and obesity are significantly associated with diabetes, high blood pressure, high cholesterol, asthma, arthritis, and poor health.

- When BMI is excessive (>30, or >25 with comorbidities), energy intake should be less than the energy expended in physical activity to reduce BMI. Energy restriction sufficient to produce weight reductions between 5% and 10% reduces the risk for heart disease and stroke.

- Target weights for persons with diabetes are based on a reasonable or healthy body weight, which is not the same as the traditionally defined desirable or ideal body weight. Reasonable body weight is the weight an individual and health professional acknowledge as achievable and maintainable, both short-term and long-term.

- The type of obesity associated with metabolic diseases (glucose intolerance, hypertension, and lipid abnormalities) is the android or abdominal distribution of adipose tissue. Intraabdominal obesity is associated with insulin resistance and hyperinsulinemia, which are both risk factors for metabolic disease.[53,54] Waist circumference (>40 in [102 cm] for men, >35 in [88 cm] for women) indicates risk for metabolic disease.[51]

- Energy restriction results in early improvements in glycemia,[45] whereas moderate weight loss results in later improvements in lipids.[49] Reducing abdominal fat improves insulin sensitivity as well as lipid profiles.

C Consistent day-to-day carbohydrate intake at meals and snacks is important because carbohydrate is the macronutrient with the greatest impact on postprandial glucose levels. Individuals need to be provided with basic guidelines for the amount of carbohydrate to eat at meals and/or snacks.

- Foods containing carbohydrate (fruits, vegetables, whole grains, low-fat dairy products) are important components of a healthy diet. They provide the glucose required by the brain to function and a readily available source of energy for everyday activities. These healthy foods should not be eliminated from the diet because of concerns of elevated glycemia.

- With the help of blood glucose monitoring, the amount of carbohydrate eaten at a particular meal or snack from day to day can be evaluated and adjustments can be made to find the amount of carbohydrate that can be tolerated by an individual (ie, carbohydrate load).

Figure 1.1. Determining Body Mass Index (BMI)

How to use this chart:

1 Find height (in feet and inches) in the left column.
2 Look across the row to find weight (in pounds).
3 Find the number at the top of the column to determine the BMI.

BMI	19	20	21	22	23	24	25	26	27	28	29	30	35	40
						Weight (lb)								
4'10"	91	96	100	105	110	115	119	124	129	134	138	143	167	191
4'11"	94	99	104	109	114	119	124	128	133	138	143	148	173	198
5'	97	102	107	112	118	123	128	133	138	143	148	153	179	204
5'1"	100	106	111	116	122	127	132	137	143	148	153	158	185	211
5'2"	104	109	115	120	126	131	136	142	147	153	158	164	191	218
5'3"	107	113	118	124	130	135	141	146	152	158	163	169	197	225
5'4"	110	116	122	128	134	140	145	151	157	163	169	174	204	232
5'5"	114	120	126	132	138	144	150	156	162	168	174	180	210	240
5'6"	118	124	130	136	142	148	155	161	167	173	179	186	216	247
5'7"	121	127	134	140	146	153	159	166	172	178	185	191	223	255
5'8"	125	131	138	144	151	158	164	171	177	184	190	197	230	262
5'9"	128	135	142	149	155	162	169	176	182	189	196	203	236	270
5'10"	132	139	146	153	160	167	174	181	188	195	202	207	243	278
5'11"	136	143	150	157	165	172	179	186	193	200	208	215	250	286
6'	140	147	154	162	169	177	184	191	199	206	213	221	258	294
6'1"	144	151	159	166	174	182	189	197	204	212	219	227	265	302
6'2"	148	155	163	171	179	186	194	202	210	218	225	233	272	311
6'3"	152	160	168	176	184	192	200	208	216	224	232	240	279	319
6'4"	156	164	172	180	189	197	205	213	221	230	238	246	287	328

BMI = weight/height^2.

D The majority of studies in animals and observational studies in humans have reported a relationship between total dietary fat, regardless of the type, and insulin resistance.[55-58] However, these studies are complicated by the impact of high-fat diets on obesity. The association between saturated fats and insulin resistance has been shown in controlled clinical trials,[59] especially when compared to monounsaturated fats.[60] Conversely, long-chain omega-3 fatty acids have generally been shown to improve insulin action in humans.[61]

- In general, low-fat diets (moderate to high carbohydrate) are associated with modest weight loss, maintained as long as the low-fat diet is continued.[62,63] The low-fat diet and modest weight loss results in decreases in cholesterol, triglycerides, and an increase in HDL cholesterol.[64,65]

- The concern has been that a low-fat, high-carbohydrate diet will cause an increase in insulin resistance and triglycerides. However, studies suggest that the ability of insulin to lower glucose is improved as total dietary carbohydrate is increased[66] and high intakes of dietary fat, especially saturated fats, are associated with a decline in insulin sensitivity. Furthermore, triglyceride levels are not increased until carbohydrate intake is >55% of total energy intake,[67] an intake that is quite unlikely in persons with type 2 diabetes. For example, in the UKPDS trial, although the recommended carbohydrate intake was 50% to 55% of total energy intake, the average percentage of energy from carbohydrate was only 43%.[68]

E The benefits of physical activity are well documented. Physical activity is known to improve insulin sensitivity and enhance cellular glucose uptake by the muscle during or shortly after exercise[69-71] (see Chapter 2, Physical Activity, in Diabetes Management Therapies). In men with type 2 diabetes, increased physical activity was associated with a reduced risk of mortality.[72] A minimum cumulative total of 1000 kcal/week from physical activity[73] or 30 minutes nearly every day (150 minutes week)[33] is recommended.

F Eating frequency (eg, having 3 meals per day or smaller but more frequent meals and snacks) is not associated with long-term differences in glucose, lipid, or insulin responses.[74] Therefore, the division of food intake should be based on individual preferences. However, due to a slowed first-phase insulin release, spacing meals and distributing food intake throughout the day may be beneficial.[75,76]

G It is important to help the person with diabetes focus on behaviors and attitudes that assist with long-term lifestyle changes.[77]

H Testing blood glucose levels premeal and postmeal provides tangible information to assist the person with diabetes in taking a more active role in evaluating food choices.

- If the person with diabetes has made all of the changes that he/she is able or willing to make and the target goals have not been achieved, a change in therapy (addition of or changes in medication and/or doses) is needed.[78]

- Persons with diabetes need to be reminded that while food has a significant impact on glucose levels, other variables such as stress, physical activity, and illness also affect blood glucose levels and may be the reason for variances in glycemia.

3 The results of lifestyle changes are evident by 6 weeks to 3 months.[18] Decisions regarding the success of MNT or the need to change therapy (nutrition and/or medical) should be made at this time. The need to add or change medications should not be viewed as a "diet failure," but rather reflects the natural progression of type 2 diabetes due to beta cell dysfunction. As the disease progresses, therapy must also change. Therapy progresses from MNT alone to MNT combined with oral glucose-lowering medications and/or insulin.

Insulin, Nutrients, and Food Sources

1 The therapeutic goals of diabetes care include not only striving toward euglycemia, but also the accompanying return of normal carbohydrate, protein, and fat metabolism.

2 Insulin is a hormone essential for the use and storage of these nutrients. The action of insulin is both anticatabolic (prevents breakdown) and anabolic (promotes storage), and it facilitates cellular transport of nutrients.

A Insulin suppresses hepatic glycogenolysis and gluconeogenesis and inhibits lipolysis and proteolysis. Insulin also stimulates glycogen synthesis and facilitates the transport of glucose into muscle cells.

B The effects of insulin are balanced by the effects of the counterregulatory hormones: glucagon, growth hormone, cortisol, epinephrine, and norepinephrine.

3 Carbohydrate is the body's primary source of energy. However, without adequate insulin to maintain euglycemia, hyperglycemia occurs. Hyperglycemia contributes to glucotoxicity.[79] In glucotoxicity, the high blood levels of glucose impair the ability of the beta cells to release insulin and contribute to the pathogenesis of type 2 diabetes.

A Carbohydrate provides 4 kcal per gram.

B The following terminology is recommended for referring to the 3 types of carbohydrates: sugars, starch, and fiber.[1] Terms such as complex carbohydrate, simple carbohydrates or sugars, and fast-acting carbohydrate should not be used because they are imprecise and cannot be defined based on chemical structure.

- Monosaccharides (glucose, fructose) and disaccharides (sucrose, lactose) are classified as sugars. Food sources include fruit, some vegetables, milk, and sweets. Fructose and galactose (from lactose) are primarily metabolized by the liver and converted into glycogen (and possibly triglycerides, in the case of fructose). Only a small amount is converted to glucose to cause increases in postprandial blood glucose levels. As a result, sugars such as fructose, lactose and sucrose produce a lower blood glucose response than starches and glucose.[80]

- Polysaccharides are classified as starch (amylopectin and amylose) or fiber. Food sources containing starch include cereal, grains, starchy vegetables (potato, winter squash, peas, corn), and legumes (peas, beans, lentils). The rate and completeness of digestion of starch depends on the structure of the starch, how it is packaged in the plant source, and how the starch-containing food is processed or cooked.[80] Nondigestible nonstarch polysaccharide carbohydrate components of plants are commonly referred to as dietary or food fiber.

- The glucose that is absorbed after digestion of the carbohydrate-containing foods is largely responsible for raising the blood glucose concentration; other food constituents play only a minor role in this process. However, the response is modified by the gastric emptying rate, intestinal motility, and factors that affect glucose removal from the circulation, such as the insulin response and/or insulin resistance. Usual intake of food fiber has little effect on the plasma glucose response, although it may result in a decrease in LDL cholesterol.[80]

C In the metabolism of carbohydrate, insulin facilitates entry of glucose into cells, stimulates glycogen synthesis in liver and muscle cells, and increases triglyceride stores by facilitating the entry of glucose into adipose tissue and its conversion to triglycerides. Without insulin, glucose production by the liver (gluconeogenesis) is accelerated and in liver and muscle glycogenolysis occurs.

4 Protein is necessary for growth and tissue maintenance and is a potential secondary source of energy.

A Protein contributes 4 kcal per gram.

B Dietary sources of protein are both animal (meat, milk, other dairy products) and vegetable (legumes, starches, nuts, seeds, vegetables). The source of the protein (essential or nonessential amino acids) is not a concern. Vegetarian diets can easily meet protein needs, and specific food combinations at meals are not necessary.

C Ingested protein has minimal, if any, effect on blood glucose levels in people with moderately well–controlled type 2 diabetes.[81] In people with type 1 diabetes who are adequately treated with insulin, ingested protein also has only a minimal effect on blood glucose concentration. (See section on protein.)

D In the metabolism of protein, insulin lowers blood amino acids while reducing blood glucose levels, facilitates incorporation of amino acids into tissue protein, and decreases gluconeogenesis. Without adequate insulin, gluconeogenesis increases and proteolysis and amino acid release occurs in muscle.

5 Fat in the form of free fatty acids (FFA) is used as an energy source. An excess of free fatty acids—lipotoxicity—also contributes to the pathogenesis of type 2 diabetes.[82] Lipotoxicity arises from insulin resistance of the fat cell, which results in an increased mobilization of FFA. Visceral or abdominal fat is particularly prone to release excess FFA. The increase in circulating FFA reduces glucose utilization by skeletal muscle and insulin secretion by the pancreas and increases glucose production by the liver. As a result, hyperglycemia is worsened.

A Fat contributes 9 kcal per gram.

B Dietary sources of fat are animal sources (meat, egg yolk, dairy-fat containing foods) and vegetable sources (margarine, oils, nuts, seeds, certain fruits [coconut, avocado]).

C Fats in foods are broken down into triglycerides (3 fatty acids attached to glycerol). Triglycerides are the form of fat that travel through the bloodstream and are stored in adipose tissue.

D In the metabolism of fat, insulin promotes lipogenesis by activating lipoprotein lipase, the enzyme that facilitates transport of triglycerides into adipose tissue for storage. Insulin also inhibits lipolysis and stimulates hepatic lipogenesis. Without adequate insulin, ketogenesis occurs in the liver, and lipolysis and fatty acid release occurs rapidly in adipose tissue, leading to excessive production of ketones and eventually ketoacidosis. Triglyceride levels also increase due to a decrease in cellular uptake of triglycerides.

6 Vitamins and minerals are involved in a wide range of vital body functions. For example, vitamins are involved in the processing of other nutrients (such as carbohydrate, protein, fat, and minerals); minerals are components of many enzyme systems. They do not contribute calories or require insulin to be metabolized, although many micronutrients are intimately involved in carbohydrate and/or glucose metabolism as well as with insulin release and sensitivity.

7 Water is also considered an essential nutrient and is an important component of body tissue, accounting for between one half to three fourths of body weight.
  A Water is important in regulating body temperature and carrying nutrients to and waste products away from the cells.
  B Water is involved in all of the chemical reactions in metabolism.
  C Daily water losses need to be replaced from dietary sources such as water, beverages, and water in food.

Carbohydrate in the Diabetes Food/Meal Plan

1 A number of factors influence glycemic responses to foods, including the amount of carbohydrate, nature of the monosaccharide components, nature of the starch, cooking and food processing, and other food components. Blood glucose levels at the start of the meal also affect the glycemic response. In persons with type 1 diabetes, hyperglycemia has been shown to slow the gastric emptying rate[83] while hypoglycemia increases the gastric emptying rates.[84] In persons with type 2 diabetes, the form of the food,[85] the severity of glucose intolerance,[86] insulin resistance or insulin deficiency, alter postmeal glycemic responses.

2 A commonly held belief was that sugars, both added and naturally occurring, are rapidly absorbed and lead to hyperglycemia. However, sucrose and other sugars do not have more of a deleterious effect on blood glucose levels and are not absorbed more rapidly than starches. Research has consistently shown that sucrose and other sugars do not have a greater impact on blood glucose levels than other carbohydrates when consumed separately or as part of a meal or snack.[87-90]
  A The ADA recommendations state that sucrose can be used as part of the total carbohydrate in the food/meal plan or if added, be covered with insulin or other glucose-lowering medication without affecting glycemic control.[1,2] Sucrose and sucrose-containing foods should be eaten in the context of a healthy diet.
  B Because many factors, often unpredictable, affect the glycemic responses to different carbohydrates in persons with diabetes, the total carbohydrate content of meals and snacks should be the first priority.
    • Evidence from studies on healthy subjects supports the importance of including carbohydrate such as fruits, vegetables, grains, and milk in the diet.
    • Foods containing significant amounts of added sugars (eg, regular soft drinks, syrups, desserts) not only contribute large amounts of carbohydrate to the diet but may be high in calories and/or fat as well.

3 The glycemic index represents the blood glucose area above the fasting glucose concentration following the ingestion of a 50-g carbohydrate portion of food compared with the blood glucose area obtained with a 50-g carbohydrate portion of either glucose or white bread as an index food. The glucose area response to the index food is considered to be 100%. The response to other foods is given as a percentage of that obtained from the index food.
  A In people with type 1 and type 2 diabetes, several studies have reported improvements in glycemic control after incorporating low glycemic index foods into the diet,

while other studies have reported no differences in long-term glycemic control or insulin requirements from a low glycemic index diet.[91] The overall effect from a low glycemic index compared to a high glycemic index diet is, at best, very modest.

B Although the use of low glycemic index foods may reduce postprandial hyperglycemia, there is not sufficient evidence of long-term benefit to recommend use of low glycemic index diets as a primary strategy in food/meal planning.[1,2] Other food/nutrition interventions report greater improvements in overall glycemic control than reported from the implementation of low glycemic index diets.[14]

C Even though the glycemic response is often unpredictable and variable, the glycemic index may be used with preprandial and postprandial glucose results for fine-tuning postmeal hyperglycemia.

4 Recommendations for fiber intake are the same for persons with diabetes as for the general population.[1,2] In persons with type 1 diabetes, a diet containing 50 g fiber/day compared to a diet containing 15 g per day reduced glycemia and the number of hypoglycemic events, but had no beneficial effect on lipids.[92] In persons with type 2 diabetes, a diet containing 50 g per day of food fiber, compared with 24 g per day, improved glycemia and lipids.[93] Conversely, diets containing more than typical amounts of food fiber (~24 g per day) showed no beneficial effect from the fiber in subjects with type 1 diabetes[36] and type 2 diabetes.[94]

A The average dietary fiber intake for adults is 10 to 20 g per day, with men averaging 19 g and women averaging 13 g.

B It is recommended that all Americans choose a variety of fiber-containing foods, such as whole grains, fruits, and vegetables, because they provide vitamins, minerals, fiber, and other substances important for good health.[4] This would also apply to persons with diabetes.

5 Nutritive (caloric) sweeteners such as fructose or sugar alcohols are included in the carbohydrate total for meals and/or snacks.

A Fructose produces a lower postprandial glucose response than sucrose or starch.[95] This potential benefit may be offset by the concern that fructose may have adverse effects on plasma lipids.[96] However, there is no reason to recommend that persons with diabetes avoid naturally occurring fructose in fruits, vegetables, and other foods.

B Sugar alcohols such as sorbitol, mannitol, xylitol, and starch hydrolysates also produce a lower glucose response than sucrose or glucose and are lower in calories (average, 2 kcal/g) than other sugars (4 kcal/g).[97] No evidence exists that these sweeteners have advantages or disadvantages over sucrose in decreasing the amount of carbohydrate or calories in the diet or in improving overall diabetes control. Consuming amounts greater than 10 g per day of some polyols, such as sorbitol, may cause diarrhea.

6 Nonnutritive (low-calorie) sweeteners currently available include saccharin, aspartame, acesulfame K, sucralose, and neotame. Approval is being sought from the US Food and Drug Administration (FDA) for alitame and cyclamates. All FDA-approved nonnutritive sweeteners undergo rigorous testing and are not allowed on the market unless they are safe for the general public to consume, including people with diabetes and pregnant women.

A The acceptable daily intake (ADI) is defined as the amount of a food additive that can be safely consumed on a daily basis over a person's lifetime without any adverse effects. Generally this determination includes a 100-fold safety factor and is determined by the FDA.

- The ADI for aspartame is 50 mg/kg/body weight/day. Aspartame consumption (14-day average) in persons with diabetes has been found to be 2 to 4 mg/kg/day.[98] The average amount of aspartame is 200 mg per 12-oz diet soft drink and 35 mg per packet of tabletop sweetener.[99]
- The ADI for acesulfame K is 15 mg/kg/body weight/day. The average amount of acesulfame K is 40 mg per 12-oz diet soft drink (based on the most typical blend with 90 mg aspartame) and 50 mg per packet of tabletop sweetener.[99]
- The ADI for sucralose is 5 mg/kg/body weight/day. The average amount of sucralose is 70 mg per 12-oz diet soft drink and 5 mg per packet of tabletop sweetener.[99]
- The US does not have an ADI for saccharin because it is not considered a food additive, but the World Health Organization's Joint Expert Committee of Food Additives (JECFA) has set an ADI of 5 mg/kg/body weight/day. The average amount of saccharin is 140 mg per 12-oz diet soft drink and 40 mg per packet of tabletop sweetener.[99]

B Nonnutritive sweeteners are safe to use during pregnancy. Aspartame use has shown no risk to the fetus when ingested in amounts at least 3 times the ADI.[100] Multigenerational studies on rats with acesulfame K and sucralose have shown no adverse effects on fertility, number of offspring, birth weight, mortality, or fetal development.[101] Although saccharin can cross the placenta to the fetus, there is no evidence that this compound is harmful if consumed during pregnancy.

Protein in the Diabetes Food/Meal Plan

1 In the United States, protein intake is between 15% and 20% of the average adult energy intake. Protein intake is fairly consistent across all ages from infancy to older age.[102]

A There is no evidence to suggest a change in usual protein intake. Although consuming 20% of calories from protein is approximately double the adult recommended daily allowance (RDA) for protein, there is limited evidence that protein intake at this level correlates with the development of nephropathy.[102]

B One gram of protein per kilogram of body weight will meet the protein needs of most adults, and 1.2 g of protein per kilogram of body weight will meet the protein needs for most children, adolescents, and athletes.

C Protein foods such as lean meats, low-fat dairy products, and/or low-fat plant protein foods should be selected for a low-fat diet.

2 The rate of protein degradation and conversion of protein to glucose in individuals with diabetes depends on the state of insulinization and degree of glycemic control.

A In persons with poorly controlled diabetes, gluconeogenesis can occur rapidly and adversely affect glycemic control.

B In persons with controlled type 2 diabetes, ingested protein does not increase plasma glucose levels. However, in individuals still able to secrete insulin, protein ingestion is just as potent as glucose in stimulating insulin.[103,104] Furthermore, the peak response to consuming carbohydrate alone or carbohydrate combined with protein is similar.[103]

C In persons with well-controlled type 1 diabetes, the addition of protein did not slow the absorption of carbohydrate, change peak glucose response, or affect glucose levels at 5 hours.[105] Furthermore, the addition of protein for the treatment of hypoglycemia did not prevent recurrent hypoglycemia.[106]

D Persons with diabetes are often taught that because 50% to 60% of protein can be converted to glucose, protein will have half the effect on glucose levels as carbohydrate, and this effect will occur 3 hours to 4 hours after ingestion, thus preventing hypoglycemia. However, the available evidence suggests this is not true.[103-105] Although approximately 50% to 60% of protein can undergo gluconeogenesis, the glucose does not increase the rate of glucose release from the liver and enter the general circulation.[104] What happens to the glucose is unknown, but it is speculated that this glucose is stored in the liver (or muscle) as glycogen.

3 Individuals with diabetes have traditionally been taught to have a food source of protein before bedtime, or to include protein with other snacks or even before exercise. It is doubtful, however, that the added protein has any beneficial effect. A study of bedtime snacks reported the need for a snack depends on the glucose levels at that time such that no snack is necessary at levels >180 mg/dL (10 mmol/L). At lower levels any type of snack can be advised.[107] Unfortunately, the study did not compare a carbohydrate alone snack to a carbohydrate plus protein snack.

A To prevent overnight hypoglycemia in insulin users, the following approaches can be used, although it is unknown which is most helpful: adjusting insulin doses appropriately, ingesting carbohydrate alone, or adding protein to the carbohydrate snack.

4 Although there is an interest in the role of low-carbohydrate, high-protein diets in both glycemic and weight control, carbohydrate foods are still important in a healthful diet. It is unknown whether individuals with diabetes can follow a diet high in protein and low in carbohydrate for an extended time. It is also unknown whether weight loss and/or improvements in glycemia are maintained better on these diets in the long term than with more conventional low-calorie diets.[1,2]

5 Currently recommended treatment for nephropathy focuses on methods that might reverse microalbuminuria or slow the rate of decline in macroalbuminuria and includes reducing blood pressure with angiotension-converting enzyme (ACE) inhibitors or angiotensin II receptor blocker (ARB), improving glycemia, or reducing protein intake.[108]

A There is no clear evidence to make specific nutrition recommendations for people with diabetes who have either microalbuminuria or clinical nephropathy. This is because of the small number of clinical studies and methodological problems in many of the studies.

- There is supportive evidence for reducing protein intake with microalbuminuria. A protein reduction of 0.8 to 1 g/kg/day is associated with renal improvement.[1,2] However, the first priority for individuals with microalbuminuria should be to maintain near-normal glycemic control and normal blood pressure.
- With the onset of clinical nephropathy, there is supportive evidence that lowering protein intake to 0.8 g/kg/day or lower may slow the progression toward end-stage renal disease.[1,2] Protein status should be monitored closely so that the patient's nutritional status is not compromised.

B The differing effects of animal and vegetable protein on renal function have been controversial. In a study comparing animal versus plant protein meals in persons with type 2 diabetes and microalbuminuria, both diets improved renal function, lipids, glycemia, and blood pressure.[109] Following a weight-maintaining, healthy diet, regardless of the protein source, appeared to be beneficial.

Fat in the Diabetes Food/Meal Plan

1 Several diabetes-related diet factors influence the risk of developing macrovascular disease (see Chapter 6, Macrovascular Disease, in Diabetes and Complications).

A Saturated and trans fats raise blood cholesterol levels. Food sources of saturated fats are animal fats (meat, butterfat, lard, bacon); coconut, palm, and palm kernel oils; dairy-fat-containing foods (whole milk, cheese); and hydrogenated vegetable oils. Trans fatty acids are found in processed foods (boxed cakes, candy bars, cookies, doughnuts, fried foods, pastries, microwave pastries), hard margarines, and shortenings. Saturated fats account for 12% to 14% of total calories while trans fatty acids account for only 2% to 3% of total calories.

B Polyunsaturated fats (n-6 or omega-6) have been shown to lower cholesterol levels but have a heterogeneous effect on HDL cholesterol levels. Food sources of polyunsaturated fats are vegetable oils (corn, safflower, soybean, sunflower, cottonseed) and walnuts.

C Monounsaturated fats lower total cholesterol but do not lower HDL cholesterol levels. Food sources of monounsaturated fats are canola, olive, and peanut oils; olives; and nuts (except walnuts).

D N-3 or omega-3 polyunsaturated fats (fish oils) have an antiplatelet clotting effect and have been shown to lower serum triglycerides. Food sources of omega-3 polyunsaturated fats are fish from cold, deep water; fatty fish such as salmon, herring, albacore tuna, mackerel, and sardines; and plant sources such as flax, walnuts, and canola oil.

E Dietary cholesterol affects the LDL cholesterol concentration by competing for the cell receptors for LDL cholesterol. Dietary cholesterol is found only in animal food sources. Some individuals are more sensitive to the cholesterol-raising effects of dietary cholesterol than others. Food sources that contribute cholesterol in the American diet include egg yolks, organ meats (especially liver), dairy-fat-containing food products, and meats.

F A diet high in total fat can increase chylomicron levels leading to atherogenic remnant particles. (Chylomicrons carry food cholesterol and triglycerides from the intestinal mucosa to the liver.)

2 Saturated fat is the principal dietary determinant of LDL cholesterol levels. There is evidence that persons with diabetes, compared with nondiabetic persons, have an increased risk of coronary heart disease with a higher intake of dietary cholesterol.[110] The debate about this topic is not whether saturated fat and cholesterol be restricted, but what is the best alternative energy source for the person with diabetes.[2]

A Diets enriched with monounsaturated fat and low-fat, high-carbohydrate diets improve glucose tolerance and lipid levels compared with diets high in saturated fat.[2]

B Only a few studies have evaluated the effects of polyunsaturated fats on lipid levels in persons with diabetes.[111] Limited evidence suggests polyunsaturated fat should be approximately 10% of energy intake.

3 Because 15% to 20% of usual daily energy intake is from protein, approximately 10% from saturated fat and 10% from polyunsaturated fat, the combined carbohydrate and monounsaturated fat intake will be about 60% to 70% of total daily calories. The division of calories depends on treatment goals such as identified lipid problems; glucose, lipid, and weight goals; and patient preferences.

A Less than 10% of total daily calories should be from saturated fats; some individuals may benefit from lowering their intake of saturated fats to less than 7% of daily calories. Dietary cholesterol intake should be 300 mg or less per day; some individuals may benefit from lowering their intake to 200 mg or less per day. Trans fatty acid intake should be minimal.[1,2]

B To lower LDL cholesterol concentration, energy derived from saturated fat can be reduced if weight loss is desirable, or if weight loss is not a goal, replaced with either monounsaturated fats or carbohydrate depending on patient preferences (eg, some ethnic groups may prefer monounsaturated fats while other groups may prefer carbohydrate replacements for saturated fat).[1,2]

• In weight maintenance diets, both high carbohydrate and high monounsaturated fat diets lower LDL cholesterol levels. However, diets with >55% of energy from carbohydrate may modestly increase fasting triglyceride levels.[67] In energy restricted diets, both low–fat (high–carbohydrate) and high–monounsaturated fat diets have been shown to have beneficial effects on lipids, including triglycerides.[112]

• The major monounsaturated fat in the diet is oleic, and major dietary sources of oleic are the same as for saturated fat: dairy, beef, pork, poultry and lamb; therefore, when saturated fat is restricted so is monounsaturated fat. To increase monounsaturated fat, individuals need to add to their diets oil and nuts; however, increasing fat intake may result in increased energy intake.

4 To lower triglyceride levels, efforts at improving glycemic control, achieving moderate weight loss, and increasing physical activity have all been shown to be beneficial. Persons with treated diabetes and with triglyceride levels greater than 1000 mg/dL (11 mmol/L) should have acute restriction of all types of dietary fat and treatment with medications to reduce the risk of pancreatitis.[1,2]

5 Although controversial, higher intake of total dietary fat in persons with type 2 diabetes, regardless of the type (saturated, monounsaturated, or polyunsaturated), has been associated with insulin resistance.[55-59]

A Fat intake should be individualized. With maintenance isocaloric intake, weight balance is the same on diets high in carbohydrate or high in monounsaturated fat.

B Low-fat diets, however, have been shown to assist with weight loss and weight maintenance.[32,33,62,63]

6 Eating 2 to 3 servings of fish per week provides dietary n-3 polyunsaturated fat and is encouraged. N-3 supplement use in persons with diabetes is associated with adverse effects on LDL cholesterol.[113,114] Therefore, effects on LDL cholesterol should be monitored, but glucose metabolism is not likely to be adversely affected. N-3 supplements may be beneficial in the treatment of severe hypertriglyceridemia.[115]

7 The FDA regulatory process provides reasonable assurance that current fat replacers/substitutes are safe to use in food.[99,116]

  A These substitutes are generally classified according to the nutrients from which they are made.

- Carbohydrate sources of fat replacements are dextrins, maltodextrins, modified food starches, polydextrose, cellulose, and gums.
- Protein sources of fat substitutes are microparticulated proteins from egg whites or milk and texturized proteins.
- Several sources of fat replacements from fat (eg, caprenin, salatrim, and olestra) currently are available in foods that are on the market, and others are under development.

  B Overt use of foods with fat replacers may help reduce dietary fat but may not reduce total energy intake or weight. People with diabetes need to be aware of the macronutrient content and energy consumption of foods containing fat replacers to determine how these foods impact their individualized treatment goals.

Vitamins and Minerals in Diabetes Management

1 People differ in their sensitivity to sodium; however, people with type 2 diabetes appear to be more sodium-sensitive than the general public.[117] In general, sodium intake should be limited to less than 2400 mg/day.[4,118] The Dietary Approaches to Stop Hypertension (DASH) sodium study provides strong support for reducing sodium intake.[119]

  A A teaspoon of salt (5 g) contains 2300 mg of sodium. The amount of sodium in food products is listed on the nutrition label as milligrams per serving.

  B Single servings of foods that contain more than 400 mg of sodium, or entrees with more than 800 mg of sodium, are considered significant sources of sodium in the diet.

  C The FDA defines a low-sodium food as having 140 mg or less of sodium per serving.

2 Evaluating the micronutrient status of people with diabetes involves a comprehensive clinical history and physical examination. In addition, a comprehensive food/nutrition history should be done, including use of health foods; over-the-counter vitamins, minerals, and herbal supplements; and methods of preparing foods.[1,2]

  A Persons with diabetes should be educated about the importance of obtaining daily vitamin and mineral requirements from natural food sources as well as the potential toxicity of megadoses of vitamin and mineral supplementation.

  B Persons who may benefit from vitamin and mineral supplements include elderly individuals, pregnant or lactating women, strict vegetarians, people on low-calorie diets, those taking medications known to alter micronutrient metabolism, persons in poor metabolic control (with glycosuria), or persons in critical care environments.[1,2]

3 Vitamin supplementation in pharmacological doses should be viewed as a therapeutic intervention and, therefore, should be subjected to stringent placebo-controlled trials to demonstrate safety and efficacy.

4 The following supplements are of special interest for persons with diabetes:

   A Deficiency of certain minerals such as potassium, magnesium, and possibly zinc and chromium may aggravate carbohydrate intolerance. Potassium and magnesium assessment can be done, but the need for zinc and chromium in persons with diabetes has not been established.[1,2]

   B Daily intake of 1000 mg to 1200 mg of elemental calcium, especially in older persons with diabetes, appears to be safe and likely will reduce the incidence of metabolic bone disease. However, the value of calcium supplementation in younger age groups is uncertain.[120]

   C The role of folate in preventing birth defects is widely accepted. However, the association between homocysteine levels and cardiovascular disease and the role of folate supplementation in reducing cardiovascular events is unclear.[121]

   D The ADA concluded that the potential benefits of chromium supplementation in persons with diabetes have not been conclusively demonstrated. Until larger clinical trials are conducted in countries similar to the United States and where chromium deficiency is not of concern, it is prudent to avoid chromium supplementation. Long-term benefits from pharmacological doses of chromium (1000 mg) on glycemia and lipids are unknown.[2] A recent meta-analysis supported by the Office of Dietary Supplements, National Institutes of Health, supported this recommendation.[122] The reviewers concluded that data from randomized controlled trials showed no effect of chromium on glucose or insulin concentrations in nondiabetic subjects. The data for persons with diabetes was inconclusive. Trials in well characterized, at-risk populations are necessary to determine the effects of chromium on glucose, insulin, and A1C.

   E Large observational epidemiological studies have shown a correlation between antioxidants and clinical outcomes. However, large placebo-controlled intervention clinical trials have failed to show benefits, and in some studies an increase in complications was observed.[123,124] The Heart Outcomes Prevention Evaluation Study (HOPE) included 9451 subjects, 38% of whom had diabetes. Supplementation with 400 IU of vitamin E for 4.5 years did not result in any significant benefits.[125] Because of the uncertainties as to the efficacy or safety of long-term supplementation, it is advisable to discourage routine supplementation with antioxidant vitamins.[1,2]

5 The impact of herbal medicines on glycemia and lipids requires long-term, placebo-controlled clinical trials to demonstrate efficacy and safety. At present, there is no evidence to suggest benefits. (See Chapter 7, Biological Complementary Therapies in Diabetes, in Diabetes in the Life Cycle and Research.)

Alcohol and Diabetes Management

1 The same precautions regarding the use of alcohol that apply to the general public also apply to persons with diabetes. Abstaining from alcohol should be advised for pregnant women and people with medical problems such as pancreatitis, advanced neuropathy, severe hypertriglyceridemia, or alcohol abuse.[1,2] Alcohol also may potentiate or interfere with the action of other medications.

2 The effect of alcohol on blood glucose levels is dependent on the amount of alcohol ingested as well as the relationship to food intake.[126]

A Alcohol is absorbed from the stomach and small intestine and, because of its toxicity, is metabolized in the liver before other nutrients are metabolized.

B Alcohol does not require insulin to be metabolized even though it is used as an energy source.

C Alcohol is not converted to glucose; excessive amounts of alcohol can potentially be converted to fats.

3 Alcohol blocks gluconeogenesis (the release of glucose from the liver) and is speculated to interfere with the counterregulation to insulin-induced hypoglycemia.

A Because alcohol cannot be used as a source of glucose, hypoglycemia can result when alcohol is consumed without food.

B Hypoglycemia can occur at blood alcohol levels that do not exceed mild intoxication, and the hypoglycemic effect may persist from 8 to 12 hours after the last drink.[127]

4 In persons with both type 1 diabetes and type 2 diabetes, alcohol ingested in moderation and with food does not affect blood glucose.[128] Chronic ingestion (~45 g/day or 3 drinks) can cause deterioration in glucose control; however, these effects from excess alcohol are reversed after abstinence for 3 days.[129]

A Daily intake should be limited to no more than 1 drink for adult women and 2 drinks for adult men and should be ingested with food.[1]

B Alcoholic drinks are an addition to the food/meal plan. No food should be omitted because of the possibility of alcohol-induced hypoglycemia.

C The type of drink does not make a difference.[130] One drink is defined as 12 oz beer, 5 oz wine, or 1½ oz hard liquor (distilled spirits).

5 Epidemiological evidence in nondiabetic adults suggests a U- or J-shaped association between light-to-moderate alcohol ingestion (~15 to 30 g/day or 1 to 2 drinks) and decreased risk of type 2 diabetes, coronary heart disease, and stroke[130-132] and increased insulin sensitivity.[133,134] In adult men and women with type 2 diabetes, population-based prospective studies have reported a decreased risk of coronary heart disease with light-to-moderate alcohol consumption,[135-137] perhaps due to increases in HDL cholesterol.[134]

A Light-to-moderate amounts of alcohol do not raise blood pressure; however, chronic, excessive amounts of alcohol (>30 to 60 g/day) do elevate blood pressure.[118]

B Only very excessive amounts of alcohol increase triglyceride concentrations by increasing VLDL synthesis, which is enhanced by genetics, high-fat diet, and diabetes.[138] Two drinks per day in persons with fasting hypertriglyceridemia resulted in no increase in triglycerides.[138] In nondiabetic women, 2 drinks per day beneficially affected triglyceride concentrations and insulin sensitivity.[139]

C Additional prospective long-term studies are needed to confirm these observations in persons with diabetes.

Expected Outcomes from Diabetes MNT

1 Randomized controlled trials and observational studies of diabetes MNT have demonstrated an expected decrease in A1C outcomes of approximately 1% to 2% (a 15% to 22% decrease) and 50 to 100 mg/dL (2.88 to 5.6 mmol/L) decrease in fasting plasma glucose concentrations from MNT.[14,140]

2 Outcomes from MNT will be known and, therefore, should be evaluated between 6 weeks to 3 months.[18]

   A In newly diagnosed persons with type 2 diabetes, the United Kingdom Prospective Diabetes Study[16] and the nutrition practice guidelines (NPG) for type 2 diabetes clinical trial[18] reported an average decrease in A1C of 2% from intensive nutrition therapy provided by dietitians.

   B In persons with type 2 diabetes with an average duration of 4 years, the NPG trial reported an average decrease in A1C of 1% from intensive nutrition therapy provided by dietitians who followed the NPG.[18]

   C In newly diagnosed persons with type 1 diabetes, a clinical trial using the NPG for type 1 diabetes reported an average decrease in A1C of 1% from intensive nutrition therapy provided by dietitians who followed the NPG.[17] The DAFNE trial reported a 1% decrease in A1C in patients with type 1 diabetes who were instructed by dietitians on how to adjust mealtime insulin based on the carbohydrate content of meals.[34]

3 Outcome studies from MNT on lipids in subjects with diabetes have not been done. Therefore, data from nondiabetic subjects must be used.

   A Meta-analysis of MNT in nondiabetic free-living subjects in which saturated fats were lowered to 7% to 10% of energy intake and dietary cholesterol to 200 to 300 mg daily demonstrate expected outcomes on lipids from MNT.[141]

     • Maximal MNT typically reduces LDL cholesterol by 15 to 25 mg/dL (0.2 to 0.7 mmol/L); a decrease of 12% to 16%.[141]

     • Maximal MNT reduces total cholesterol by 24 to 32 mg/dL (0.6 to 0.8 mmol/L); a decrease of 10% to 13%.

     • Maximal MNT reduces triglycerides by 15 to 17 mg/dL (~0.2 mmol/L); a decrease of 8%.

     • Without exercise, HDL cholesterol decreased by 3 mg/dL (0.1 mmol/L); a 7% decrease. With exercise, no decrease in HDL cholesterol was observed.

   B The American Diabetes Association recommends that for patients with diabetes, if the LDL cholesterol exceeds the goal by >25 mg/dL (0.7 mmol/L), pharmacological therapy may be started at the same time as MNT for high-risk patients (ie, patients with prior myocardial infarction and/or other cardiovascular risk factors).[23] In other patients with diabetes, MNT may be evaluated at the 6-week interval, with consideration of pharmacological therapy between 3 and 6 months.

   C The National Cholesterol Education Program (NCEP) Adult Treatment Panel III recommends that after 6 weeks of therapeutic lifestyle changes (TLC), LDL cholesterol response be determined.[142] If the LDL cholesterol goal has not been achieved, TLC is intensified and after another 6 weeks (3 months after the initial session), the LDL cholesterol is evaluated again. If the LDL goal has not been achieved, medications should be considered.

4 MNT outcome data on blood pressure is also from subjects without diabetes.

   A A lowering of sodium intake to 2400 mg/day is associated with a decline in systolic blood pressure of 6 mm Hg and in diastolic blood pressure of 2 mm Hg in hypertensive patients, and of 3 mm Hg systolic and 1 mm Hg diastolic in normotensive patients.[143]

     • Although there are wide variations in blood pressure responses, the lower the sodium intake, the greater is the lowering of blood pressure. Responses to sodium restriction may be greater in persons who are "salt sensitive," a characteristic of many persons with diabetes.

B Weight reduction of 10 lb (4.5 kg) has been shown to be as effective as first-level drugs in controlling blood pressure.[144]

C The Dietary Approach to Stop Hypertension (DASH) trial reported that a low-fat diet that includes fruits, vegetables, and low-fat dairy products also effectively lowers blood pressure.[145]

D Blood pressure should be monitored at every medical visit.[21]

Translating Diabetes Nutrition Recommendations Into Clinical Practice

1 MNT includes recommendations for food/nutrition and physical activity and the process or system for providing nutrition care.[146]

2 The process of providing nutrition therapy for diabetes has shifted from nutrition prescriptions based on formulas for caloric requirements and percentage of calories from macronutrients to individualized recommendations based on assessment and mutual goal setting.

A The goal is to assist individuals in acquiring and maintaining the knowledge, skills, attitudes, behaviors, and commitment to meet the challenges of daily diabetes self-management successfully.

B Furthermore, a system for providing ongoing nutrition care is essential.

3 The process of providing MNT consists of 4 steps:

A An assessment of the individual's food/nutrition and diabetes self-management knowledge and skills (at follow-up sessions this step includes an evaluation of outcomes)

B Intervention involving matching both a food/meal planning approach and educational materials to the individual's needs and self-management training

C Identification and negotiation of individualized mutually designed lifestyle goals

D Documentation and plans for ongoing follow-up and education

4 Certain assessments are needed for developing the nutrition intervention and to develop a nutrition prescription (food/meal plan).[146,147]

A The following minimum referral data are needed before beginning a nutrition assessment:
- Diabetes treatment regimen
- Laboratory data: A1C (date of test), fasting/nonfasting plasma glucose, total cholesterol and fractionations, fasting triglycerides, and microalbumin (when appropriate)
- Blood pressure
- Goals for patient care
- Medical history including medications that affect nutrition therapy
- Medical clearance and/or limitations for exercise

B The following patient parameters need to be assessed:
- Anthropometric measures
- Social history
- Diabetes history

- Food/nutrition history
- Learning style, cultural heritage, religious practices, food-related beliefs, attitudes and concerns, and socioeconomic status
- Medications/supplements

C A complete food/nutrition history is needed. Two methods that can be used to assess eating patterns and food choices are a food history taken by the dietitian or food records (for 1 to 3 days) kept by the individual. An example of a daily food record is given in Figure 1.2.

D A preliminary meal plan can be designed using the food history and the food/nutrition assessment information. Keeping the food/meal plan flexible makes it doable for the individual. The nutrition history form shown in Figure 1.3 can be used to record and modify usual food intake. This can be completed from the food history. Calculations and mutually agreed upon changes in the food/meal plan can then be done based on these data (Figure 1.4).

- A registered dietitian has the major responsibility for working with the patient to develop an appropriate meal plan. Although the nutrition history form in Figure 1.3 is based on the exchange system, the use of exchanges is not necessarily the preferred meal planning approach. The advantage of this form is that it allows the meal plan to be based on the modification of usual eating habits instead of beginning with a predetermined calorie level that is usually not appropriate and calculating the percentages of calories for macronutrients.
- Nutrient values from the exchange lists (Table 1.4) are useful for evaluating the nutrition assessment and making calculations for the meal plan.[148,149] After completing an assessment, the dietitian may determine that the food/meal planning and blood glucose goals can be best achieved by using basic nutrition guidelines or by using carbohydrate counting.
- Adult calorie needs vary depending on the level of activity, age, and desired weight change. General guidelines for estimating adult energy requirements are shown in Table 1.5.
- Energy should be prescribed to provide for normal growth and development in children and adolescents. To determine normal growth and weight profiles, the growth of children and adolescents should be monitored on a weight and height growth grid at a minimum of every 3 to 6 months. The meal plan is not intended to restrict calories but to ensure a reasonably consistent food intake and nutritionally balanced eating pattern. Table 1.6 is one method that can be used to evaluate the adequacy of energy intake. Parents of young children and adolescents need to be taught to adjust the insulin dose rather than restrict food intake to control blood glucose levels. (For more information, see Chapter 2, Type 1 Diabetes in Youth, in Diabetes in the Life Cycle and Research.)
- For more accurate methods of determining energy requirements in adults and children, see the 2002 Dietary Reference Intakes: Energy, Carbohydrate, Fiber, Fat, Fatty Acids, Cholesterol, Protein, Amino Acids.[150] Estimated Energy Requirement (EER) are defined as the dietary energy intake that is predicted to maintain energy balance in healthy persons of a defined age, gender, weight, height, and level of physical activity consistent with good health. To calculate EER, prediction equations were developed from data on total daily energy expenditure measured by doubly labeled water technique. In children and adolescents, the EER also included the requirements for growth. For overweight/obese individuals,

Figure 1.2. Example of Diabetes Daily Record

Name: JD
BG Goal: 80 to 150 mg/dL

Day/Date	Time	Med/Insulin Type/Dose	BG, mg/dL Premeal	Postmeal	Food Intake Amt.	Type (food/drink)	Carbohydrate Info Servngs	Grams	Exercise Type/Amount
Tues. 4/15	5:30 PM	Glucotrol/2.5 mg	160		4 oz	Ground beef	0	0	Watch TV
					8 oz	Baked potato	3	43 g	
					1 c	Corn	2	30 g	
							5 Total	73 g Total	
	10:30 PM			212					
Wed. 4/16	5:30 PM	Glucotrol/2.5 mg	141		2 c	Macaroni and cheese	4	60 g	Shop, walk in mall 1 hour at 7:00 PM
					1 c	Green peas	2	30 g	
					1 pc	Bread	1	12 g	
							7 Total	102 g Total	
	10:00 PM			163					
Thurs. 4/17	5:45 PM	Glucotrol/2.5 mg	170		3 pc	Fried chicken	2	27 g	Walk 15 minutes at 7:30 PM
					1 c	Mashed potatoes	2	30 g	
					1/2 c	Gravy	0	6 g	
					3 oz	Biscuit	2	34 g	
							6 Total	97 g Total	
	11:00 PM			192					

Figure 1.3. Example of Nutrition History Form

Food Group	MEAL/SNACK/TIME						Total servings/ day	CHO (g)	Protein (g)	Fat* (g)	Calories
	Breakfast	Snack	Lunch	Snack	Dinner	Snack					
Starch								15	3	1	80
Fruit								15			60
Milk, Skim								12	8	1	90
Vegetables								5	2		25
Meats/Substitutes									7	(8)(5)(3)(1)	(100)(75)(55)(35)
Fats										5	45
Carbohydrate Choices											
TOTAL											
Calories								x 4 =	x 4 =	x 9 =	Total =
Percent Calories											

*Calculations are based on medium-fat meats and skim/very-low-fat milk. If diet consists predominantly of lean meats, use the factor 3 g fat instead of 5 g fat; if predominantly very lean meats, use 1 g fat; if predominantly high-fat meats, use 8 g fat. If low-fat (2%) milk is used, use 5 g fat; if whole milk is used, use 8 g fat.

Source: Adapted from Franz M. A new era in nutrition therapy for diabetes. On the Cutting Edge [Newsletter]. 1995;16(2):6.

Figure 1.4. Example of Completed Nutrition History Form

Food Group	MEAL/SNACK/TIME						Total servings/day	CHO (g)	Protein (g)	Fat* (g)	Calories
	Breakfast 7:30	Snack 10:00	Lunch 12:00	Snack 3:00	Dinner 6:30	Snack 10:00					
Starch	3		2-3	0-1	2-3	1-2	10	15 / 150	3 / 30	1 / 10	80
Fruit	1		1		1		3	15 / 45			60
Milk, Skim	1				1		2	12 / 24	8 / 16	1	90
Vegetables			0-1		1-2		2	5 / 10	2 / 4		25
Meats/Substitutes			2		3		5		7 / 35	(8)(5)(3)(1) / 25	(100)(75)(55)(35)
Fats	0-1		1	0-1	1-2	0-1	5			5 / 25	45
Carbohydrate Choices	4	0	3-4	0-1	4-5	1-2					

		CHO	Protein	Fat	
TOTAL		230	85	60	
Calories		×4 = 920	×4 = 340	×9 = 540	Total = 1800
Percent Calories		51%	19%	30%	

*Calculations are based on medium-fat meats and skim/very-low-fat milk. If diet consists predominantly of lean meats, use the factor 3 g fat instead of 5 g fat; if predominantly very lean meats, use 1 g fat; if predominantly high-fat meats, use 8 g fat. If low-fat (2%) milk is used, use 5 g fat; if whole milk is used, use 8 g fat.

Source: Adapted from Franz M. A new era in nutrition therapy for diabetes. On the Cutting Edge [Newsletter]. 1995;16(2):6.

equations to predict Total Energy Expenditure (TEE) from age, height, weight, gender, and activity level were developed. Energy expenditure decreases when energy intake is less than the TEE, with the result that weight loss is less than anticipated based on the reduction in energy intake. The coefficient of 16.6 kcal/kg weight loss can be utilized to anticipate the reduction in energy intake required for maintaining lower body weights.

Table 1.4. Macronutrient and Calorie Values per Serving for 2003 Exchange List

Groups/Lists	Carbohydrate (g)	Protein (g)	Fat (g)	Calories
Carbohydrates				
Starch	15	3	0-1	80
Fruit	15	—	—	60
Milk				
Fat-free, low-fat	12	8	0-3	90
Reduced-fat	12	8	5	120
Whole	12	8	8	150
Sweets, Desserts and Other Carbohydrates	15	Varies	Varies	Varies
Nonstarchy Vegetables	5	2	—	25
Meat and Substitutes				
Very lean	—	7	0-1	35
Lean	—	7	3	55
Medium-fat	—	7	5	75
High-fat	—	7	8	100
Fat Group	—	—	5	45

Source: Reprinted with permission from the American Diabetes Association.[148]

Table 1.5. Estimating Approximate Energy Requirements in Adults

Estimating approximate energy requirements for adults based on actual weight

Obese or very inactive individuals and chronic dieters	•10 to 12 kcal/lb (20 kcal/kg)
Individuals >55 years, active women, sedentary men	•13 -kcal/lb (25 kcal/kg)
Active men, very active women	•15 kcal/lb (30 kcal/kg)
Thin or very active men	•20 kcal/lb (40 kcal/kg)

Table 1.6. Estimating Minimum Energy Requirements for Youth

Age 1 year	• 1000 kcal for 1st year
Age 2 to 10 years	• Add 100 kcal/y to 1000 kcal up to 2000 kcal at age 10
Girls ages 11 to 15 years	• 2000 kcal plus 50 to 100 kcal/y after age 10
Girls >15 years	• Calculate as an adult (Table 1.5)
Boys ages 12 to 15 years	• 2000 kcal plus 200 kcal/y after age 10
Boys >15 years	• Sedentary: 16 kcal/lb (30-35 kcal/kg) • Moderate physical activity: 18 kcal/lb (40 kcal/kg) • Very physically active: 23 kcal/lb (50 kcal/kg)

E For persons requiring insulin therapy, once the food/meal plan has been mutually determined, insulin regimens can be planned and adjusted to match the individual's customary food intake and activity schedule.

F For persons with type 2 diabetes, having smaller meals and snacks spaced throughout the day may assist in controlling postmeal hyperglycemia.

G The preliminary food/meal plan can be evaluated by asking the following questions.
- Is the food/meal plan appropriate for reaching blood glucose and other metabolic goals?
- Does the food/meal plan take into account personal preferences, cultural background, and religious practices?
- Does the food/meal plan encourage healthful eating?
- Are the calories appropriate?

5 Interventions using a patient-centered or empowerment approach can improve adherence to MNT. Successful nutrition therapy involves a process of problem solving, adjustment, and readjustment.[151] Nutrition self-management training occurs in 2 phases and consists of basic or survival education followed by more in-depth and continuing education.

A Basic or initial education provides the information needed at the time of diagnosis, when the treatment program changes or the person's lifestyle changes, or at the time of initial contact with a dietitian (Table 1.7). Initial skill topics provide information about basic nutrition guidelines or basic carbohydrate counting and beginning strategies for altering eating patterns; these are considered basic nutrition therapy skills for all persons with diabetes.
- Identify and monitor outcomes after the second or third visit (approximately 6 weeks after the initial nutrition consult) to determine whether the individual is making progress toward personal goals.
- If no progress is evident, the individual and educator need to reassess and consider making possible revisions to the food/nutrition plan.
- If the person has done all that he/she can do or is willing to do and blood glucose levels are not in the target range, notify the healthcare provider that medications need to be added or adjusted.

Table 1.7. Basic and Initial Self-Management Skills

- Basic food/meal guidelines
- Blood glucose monitoring skills, if not already known
- Signs, symptoms, treatment, and prevention of hypoglycemia if on insulin or insulin secretagogues
- Guidelines for short-term illness management
- Guidelines for safe physical activity
- Plans for continuing nutrition care and education

Source: Adapted from Monk, Barry, McClain, et al.[78]

- Food diaries can be helpful for all phases of self-management training. Food diaries have been shown to be an effective strategy for helping individuals make positive changes in their eating patterns as well as reach and maintain weight goals. Users record everything they eat, including approximate amounts and the circumstances under which the food was eaten, over a specified time. Food diaries can be kept for 1 day each week, a few days each month, or longer periods. See Table 1.8 for suggestions on how to use food diaries.

Table 1.8. Using Food Diaries

Patients who might benefit from keeping food diaries
- Those starting a new food/meal plan
- Those initiating intensive insulin therapy or insulin pumps
- Those having problems with blood glucose control
- Those needing motivation to follow their food/meal plan
- Those wanting to lose weight
- Those needing help in setting short-term and long-term goals

What can be learned from food diaries
- How much carbohydrate is usually eaten at meals or for snacks
- Portion sizes
- Unconscious eating or nibbling patterns
- Eating from boredom, being tired, being under stress, etc
- Skipping planned meals and/or snacks
- Eating food in places other than at the table
- Food choices, such as foods high in fat, foods with hidden fats, excessive sweets
- Level of exercise

How information from food diaries can be used
- To determine what, where, and how much food was eaten
- To identify improvements that can be made
- To identify progress made toward short-term goals
- To determine the effect of food intake and activity on blood glucose levels (correlations can be made between foods eaten and blood glucose records)

B Continuing self-management training provides essential education and includes both management and lifestyle skills (Table 1.9). Topics emphasized or chosen are based on the individual's choice; lifestyle; level of nutrition knowledge; and experience in planning, purchasing, and preparing food and meals. Individuals are taught to make adjustments in food planning or medications for a number of situations.

Table 1.9. Topics for Continuing Self-Management Training

Management Skills *(Information required to make decisions to achieve management goals)*
- Food sources of carbohydrate, protein, fat
- How to use Nutrition Facts on food labels
- Food planning (and insulin adjustments) for
  Short-term illness
  Delay or changes in meal times
  Drinking alcoholic beverages
  Physical activity
  Travel
  Competitive athletics
  Holidays
- Treatment and prevention of hypoglycemia
- How to use blood glucose monitoring data for problem solving and identifying blood glucose patterns
- Behavior change strategies
- Vitamin, mineral, other nutritional supplements
- Working rotating shifts, if needed

Improvement of Lifestyle *(Problem-solving skills)*
- Eating away from home
- Eating lunch in school cafeterias
- Fast-food choices
- Special occasions, birthdays, holidays
- Grocery shopping guidelines
- Reducing and modifying fat intake
- Reducing sodium intake
- Vegetarian food choices
- New ideas for snacks
- Recipe modifications, menu ideas, cookbooks
- Ethnic foods
- Use of convenience food

Source: Adapted from Monk, Barry, McClain, et al.[78]

6 Goal setting is done mutually with the individual with diabetes and the professional and identifies specific behavioral goals. The individual's interests and concerns can be discerned from the assessment and specific short-term behavioral goals reviewed at the end of each session.

A Goals should be realistic and specific.

B In general, no more than 1 or 2 behavioral goals should be identified at a time.

7 Appropriate documentation of nutrition self-management training includes summaries of history and assessment, nutrition problem list, food/meal plan, educational topics addressed, assessment of patient acceptance and understanding, behavior changes, additional skills or information needed, short-term and long-term goals, additional recommendations, and plans for ongoing care. Effectiveness (outcomes) of nutrition interventions also need to be documented.

8 Follow-up and ongoing self-management training and nutrition care are essential parts of MNT.

A Patients and team members need to understand that persons with diabetes need follow-up and ongoing, long-term nutrition care.

B It is recommended that persons with diabetes be seen periodically for continuing education, updating of the food/meal plan, and support.

- Adults should be seen every 6 months to 1 year or when there are any major changes in work schedule, activity level, type of diabetes medication (especially insulin), blood glucose control, or medical status (development of complications). Weight management may require more frequent visits.[78]
- Children should be seen a minimum of every 6 months, preferably every 3 months. Energy intake needs to be adjusted to accommodate growth and development requirements.[152]

Methods for Teaching Food/Meal Planning

1 No single meal-planning approach works for every patient. For each phase of education, different educational resources may be needed. Basic nutrition interventions are needed for beginning education, and more in-depth tools may be needed as the counseling process continues. Preplanned printed diet sheets are ineffective and should not be used.[1,2]

2 Several meal-planning approaches are available to teach basic diabetes nutrition guidelines as well as more in-depth nutrition interventions. The person with diabetes and the educator may begin with one meal-planning approach and try other resources as the counseling process continues.

3 Carbohydrate counting has become the preferred approach for food and meal planning. This approach is described in the next section.

Carbohydrate Counting

1 Carbohydrate counting is useful for all persons with diabetes. Some individuals will benefit from simply knowing which foods are carbohydrates and how many servings of foods containing carbohydrate to select for meals and/or snacks. Other individuals, usually those using flexible or intensive insulin therapy, will move on and use insulin-to-carbohydrate ratios to determine their mealtime insulin doses.

2 Emphasis is placed on the total amount of carbohydrate rather than the source or type. Sucrose and other sugars may be substituted for other carbohydrates as part of the food/meal plan. Healthy eating remains the bottom line.

3 Foods are divided into 3 food groups: carbohydrate, meat and meat substitutes, and fat.
   A One carbohydrate serving or choice contains 15 g of carbohydrate.
   - Foods that contain carbohydrate are starches, starchy vegetables, fruits, milk, and desserts. Table 1.10 lists examples of common carbohydrate servings.[153]
   - Vegetables also contain carbohydrate but generally in smaller amounts. The green and leafy vegetables only count as a carbohydrate if large amounts are eaten, such as a lunch that consists primarily of a large salad or a plate of cooked vegetables. However, starchy vegetables such as potatoes, corn, peas, or winter squash are considered carbohydrate servings.
   - A free food is defined as any food or drink that contains less than 20 calories and 5 g or less of carbohydrate per serving.
   B An average serving of meat, fish, or poultry is 3 oz or about the size of a deck of cards. An average serving of a meat substitute is 1 oz cheese, ½ cup cottage cheese, 1 egg, or 1 Tb peanut butter.
   C Each fat serving has approximately 5 g of fat. Examples are 1 tsp of butter, margarine, mayonnaise, or oil; 1 Tb of reduced-fat mayonnaise or regular salad dressings; and 2 Tb of reduced-fat salad dressings, cream cheese, or sour cream.

Table 1.10. Examples of Carbohydrate Servings[153]

1 carbohydrate serving = 15 g of carbohydrate

Starch	*Milk*
• 1 slice bread	• 1 cup fat-free or reduced-fat milk
• ⅓ cup pasta or rice	• 6 oz. cup yogurt, plain or flavored, sweetened
• ¾ cup dry cereal	with nonnutritive sweetener
• 4-6 crackers	
• ¼ large baked potato	*Sweets and Desserts*
	• 2 small cookies
Fruit	• 1 Tb jam, honey, syrup
• 1 small fresh fruit	• ½ cup ice cream or frozen yogurt
• ½ cup juice	• 2-in-square cake or brownie

4 Individuals need to know how many carbohydrate servings to choose for meals or snacks, if needed or desired. A typical food/meal plan for adults with type 2 diabetes may start with 3 to 4 carbohydrate servings (45 to 60 g) per meal for women, 4 to 5 carbohydrate servings (60 to 75 g) per meal for men, and 1 to 2 servings (15 to 30 g) for 1 snack. Food records and blood glucose monitoring data can then be used to determine if this amount is appropriate for the individual to consume.
   A Self-monitoring of blood glucose provides the information needed by the individual and the healthcare team to determine the plan's effectiveness in reaching target blood glucose goals.

B In most cases, consistency of carbohydrate intake will reduce fluctuations in postprandial glucose levels. When variation in carbohydrate intake is desired, individuals can be taught to adjust medication to maintain target blood glucose levels.

C As individuals gain more experience with the basics of carbohydrate counting, they become more skilled at estimating and recording carbohydrate intake using either the serving or gram method.

5 Teach persons with diabetes how to prioritize information on the food label.

A The serving size should be considered first. All of the information on the food label is based on the serving size.

B The next information that should be reviewed is total carbohydrate. This number shows the total grams of carbohydrate in 1 serving. Total carbohydrate includes all starches, sugars, and fiber; 15 g of carbohydrate equals 1 carbohydrate serving.

C Grams of sugar can be ignored because they are included in the total grams of carbohydrate.

D If a food has 5 g or more of fiber in a serving, the grams of fiber can be subtracted from the total carbohydrate before converting the total grams of carbohydrate into servings. This applies primarily to nonsoluble fiber and is usually only necessary for persons using insulin-to-carbohydrate ratios.

6 When using carbohydrate counting, the protein and fat content of foods must be considered because of the calories they contribute and, therefore, the potential for weight gain. In usual amounts, however, protein and fat have minimal effects on blood glucose levels.

7 Insulin-to-carbohydrate ratios are important for flexible or intensive insulin regimens or for insulin pump therapy. The goal is to provide accurate rapid-acting bolus (mealtime) insulin doses to cover the amount of carbohydrate that will be eaten.

A Individuals need to eat a consistent amount of carbohydrate at meals for at least 3 days and determine the amount of meal rapid-acting insulin needed to cover that amount of carbohydrate. Furthermore, their diabetes must be relatively well controlled (average glucose <200 mg/dL [11.1 mmol/L]). After the amount of insulin has been determined, the insulin dose is divided into the usual carbohydrate intake. For example, if 60 g of carbohydrate are eaten at breakfast and 4 units of rapid-acting insulin are used before breakfast to cover the carbohydrate consumed, the insulin-to-carbohydrate ratio is 1:15.

B To make insulin adjustments for consuming more or less carbohydrate, the bolus insulin dose can be adjusted accordingly. For more information on insulin-to-carbohydrate ratios, see Chapter 7, Insulin Pump Therapy and Carbohydrate Counting for Pump Therapy: Insulin-to-Carbohydrate Ratios, in Diabetes Management Therapies.

Food/Meal Planning Resources

1 The following resources are some of the materials available from different organizations that can be used in teaching food/meal planning for diabetes.[154]

A *Dietary Guidelines for Americans*[4] and *The Food Guide Pyramid*[155] can be used as an introduction to basic nutrition and to begin the process of changing eating behaviors; these resources do not address issues specific to diabetes.

B *The First Step in Diabetes Meal Planning* (English and Spanish)[25] is a basic, self-contained nutrition pamphlet based on the Food Guide Pyramid. It is designed to be given to persons with diabetes for use until an individualized meal plan can be developed by a dietitian. General guidelines are provided for the recommended number of servings from each food group, and space is provided for the client to identify health goals and steps for reaching goals and to write in an individualized food/meal plan. Foods containing carbohydrate are grouped to facilitate the introduction of this concept, and guidelines for increasing physical activity are included.

C *Healthy Food Choices*[156] is a pamphlet that illustrates the basics of good nutrition and the exchange lists. It opens into a mini-poster that provides a general overview of what to eat and when. Space is provided to write in a detailed meal plan in any "meal planning language" (ie, carbohydrate servings, exchange groups, or actual menu items).

D *Eating Healthy with Diabetes: Easy Reading Guide*[157] is intended for persons with diabetes and limited reading skills or impaired vision. It offers larger print, more photos, and very little text. Food lists are presented in the context of breakfast, lunch, dinner, and snack choices.

E *Exchange Lists for Meal Planning* (English and Spanish)[148] lists groups of measured foods of approximately the same nutritional value; foods in each list can be substituted or exchanged for other foods in the same list. It continues to be the most complete set of food lists that all other diabetes nutrition resources are based on. The exchange lists are used with an individualized meal plan that specifies when and how many exchanges from each group are to be eaten for meals and/or snacks.

F *Basic Carbohydrate Counting*[153] is a foldout pamphlet that introduces basic concepts of carbohydrate counting and encourages consistency of carbohydrate intake using abbreviated food lists.

G *Advanced Carbohydrate Counting*[158] is a booklet that is designed to teach pattern management and how to use insulin-to-carbohydrate ratios. An advanced carbohydrate counting vocabulary list, a list of needed skills, practice exercises, and questions and answers are included. This booklet is intended to be used in conjunction with the *Exchange Lists for Meal Planning* or other carbohydrate-counting nutrition references, as food lists are not included.

H *My Food Plan*[159] is a brochure that provides a simplified approach to carbohydrate counting and meal planning. Common foods are grouped by approximate portion sizes. A personalized food plan provides for individualization; general guidelines for making healthful food choices are included. The booklet is also available in Spanish, *Mi Plan de Comidas.*[159]

I *My Food Plan for Kids & Teens*[160] teaches carbohydrate counting and good nutrition for youth with diabetes and includes fast foods, snack foods, and other favorites. *My Food Plan for Early Kidney Disease*[161] provides simple information about protein, phosphorous, and sodium. *My Food Plan Made Easy*[162] is a simplified, large-print version of *My Food Plan.*

J *Being Healthy Rocks*[163] is a hands-on, educational tool for children and teens who have type 2 diabetes or are at risk. It encourages physical activity and healthier food choices by using engaging characters, lively graphics, and interactive implementation activities.

Ethnic and Cultural Appropriateness

1 Successful diabetes prevention and treatment in diverse ethnic populations requires sensitivity to cultural differences in health beliefs and eating habits.

2 Food choices and eating habits must be understood within the context of culture. Eating is a personal matter that may carry great cultural significance.

3 Health professionals can use a 4-step process to improve cross-cultural counseling: (1) self-evaluation of their own cultural heritage; (2) pre-interview research on the cultural background of each client; (3) in-depth, cross-cultural interview to establish client's personal preferences and cultural background and eating habit adaptations made in the United States; and (4) unbiased analysis of the data[164] (See Chapter 4, Cultural Competence in Diabetes Education and Care, in Diabetes Education and Program Management.)

Celiac Disease and Diabetes

1 Celiac disease is a chronic immunological disorder that affects approximately 2% to 7% of people with type 1 diabetes, which is approximately tenfold the risk compared to the general population.[165,166] People with type 2 diabetes have the same risk as the general population. The association of celiac disease and type 1 diabetes is at least partly explained by similar genetic involvement—HLA-DR3-DQ2 extended haplotype.[166]

2 The mucosa of the small intestine is composed of millions of finger-like projections called villi. The villi produce enzymes necessary to complete the digestion and absorption of food nutrients. In people with celiac disease, gliadin or gluten ingestion causes the villi to atrophy, decreasing their ability to absorb nutrients.

A In the early stage of the disease, the person may experience diarrhea (constant or off-and-on), stomach pains, cramping and bloating, and a feeling of tiredness.

B With repeated exposure to gliadin or gluten, the mild irritation turns into an inflammation. Malabsorption at this point becomes severe. Undiagnosed celiac disease can result in osteoporosis, lymphoma of the small intestine, and serious vitamin and mineral deficiencies. Iron, calcium, and folic acid deficiencies are common in undiagnosed or untreated celiac disease.

C In persons with diabetes, celiac disease may result in poor metabolic control and problems with hypoglycemia.[167,168] However, in a study of 22 persons with type 1 diabetes and celiac disease, there were no significant differences in metabolic control, weight, or hypoglycemic episodes before and after treatment with a gluten-free diet.[169]

3 There is no cure for celiac disease. Treatment is a strict gluten-free diet. Gluten is the protein found in grains, such as wheat, barley, rye, spelt, kamut, graham flour, triticale, millet, buckwheat, and US-grown or processed oats.

A Gluten is the ingredient in flour that gives foods elasticity and a smooth texture. Gluten-free foods tend to be flat and heavy.

B The obvious sources of gluten include wheat, rye, barley and foods processed with these items. The less obvious sources include malt, grain-derived vinegar, modified food starch, hydrolyzed vegetable or plant proteins, stabilizers, gums, artificial colorings or flavorings that have a gluten base, extracts, grain-processed alcohol, and gluten-containing medications. Although consumption of oats has been controversial, the body of research on oats suggests individuals with celiac disease can consume moderate amounts of oats that are not contaminated with wheat, rye, or barley.[170]

C Corn, rice, soybean, tapioca, and potato flours do not contain gluten and are safe to consume. Starches that can be consumed are potatoes, rice, and corn products. There are commercially available pastas made from these starches. Alternative flours include rice, potato, corn, tapioca, bean, nut, soy, arrowroot, and chick peas. Texture is often improved by using a combination of these flours.

Cystic Fibrosis-Related Diabetes

1 Cystic fibrosis is an inherited disease of the exocrine glands resulting in thick, sticky secretions in many organs, including the lung, liver, gastrointestinal tract, and pancreas. The obstructive nature of this mucus predisposes to infection, particularly in the respiratory tract.[171]

A Life expectancy of individuals with cystic fibrosis has improved, with many individuals now reaching adulthood. As survival has increased, cystic fibrosis–related diabetes, has become the leading comorbidity in the population.[172]

B There are four categories of cystic fibrosis–related diabetes based on a standard glucose tolerance test:[173]

- Normal glucose tolerance (NGT)
- Impaired glucose tolerance (IGT)
- Cystic fibrosis–related diabetes without fasting hyperglycemia (CFRD without FH)
- Cystic fibrosis–related diabetes with fasting hyperglycemica (CFRD with FH)

C A1C is not useful for diagnosing CFRD because increased red blood cell turnover in individual's with cystic fibrosis may falsely lower A1C levels. However, it can be useful in monitoring control in established CFRD patients.[173]

D Patients in their baseline state of health are usually insulin sensitive. However, pulmonary exacerbations, severe chronic inflammation, and/or use of high-dose steroids make these individuals highly insulin resistant.

E Currently insulin is the only recommended medication for treatment of CFRD.

- Individuals with CFRD are at risk for the microvascular complications of diabetes, so optimal control of glucose is imperative to prevent these complications and to normalize nutrient metabolism and optimize weight and nutritional status.[171]
- Energy intake may vary widely from day to day depending on the individual's state of health. Therefore, the CFRD consensus guidelines recommend matching insulin to carbohydrates for maximum flexibility.[173]

F The complexity of the daily cystic fibrosis regimen—pulmonary treatments at least 2 times per day; ingestion of pancreatic enzymes with each meal and snack; multiple medications; vitamins—is compounded by the demands of CFRD.

2 Medical nutrition therapy recommendations for type 1 or type 2 diabetes are generally not applicable to patients with CFRD. A high-calorie, high-fat, high-sodium diet is essential to maintaining weight and nutritional status in cystic fibrosis.[174]

A In all cases including those with normal glucose tolerance, caloric restriction is never appropriate. A high-sodium diet is essential in CFRD because of the increased sodium losses via sweat, illness, and exercise. Hyponatremia can result in seizures and death.

B Individuals with IGT are at high risk for progressing to CFRD; however, weight loss and a low-fat diet would never be appropriate for individuals with cystic fibrosis.[171] The only potentially beneficial dietary restriction may be to minimize excessive consumption of regular soda or other sweetened beverages and to maximize intake of nutrient-dense foods to prevent weight loss. Spreading carbohydrate throughout the day may also be beneficial.

C Individuals with CFRD without FH may have elevated postprandial glucose caused by illness, chronic steroid use, and insulin resistance. This can result in malnutrition and weight loss, and this nutritional decline may warrant mealtime insulin therapy. Those not treated with insulin may do better by minimizing large carbohydrate loads; spreading carbohydrate intake throughout the day without reducing caloric intake.[171]

D Individuals with CFRD with FH typically produce adequate amounts of basal insulin during the day but require exogenous insulin for meals and large snacks. They may also require modest doses of nighttime insulin to cover morning fasting hyperglycemia.[173] Reviewing food and blood glucose monitoring records is recommended to confirm the insulin-to-carbohydrate ratio.

3 Pregnancy in women with cystic fibrosis is now commonplace. During pregnancy in women with CFRD or gestational diabetes, adequate weight gain is imperative for the best outcomes and the use of oral supplements may be necessary to ensure proper weight gain. Monitoring of blood glucose and aggressive use of insulin assist in achieving blood glucose goals.[171]

Translating Diabetes Nutrition Recommendations for Use in Healthcare Facilities

1 Standardized calorie-level meal patterns based on exchange lists have traditionally been used to plan meals for hospitalized patients.

A The nutrition prescription was usually determined by a physician and ordered as an ADA diet with a specified calorie level and/or percentage of carbohydrate, protein, and fat.

B The term ADA diet is no longer appropriate since the American Diabetes Association does not endorse any single meal plan or specified percentages of macronutrients.[175,176]

2 A number of alternative meal planning systems are available, each with various advantages and disadvantages. A preferred method of meal planning is to implement a consistent day-to-day carbohydrate diabetes meal plan. This method uses meal plans that incorporate consistent carbohydrate intake at meals and snacks, appropriate fat modifications, and consistent timing of meals and snacks instead of specific calorie levels.

3 Meal plans that are labeled "no concentrated sweets," "no sugar added," "low sugar," and "liberal diabetic diets" are no longer appropriate. These diets do not reflect the current diabetes nutrition recommendations and unnecessarily restrict sucrose.

4 Patients requiring clear-liquid or full-liquid diets should receive approximately 150 to 200 g of carbohydrate per day spread evenly throughout the day at meal and snack times to prevent starvation ketosis. Liquids included should not be sugar-free.

5 Providing adequate nutrition is the primary concern for residents of long-term care facilities. It is appropriate to use the regular menu for residents with fairly consistent day-to-day amounts of carbohydrate at meals and snacks (+ 15 g). Low-calorie meal plans are not generally appropriate.

6 For the hospitalized patient with diabetes who requires parenteral or enteral nutrition, the nutritional assessment, indications for nutrition support, estimate of nutritional needs, and guidelines for metabolic monitoring are similar to those of the nondiabetic patient.[177]

   A Once it is determined that nutrition support is necessary, the optimal route for nutrient delivery should be determined. The enteral route is preferred if the gastrointestinal tract is functional.

   B A major goal of glucose management is to avoid the extremes of hyper- and hypoglycemia. Avoidance of overfeeding is important because an excess of calories can exacerbate hyperglycemia. Studies have shown that the actual energy expenditure of most hospitalized patients is between 100% and 120% of usual calorie expenditure.[177] No consensus exists concerning nutritional requirements of obese patients. One suggestion is to provide approximately 75% of basal energy requirements calculated on the basis of the obese weight.[177]

   C In general, the malnourished patient with normal renal and hepatic function should receive 1.0 to 1.5 g protein/kg body weight; the higher end of the range is for more stressed patients.

Key Educational Considerations

1 Emphasize the goals of nutrition therapy for persons with either type 1 or type 2 diabetes: improve blood glucose control, lipids, and blood pressure. To prevent hyperglycemia and maintain euglycemia, food intake is balanced with insulin(s) taken by injection or insulin still being produced by the pancreas and with physical activity. Strategies for improving blood glucose control for persons with type 2 diabetes that can be helpful include

   A Decreasing energy intake, fat, and carbohydrate through food selection and eating smaller portion sizes

   B Achieving moderate weight loss; the biggest improvement in blood glucose levels occurs with a modest weight loss

   C Increasing physical activity levels

   D Improving eating behaviors (eg, eating breakfast and lunch instead of consuming all calories late in the day)

   E Using blood glucose monitoring results to evaluate the relationships between food, physical activity, medication, coping skills, and the effectiveness of food/meal and physical activity changes.

2 Emphasize to individuals that they have not failed if their meal-planning strategies have not improved their blood glucose control. A change in therapy may be needed to meet blood glucose goals; changing medications is a natural progression in the management of diabetes.

3 To encourage participation in nutrition education, show individuals a list of the nutrition-related topics that are offered and let them choose what they want to learn at each session. This technique also relieves the educator of the unrealistic burden of trying to teach everything in a single session.

4 To elicit past experiences with dietitians or weight loss, ask individuals or use examples of former patients (without identifying source of information). For example, start the discussion with the following patient history: "I worked with a woman who resisted making the initial appointment because her previous experience with dieting was in a program where she had to weigh in at every visit, measure her food at all times, and eat foods that she did not like. She was amazed that meal planning for blood glucose control could be so flexible. What's been your experience?"

5 Use the Nutrition Facts label on food packages to point out the grams of carbohydrate, protein, fat, and number of calories per serving. Help individuals understand that carbohydrate servings are based on 15 g of carbohydrate and fat servings are based on 5 g of fat. Use an actual food label to illustrate that the serving size on the food label may differ from the exchange value. For example, a label for brown rice lists a serving size of 1 cup while the serving size from the starch list for brown rice is ⅓ cup.

6 Invite the individual to teach the educator(s) about the ingredients in and preparation of cultural/ethnic foods. Combining the individual's cultural expertise with the diabetes and nutrition knowledge of the educator allows for a true exchange of information that will benefit the person being counseled.

7 Use menus from local restaurants or fast-food chains to help individuals plan a meal according to their food/meal plan. Using a menu allows for individual preferences and variety and often brings some humor and realism to the teaching session. Through role playing, individuals can also practice their assertiveness skills by asking their "waiter" partner questions about ingredients, preparation, and presentation of food.

8 Conduct a supermarket tour to teach flexibility and variety in meal planning. Participants can read the food labels, learn where to find the recommended foods in the supermarket, learn the aisles to avoid, and compare the nutritional content of different brands of foods.

9 Display a chart or test tubes showing the amounts of sucrose or fat in common foods.
   A Compare small portions of common foods such as a cookie, frozen yogurt, or ice milk with the sucrose in a 12-oz can of regular soft drink, Jello®-type gelatins, fruited yogurt, and other foods.
   B Point out that small portions of sucrose-containing foods can be used as a carbohydrate serving in the meal plan, but that the calorie and fat content of sucrose-containing foods also need to be considered.

10 Offer samples of products or coupons to encourage people to try some new foods. Helping an individual change from the usual egg-and-bacon-on-a-roll breakfast may be more successful if the person has tried and liked a new whole-grain cereal.

11 The terms sugar-free, fat-free, and lite on foods do not mean that these foods are "free" or contain fewer calories than regular foods. To teach this concept, use food labels to demonstrate the number of calories in and the fat and carbohydrate content of a common sugar-free or fat-free product.

12 To teach people with diabetes how to consider the total amount of carbohydrate when selecting a piece of cake, the educator can offer a rule of thumb that a 2-in square contains approximately 15 g of carbohydrate and 5 g of fat (1 carbohydrate and 1 fat serving). One piece (1/6) of a frosted, 2-layer cake, however, contains approximately 45 g of carbohydrate and 10 g of fat (3 carbohydrate and 2 fat servings).

13 Emphasize the importance of accurate portion skills. Encourage use of a food scale, measuring spoons, and measuring cups. Consider using food labs to improve your own skills as well as the skills of those you educate. Practice repeatedly. Explain that periodic measuring and weighing needs to be an ongoing activity for accurate carbohydrate counting.

14 Use the individual's records to demonstrate patterns in food, medication, activity, and blood glucose levels. Ask the individual's opinion of what is happening. Initially, the educator can interpret the results. The individual can assume increasing responsibility for this over time.

15 After determining individual insulin-to-carbohydrate ratios, provide ample opportunities for the individual to complete paper-and-pencil exercises that simulate situations in which insulin adjustments would be needed for larger- or smaller-than-usual meals or snacks. Examples include weekend brunch, pizza parties, or a light lunch.

16 Monitor the individual's weight. If weight gain is a problem, emphasize portion control, limiting meat and fat intake, and using weight-management behaviors.

Self-Review Questions

1 What are the major goals of medical nutrition therapy (MNT) for persons with diabetes?

2 How many calories per gram do carbohydrate, protein, fat, and alcohol contribute to the energy content of the diet?

3 What factors determine the postmeal glycemic response of foods?

4 What are 2 priorities related to the carbohydrate content of the food/meal plan?

5 How are foods containing sucrose used in a food/meal plan?

6 Name 4 types of nonnutritive sweeteners currently available on the market and 4 nutritive sweeteners that are frequently substituted for sucrose in food products.

7 What is the effect of protein on the postmeal blood glucose response?

8 List 3 types of fatty acids found in foods and list 3 examples of foods containing each type of fatty acid. What is the major effect of each type of fatty acid on blood lipid levels?

9 What are recommendations for the use of alcoholic beverages for persons with diabetes?

10 What information is needed prior to the first nutrition visit?

11 How is the nutrition prescription determined?

12 List the 4 groups of foods that contain carbohydrate. What are average portion sizes for common foods in each group?

13 List the exchange lists. Each list is based on how many calories and grams of carbohydrate, protein, and fat? Why is it helpful to know these values?

14 Distinguish between basic/initial versus continuing self-management training. How are food diaries used?

15 Determine the approximate range of caloric requirement per day for an inactive man weighing 195 lb (89 kg).

16 Determine the approximate range of caloric requirement per day for an inactive woman weighing 165 lb (75 kg).

17 List 2 meal-planning tools that can be used to teach basic diabetes nutrition.

18 How can the values on food labels be prioritized?

19 What is the definition of a "free food" for carbohydrate counting?

20 State 2 primary principles of insulin-to-carbohydrate ratios.

21 Calculate how much insulin would be needed to cover 90 g of carbohydrate for someone using an insulin-to-carbohydrate ratio of 1 unit of insulin to 15 g of carbohydrate.

22 Why do individuals using insulin-to-carbohydrate ratios also need to be concerned about intake of dietary fat and meat?

Learning Assessment: Case Study 1

AJ is a 45-year-old woman who was diagnosed with type 2 diabetes 5 years ago. She has not been in for a medical checkup for 3 years. She decided to return at this time because of chronic fatigue and blurry vision. Her A1C value is 8.3% (normal = 4% to 6%), cholesterol is 214 mg/dL (5.5 mmol/L), and triglycerides are 275 mg/dL (3.1 mmol/L). Her current weight is 175 lb (79.5 kg), height 5 ft 4 in (162 cm); body mass index (BMI) = 30 kg/m². She states that she hasn't returned for any follow-up visits because the only advice she gets is to lose weight and not eat sugar, neither of which she is able to do.

Questions for Discussion

1 How should you deal with AJ's negative feelings about diabetes food/meal planning?

2 What are possible initial educational topics for AJ?

3 What are short-term food/meal planning strategies for AJ?

4 What information and educational tools might be helpful for AJ at this time?

5 How can continued education and counseling be planned and provided for AJ?

Discussion

1 Start the session by asking AJ about her concerns about diabetes and the symptoms she is experiencing. Ask how she believes you can be most helpful to her.

2 The initial educational approaches that can be discussed with AJ include reviewing lifestyle strategies besides weight loss she can implement to improve her diabetes control. Explain to her the changes in the understanding of diabetes and management that have occurred since she was diagnosed. Diabetes is a progressive disease and the symptoms she is experiencing may be the result of a failing pancreas. It is important to start with lifestyle changes, and then decide whether medication(s) also needs to be added. She needs to understand she is not to blame herself. Ask if she is willing to identify a strategy to implement, and then review blood glucose monitoring and blood glucose goals with her.

3 Short-term meal planning options for AJ include learning to count carbohydrate servings at meals and snacks and beginning some type of regular physical activity.

4 AJ was introduced to carbohydrate counting. A simplified educational tool was used to help her understand that foods are grouped into carbohydrate, meat, and fat servings. Average portion sizes for different types of food were discussed. She felt that 3 to 4 carbohydrate servings at breakfast, 2 to 3 at lunch, 3 to 4 at dinner, and 1 to 2 for a snack (evening), 1 oz to 2 oz of meat at lunch, 3 oz to 4 oz of meat at supper, and 1 to 2 fat servings per meal would be a reasonable food plan. She also stated she would like to begin a walking program.

  A AJ agreed to keep food and blood glucose records and return in 2 weeks for a follow-up visit. At that visit she will have the opportunity to identify problems she is having with the strategies she chose. The dietitian and AJ can also evaluate the effect of the food and exercise changes on her blood glucose levels. Changes will be made as needed.

  B As an educator you realize that, depending on her previous eating habits and with her 5-year duration of diabetes, the expected outcome from MNT is approximately a 1% decrease in A1C. Therefore, you need to evaluate if lifestyle changes alone will be adequate for AJ or whether medications need to be combined with MNT.

5 At 3 months AJ is to return for an A1C test. At that time, the decision can be made as to whether MNT and physical activity alone are adequate or if there is a need to add an oral agent or other medications. Her lipids should be retested in 3 to 6 months. At each visit, the emphasis should be on reaching blood glucose goals and not on weight loss.

Learning Assessment: Case Study 2

JD is a 52-year-old male diagnosed with type 2 diabetes 6 years ago. His A1C value is 9.6% (normal = 4.4% to 6.1%). He has hypertension and is on antihypertensive medication and has elevated triglycerides and low HDL cholesterol. He is currently taking glipizide 2.5 mg, tid. JD has been asked to test his blood glucose before breakfast and dinner and at bedtime. His readings are consistently above his target goal ranges. He reports that over the years his blood glucose levels have continued to go up even though he hasn't changed what he eats. Lately, he has stopped testing because he reports that no matter what he does and how hard he tries to follow his diet, his blood glucose levels do not improve.

JD is 5 ft 10 in (178 cm) and weighs 195 lb (89 kg) (BMI is 28). His weight has been stable over the past 5 years. The food/nutrition assessment shows that JD eats 3 meals daily and a midafternoon and evening snack. His current estimated daily caloric intake is 2300 to 2500 calories. He eats breakfast at home, brings a lunch to work, and has his evening meal at home. He used to drink 2 to 3 beers per day but has been avoiding alcohol the past year. He is physically active in his job as a school custodian and walks to and from work Monday through Friday (2 miles round trip).

JD's doctor wants him to begin taking insulin and has recommended he start with 2 injections a day, taking rapid-acting insulin and NPH insulin before breakfast and before his evening meal. JD states that he attended diabetes classes when he was first diagnosed with diabetes. Three months ago he had a consult with a dietitian who introduced him to carbohydrate counting. He has been keeping a record of his food intake, blood glucose levels, and physical activity, but has been frustrated because they have not improved, so he is willing to try insulin.

Questions for Discussion

1 Why have JD's blood glucose levels increased even though his lifestyle has not changed and his food habits and physical activity level are better than a year ago?

2 What food/meal planning skills will be important for JD as he starts taking insulin?

3 What resources or tools can you recommend to JD to help him be more successful with carbohydrate counting?

4 How can you determine JD's interest in his wife's involvement and her willingness to assist JD?

Discussion

1 Explain to JD about the progressive nature of type 2 diabetes and why at this time it is important for him to begin taking insulin. He appears to have mastered the basics of carbohydrate counting. He is willing to keep records of his food intake, blood glucose levels, and insulin so that his insulin dose can be adjusted to cover his preferred lifestyle. He plans to highlight blood glucose levels outside the target range and will focus on the influence of carbohydrate foods.

2 It will be beneficial for JD to purchase a carbohydrate reference book and measuring cups so he can better determine portion sizes. He also needs to be alerted to the possibility of weight gain as his blood glucose levels improve and, therefore, to watch his meat and fat portions. He feels that he can eat a smaller midafternoon snack. On weekends he will also test his blood glucose levels before lunch. By using his food and testing information, JD hopes to determine what type of insulin regimen would be best for him.

3 JD states that his wife is willing to alter her cooking and he needs her help and support. He is also willing to help with some of the cooking and grocery buying. How to read food labels, prevention and treatment of hypoglycemia, and how to deal with sick days should be reviewed with JD and his wife.

4 JD and his wife plan to develop a list of dinner menus and bedtime snacks. He is also anxious to learn about insulin-to-carbohydrate ratios so eventually he can do more adjusting of his insulin doses. JD and his wife agreed to a follow-up visit in 3 weeks, at which time JD will bring his food and glucose data. JD will probably do better with a longer acting insulin such as glargine at bedtime and rapid-acting insulin before meals to give him the flexibility he wants.

References

1 American Diabetes Association. Evidence-based nutrition principles and recommendations for the treatment and prevention of diabetes and related complications (position statement). Diabetes Care. 2003;26(suppl 1):S51-S61.

2 Franz MJ, Bantle JP, Beebe CA, et al. Evidence-based nutrition principles and recommendations for the treatment and prevention of diabetes and related complications (technical review). Diabetes Care. 2002;25:148-198.

3 Franz MJ, Bantle JP, eds. The American Diabetes Association's Guide to Medical Nutrition Therapy for Diabetes. Alexandria, Va: American Diabetes Association; 1999.

4 US Department of Agriculture and US Department of Health and Human Services. Nutrition and Your Health: Dietary Guidelines for Americans 2000. 5th ed. Hyattsville, Md: USDA Human Nutrition Information Service; 2000. Home and Garden Bulletin No. 232.

5 Krauss RM, Eckel RH, Howard B, et al. AHA dietary guidelines. Revision 2000: a statement for healthcare professionals from the Nutrition Committee of the American Heart Association. Circulation. 2000; 102:2284-2299.

6 de Chavez M, Chavez A. Diet that prevents cancer: recommendations from the American Institute for Cancer Research. Int J Cancer. 1998;11(suppl):85-89.

7 Kant AK, Schatzkin A, Graubard BI, Schairer C. A prospective study of diet quality and mortality in women. JAMA. 2000;283:2109-2115.

8 Huijbregts P, Feskens E, Rasanen L, et al. Dietary patterns and 20 year mortality in elderly men in Finland, Italy, and The Netherlands: longitudinal cohort study. BMJ. 1997;315:13-17.

9 Appel LJ, Moore TJ, Obarzanek E, et al. A clinical trial of the effects of dietary patterns on blood pressure. N Engl J Med. 1997;336:1117-1124.

10 Anderson JW, Hanna TJ, Peng X, Kryscio RJ. Whole grain foods and heart disease risk. J Am Coll Nutr. 2000;19:291S-299S.

11 Liu S, Manson JE, Lee I-M, et al. Fruit and vegetable intake and risk of cardiovascular disease: the Women's Health Study. Am J Clin Nutr. 2000;72:922-928.

12 Hu FB, Rimm EB, Stampfer MJ, Ascherio A, Spiegelman D, Willett WC. Prospective study of major dietary patterns and risk of coronary heart disease in men. Am J Clin Nutr. 2000;72:912-921.

13 Ary DV, Toobert D, Wilson W, Glasgow RE. Patient perspective factors contributing to nonadherence to diabetes regimen. Diabetes Care. 1986;9:168-172.

14 Pastors JG, Warshaw H, Daly A, Franz M, Kulkarni K. The evidence for the effectiveness of medical nutrition therapy in diabetes management. Diabetes Care. 2002;25:608-613.

15 Delahanty LM, Halford BN. The role of diet behaviors in achieving improved glycemic control in intensively treated patients in the Diabetes Control and Complications Trial. Diabetes Care. 1993;16:1453-1458.

16 UK Prospective Diabetes Study (UKPDS) Group: UK Prospective Diabetes Study 7: response of fasting plasma glucose to diet therapy in newly presenting type II diabetic patients. Metabolism. 1990;39:905-912.

17 Kulkarni K, Castle G, Gregory R, et al. Nutrition practice guidelines for type 1 diabetes mellitus positively affect dietitian practices and patient outcomes. J Am Diet Assoc. 1998;98:62-70.

18 Franz MJ, Monk A, Barry B, et al. Effectiveness of medical nutrition therapy provided by dietitians in the management of non-insulin-dependent diabetes mellitus: a randomized, controlled clinical trial. J Am Diet Assoc. 1995;95:1009-1017.

19 Diabetes Control and Complications Trial Research Group. The effect of intensive treatment of diabetes on the development and progression of long-term complications in insulin-dependent diabetes mellitus. N Engl J Med. 1993;329:977-986.

20 UK Prospective Diabetes Study (UKPDS) Group. Intensive blood-glucose control with sulphonylureas or insulin compared with conventional treatment and risk of complications in patients with type 2 diabetes (UKPDS 33). Lancet. 1998;352:837-853.

21 American Diabetes Association. Standards of medical care for patients with diabetes mellitus (position statement). Diabetes Care. 2003;26(suppl 1):S33-S50.

22 ACE Consensus Development Conference on Guidelines for Glycemic Control. Endocr Pract. 2001;suppl. Nov/Dec.

23 American Diabetes Association. Management of dyslipidemia in adults with diabetes (position statement). Diabetes Care. 2003;26(suppl 1):S83-S86.

24 American Academy of Pediatrics, Committee on Nutrition. Cholesterol in children. Pediatrics. 1998;101:141-147.

25 The First Step in Diabetes Meal Planning. Alexandria, Va and Chicago: American Diabetes Association and American Dietetic Association; 2003.

26 American Diabetes Association. Type 2 diabetes in children and adolescents (consensus statement). Diabetes Care. 2000;23:381-389.

27 Helmrich SP, Ragland DR, Leung RW, Paffenbarger RS. Physical activity and reduced occurrence of non-insulin dependent diabetes mellitus. N Eng J Med. 1991;325:147-152.

28 Wei M, Gibbons LW, Mitchell TL, Kampert JG, Lee CD, Blair SN. The association between cardiorespiratory fitness and impaired fasting glucose and type 2 diabetes in men. Ann Intern Med. 1999;130:89-96.

29 Hu FB, Sigal RJ, Rich-Edwards JW, et al. Walking compared with vigorous physical activity and risk of type 2 diabetes in women. JAMA. 1999;282:1433-1439.

30 Moore LL, Visioni AJ, Wilson PWF, D'Agostino RB, Finkle WD, Ellison RC. Can sustained weight loss in overweight individuals reduce the risk of diabetes mellitus? Epidemiology. 2000;11:269-273.

31 Will JC, Williamson DF, Ford ES, Calle EE, Thun MJ. International weight loss and 13-year diabetes incidence in overweight adults. Am J Public Health. 2002;92:1245-1248.

32 Tuomilehto J, Lindstom J, Eriksson JG, et al. For the Finnish Diabetes Prevention Study Group. Prevention of type 2 diabetes mellitus by changes in lifestyle among subjects with impaired glucose tolerance. N Engl J Med. 2001;344:1343-1350.

33 Diabetes Prevention Program Research Group. Reduction in the incidence of type 2 diabetes with lifestyle intervention or metformin. N Engl J Med. 2002;346:393-403.

34 DAFNE Study Group. Training in flexible, intensive insulin management to enable dietary freedom in people with type 1 diabetes: dose adjustment for normal eating (DAFNE) randomized controlled trial. BMJ; 2002;325:746-752.

35 Rabasa-Lhoret R, Garon J, Langlier H, Poisson D, Chiasson J-L. Effects of meal carbohydrate on insulin requirements in type 1 diabetic patients treated intensively with the basal-bolus (Ultralente-regular) insulin regimen. Diabetes Care. 1999;22:667-673.

36 Lafrance L, Rabasa-Lhoret R, Poisson D, Ducros F, Chiasson J-L. The effects of different glycaemic index foods and dietary fibre intake on glycaemic control in type 1 diabetic patients on intensive insulin therapy. Diabetic Med. 1998;15:972-978.

37 Wolever TMS, Hamad S, Chiasson J-L, et al. Day-to-day consistency in amount and source of carbohydrate intake associated with improved glucose control in type 1 diabetes. J Am Coll Nutr. 1999;18:242-247.

38 Chaturvedi N, Stevens LK, Fuller JH. The WHO Multinational Study of Vascular Disease in Diabetes. Mortality and morbidity associated with body weight in people with IDDM. Diabetes Care. 1995;18:761-765.

39 Purnell JQ, Hokanson JE, Marcovina SM, Steffes MW, Cleary PA, Brunzell JD. Effect of excessive weight gain with intensive therapy of type 1 diabetes on lipid levels and blood pressure. JAMA. 1998;280:140-146.

40 Williams KV, Erbey JR, Becker D, Orchard TJ. Improved glycemic control reduces the impact of weight gain on cardiovascular risk factors in type 1 diabetes. Diabetes Care. 1999;22:1084-1091.

41 Rabasa-Lhoret R, Bourque J, Ducros F, Chiasson J-L. Guidelines for premeal insulin dose reduction for postprandial exercise of different intensities and durations for type 1 diabetic subjects (Ultralente-lispro). Diabetes Care. 2001;24:635-640.

42 Brownell KD, Wadden TA. Etiology and treatment of obesity: understanding a serious, prevalent, and refractory disorder. J Consult Clin Psychol. 1992;60:505-517.

43 Maggio CA, Pi-Sunyer FX. The prevention and treatment of obesity. Application to type 2 diabetes (technical review). Diabetes Care. 1997;20:1744-1766.

44 Foreyt JP, Goodrick GK. Evidence for success of behavior modification in weight loss and control. Ann Intern Med. 1993;119:698-701.

45 Markovic TP, Jenkins AB, Campbell LV, Furler SM, Kraegen EW, Chisholm DJ. The determinants of glycemic responses to diet restriction and weight loss in obesity and NIDDM. Diabetes Care. 1998;21:687-694.

46 Wing RR, Blair EH, Bononi P, et al. Caloric restriction per se is a significant factor in improvements in glycemic control and insulin sensitivity during weight loss in obese NIDDM patients. Diabetes Care. 1994;17:30-36.

47 Kelley DE, Wing R, Buonocore C, Sturis J, Polonsky K, Fitzsimmons M. Relative effects of calorie restriction and weight loss in non-insulin-dependent diabetes mellitus. J Clin Endocrinol Metab. 1993;77:1287-1293.

48 Wing RR, Koeske R, Epstein LH, et al. Long-term effects of modest weight loss in type II diabetic patients. Arch Intern Med. 1987;147:1749-1753.

49 Markovic TP, Campbell LV, Balasubramanian S, et al. Beneficial effect on average lipid levels from energy restriction and fat loss in obese individuals with or without type 2 diabetes. Diabetes Care. 1998;21:695-700.

50 Watts NB, Spanheimer RG, DiGirolamo M, et al. Prediction of glucose response to weight loss in patients with non-insulin-dependent diabetes mellitus. Arch Intern Med. 1990;150:803-806.

51 National Institutes of Health, National Heart, Lung, and Blood Institute. Clinical guidelines on the identification, evaluation, and treatment of overweight and obesity in adults—the evidence report. Obes Res. 1998;6:51S-209S.

52 Mokdad AH, Ford ES, Bowman BA, et al. Prevalence of obesity, diabetes, and obesity-related health risks factors, 2001. JAMA. 2003;289:76-79.

53 Yamashita S, Nakamura T, Shimonura I, et al. Insulin resistance and body fat distribution. Diabetes Care. 1996;19:287-291.

54 Fujimoto WY, Bergstrom RW, Boyko EJ, et al. Visceral adiposity and incident coronary heart disease in Japanese-American men. Diabetes Care. 1999;22:1808-1812.

55 Tsunehara CH, Leonetti DL, Fujimoto WY. Diet of second-generation Japanese American men with and without noninsulin-dependent diabetes. J Am Clin Nutr. 1990;52:731-738.

56 Lovejoy JC, Windhauser MM, Rood JC, de la Bretonne JA. Effect of a controlled high-fat versus a low-fat diet on insulin sensitivity and leptin levels in African-American and Caucasian women. Metabolism. 1998;47:1520-1524.

57 Marshall JA, Bessesen DH, Hamman RF. High saturated fat and low starch and fiber are associated with hyperinsulinemia in a non-diabetic population: the San Luis Valley Diabetes Study. Diabetologia. 1997;40:430-438.

58 Mayer-Davis EJ, Monacao JH, Hoen HM, et al. Dietary fat and insulin sensitivity in a triethnic population: the role of obesity. The Insulin Resistance Atherosclerosis Study (IRAS). Am J Clin Nutr. 1997;65:79-87.

59 Louheranta AM, Schwab US, Sarkkinen ES. Insulin sensitivity after a reduced-fat diet and a mono-enriched diet in subjects with elevated serum cholesterol and triglyceride concentrations. Nutr Metab Cardiovasc Dis. 2000;10;177-187.

60 Riccardi G, Rivellese AA. Dietary treatment of the metabolic syndrome—the optimal diet. Br J Nutr. 2000;83(suppl 1):S143-S148.

61 Denkins YM, Lovejoy JC, Smith SR. Omega-3 PUFA supplementation and insulin sensitivity. FASEB J. 2002;16:A24.

62 Lissner L, Levitsky DA, Strupp BJ, Kalkwarf HJ, Roe DA. Dietary fat and the regulation of energy intake in human subjects. Am J Clin Nutr. 1987;46:886-892.

63 Schaefer EJ, Lichtenstein AH, Lamon-Fava S, et al. Body weight and low-density lipoprotein cholesterol changes after consumption of a low-fat ad libitum diet. JAMA. 1995;274:1450-1455.

64 Turley ML, Skeaff CM, Mann JI, Cox B. The effect of a low-fat, high-carbohydrate diet on serum high density lipoprotein cholesterol and triglycerides. Eur J Clin Nutr. 1998;52:728-732.

65 Tourbro S, Astrup A. Randomized comparison of diet for maintaining obese subjects' weight after major weight loss: ad lib, low fat, high carbohydrate diet vs. fixed energy intake. BMJ. 1997:314:29-34.

66 Bessesen DH. The role of carbohydrate in insulin resistance. J Nutr. 2001;131:2782S-2786S.

67 Garg A, Bantle JP, Henry RR, et al. Effects of varying carbohydrate content of diet in patients with non-insulin dependent diabetes mellitus. JAMA. 1994;271:1421-1428.

68 Eely EA, Stratton IM, Hadden DR, on behalf of the UKPDS. Estimated dietary intake in type 2 diabetic patients randomly allocated to diet, sulfonylurea, or insulin therapy (UKPDS). Diabetic Med. 1996;13:656-662.

69 Mayer-Davis EJ, D'Agostino RJ, Karter AJ, et al. Intensity and amount of physical activity in relation to insulin sensitivity. The Insulin Resistance and Atherosclerosis Study (IRAS). JAMA 1998;270:669-674.

70 Schneider SH, Khachadurian AK, Amorosa LF, et al. Ten-year experience with exercise-based outpatient life-style modification program in the treatment of diabetes mellitus. Diabetes Care. 1992;15:1800-1810.

71 Yamanouchi K, Shinozaki T, Chikada K, et al. Daily walking combined with diet therapy is a useful means for obese NIDDM patients not only to reduce body weight but also to improve insulin sensitivity. Diabetes Care. 1995;18:775-778.

72 Wei M, Gibbons LW, Kampert JB, Nichaman MZ, Blair SN. Low cardiorespiratory fitness and physical inactivity as predictors of mortality in men with type 2 diabetes. Ann Intern Med. 2000;132:605-611.

73 Albright A, Franz M, Hornsby G, et al. American College of Sports Medicine position stand. Exercise and type 2 diabetes. Med Sci Sports Exerc. 2000;32:1345-1350.

74 Arnold L, Mann J, Ball M. Metabolic effects of alterations in meal frequency in type 2 diabetes. Diabetes Care. 1997;20:1651-1654.

75 Jenkins DJ, Ocana A, Jenkins AL, et al. Metabolic advantages of spreading the nutrient load: effects of increased meal frequency in non-insulin-dependent diabetes. Am J Clin Nutr. 1992;55:461-467.

76 Bertelsen J, Christiansen C, Thomsen C, et al. Effect of meal frequency on blood glucose, insulin, and free fatty acids in NIDDM subjects. Diabetes Care. 1993;16:4-7.

77 Vallis M, Ruggiero L, Greene G, et al. Stages of change for healthy eating in diabetes. Diabetes Care. 2003;26:1468-1474.

78 Monk A, Barry B, McClain K, et al. Practice guidelines for medical nutrition therapy provided by dietitians for persons with non-insulin-dependent diabetes mellitus. J Am Diet Assoc. 1995;95:999-1006.

79 Rossetti L, Giaccari A, DeFronzo RA. Glucose toxicity. Diabetes Care. 1990; 13:610-630.

80 Nuttall FQ, Gannon MC. Carbohydrates and diabetes. In: Franz MJ, Bantle JP, eds. American Diabetes Association Guide to Medical Nutrition Therapy for Diabetes. Alexandria, Va: American Diabetes Association; 1999:85-106.

81 Gannon MC, Nuttall FQ. Protein and diabetes. In: Franz MJ, Bantle JP, eds. American Diabetes Association Guide to Medical Nutrition Therapy for Diabetes. Alexandria, Va: American Diabetes Association; 1999:107-125.

82 Boden G, Chen X. Effects of fat on glucose uptake and utilization in patients with non-insulin-dependent diabetes. J Clin Invest. 1995;96:1251-1268.

83 Fraser RJ, Horowitz M, Maddox AF, Harding PE, Chatterton BE, Dent J. Hyperglycemia slows gastric emptying rate in type I (insulin-dependent) diabetes mellitus. Diabetologia. 1990;33;675-680.

84 Schvarcz E, Palmer M, Aman J, Lindkvist B, Beckman K-W. Hypoglycemia increases gastric emptying rate in patients with type I diabetes mellitus. Diabetic Med. 1993; 10:660-663.

85 Jarvi A, Karlstrom B, Grandfeldt Y, Bjorck I, Vesby B. The influence of food structure on postprandial metabolism in patients with NIDDM. Am J Clin Nutr. 1995; 61:837-842.

86 Parillo M, Giacco R, Ciardullo AV, Rivellese AA, Riccardi G. Does a high-carbohydrate diet have different effects in NIDDM patients treated with diet alone or hypoglycemic drugs. Diabetes Care. 1996; 19:498-500.

87 Bantle JP, Swanson JE, Thomas W, Laine DC. Metabolic effects of dietary sucrose in type II diabetic subjects. Diabetes Care. 1993;16:1301-1305.

88 Peterson DB, Lambert J, Gerring S, et al. Sucrose in the diet of diabetic patients - just another carbohydrate? Diabetologia. 1986;29:216-220.

89 Rickard KA, Loghmani E, Cleveland JL, Fineberg NS, Greidenberg GR. Lower glycemic response to sucrose in the diets of children with type 1 diabetes. J Pediatr. 1998;133:429-432.

90 Malerbi DA, Paiva ES, Duarte AL, Wajchenberg BL. Metabolic effects of dietary sucrose and fructose in type II diabetic subjects. Diabetes Care. 1996;19:1249-1256.

91 Franz MJ. Carbohydrate and diabetes: is the source or the amount of more importance? Current Diabetes Reports. 2002;1:177-186.

92 Giacco R, Parillo M, Rivellese AA, et al. Long-term dietary treatment with increased amounts of fiber-rich low-glycemic index natural food improves blood glucose control and reduces the number of hypoglycemic events in type 1 patients with diabetes. Diabetes Care. 2000;23:1461-1466.

93 Chandalia M, Garg A, Luthohann D, vonBergmann K, Grundy SM, Brinkley LJ. Beneficial effects of a high dietary fiber intake in patients with type 2 diabetes. N Engl J Med. 2000;342:1392-1398.

94 Hollenbeck CG, Coulston AM, Reaven GM. To what extent does increased dietary fiber improve glucose and lipid metabolism in patients with noninsulin-dependent diabetes mellitus (NIDDM)? Am J Clin Nutr. 1986;43:16-24.

95 Bantle JP, Swanson JE, Thomas W, Laine DC. Metabolic effects of dietary fructose in diabetic subjects. Diabetes Care. 1992;15:1468-1476.

96 Bantle JP, Raatz SK, Thomas W, Georgopoulos A. Effects of dietary fructose on plasma lipids in healthy subjects. Am J Clin Nutr. 2000;72:1128-1134.

97 Akgum S, Ertel NH. A comparison of carbohydrate metabolism after sucrose, sorbitol, and fructose meals in normal and diabetic subjects. Diabetes Care. 1980;3:582-585.

98 Butchko HH, Stargel WW. Aspartame: scientific evaluation in the postmarketing period. Regulatory Toxicol and Pharmacol. 2001;34:221-233.

99 Powers M. Sugar alternatives and fat replacers. In: Franz MJ, Bantle JP, eds. American Diabetes Association Guide to Medical Nutrition Therapy for Diabetes. Alexandria, Va: American Diabetes Association; 1999:148-164.

100 London R. Saccharin and aspartame. Are they safe to consume during pregnancy? J Reprod Med. 1988;33:17-21.

101 World Health Organization Expert Committee on Food Additives. Toxicological Evaluation of Certain Food Additives and Food Contaminants. Geneva, Switzerland: World Health Organization. 1981;16:11-27 and 1983; 18:12-14.

102 Franz MJ. Protein controversies in diabetes. Diabetes Spectrum. 2000;13: 132-141.

103 Nuttall FQ, Mooradian AD, Giannon MC, Billington C, Krezowski P. Effect of protein ingestion on the glucose and insulin response to a standardized oral glucose load. Diabetes Care. 1984;7:465-470.

104 Gannon MC, Nuttall JA, Damberg G, Gupta V, Nuttall FQ. Effect of protein ingestion on the glucose appearance rate in people with type 2 diabetes. J Clin Endocrinol Metab. 2001;86:1040-1047.

105 Peters AL, Davidson MB. Protein and fat effects on glucose responses and insulin requirements in subjects with insulin-dependent diabetes mellitus. Am J Clin Nutr. 1993;58:555-560.

106 Gray RO, Butler PC, Beers TR, Kryshak EJ, Rizza RA. Comparison of the ability of bread versus bread plus meat to treat and prevent subsequent hypoglycemia in patients with insulin-dependent diabetes mellitus. J Clin Endocrinol Metab. 1996;81:1508-1511.

107 Kalergis M, Schiffrin A, Gougeon R, Jone PJH, Yale J-F. Impact of bedtime snack composition on prevention of nocturnal hypoglycemia in adults with type 1 diabetes undergoing intensive insulin management using lispro insulin before meals. A randomized, placebo-controlled, crossover trial. Diabetes Care. 2003;26:9-15.

108 American Diabetes Association. Diabetic nephropathy (position statement). Diabetes Care. 2003;26(suppl 1):S94-S98.

109 Wheeler ML, Fineberg SE, Fineberg NS, Gibson RG, Hackward LL. Animal versus plant protein meals in individuals with type 2 diabetes and microalbuminuria. Diabetes Care. 2002;15:1277-1282.

110 Hu FB, Stampfer MJ, Rimm EB, et al. A prospective study of egg consumption and risk of cardiovascular disease in men and women. JAMA. 1999;281:1387-1394.

111 Madigan C, Ryan M, Owens D, Collins P, Tomkin GH. Dietary unsaturated fatty acids in type 2 diabetes. Diabetes Care. 2000;23:1472-1477.

112 Heilbronn L, Noakes M, Clifton P. Effect of energy restriction, weight loss, and diet composition on plasma lipids and glucose in patients with type 2 diabetes. Diabetes Care. 1999;22:889-895.

113 Friedberg CE, Janssen MJEM, Heine RJ, Grobbee DE. Fish oil and glycemic control in diabetes: a meta-analysis. Diabetes Care. 1998;21:494-500.

114 Montori VM, Farmer A, Wollan PC, Dinneen SF. Fish oil supplementation in type 2 diabetes: a quantitative systematic review. Diabetes Care. 2000;23:1407-1415.

115 Santamarina-Fogo S. The familial chylomicronemia syndrome. Endocrinol Metab Clin North Am. 1998;27:551-567,viii.

116 Warshaw H, Franz M, Powers MA, Wheeler M. Fat replacers: their use in foods and role in diabetes medical nutrition therapy (technical review). Diabetes Care. 1996;19:1294-1301.

117 Tuck M, Corry D, Trujillo A. Salt-sensitive blood pressure and exaggerated vascular reactivity in the hypertension of diabetes mellitus. Am J Med. 1990;88:210-216.

118 The sixth report of the Joint National Committee on Prevention, Detection, Evaluation, and Treatment of High Blood Pressure. Arch Intern Med. 1997;2413-2446.

119 Sacks FM, Svetkey LP, Vollmer WM, et al. Effects on blood pressure of reduced dietary sodium and the Dietary Approaches to Stop Hypertension (DASH) diet. N Engl J Med. 2001;344:3-10.

120 Kanis JA. The use of calcium in the management of osteoporosis. Bone. 1999;24:279-290.

121 Koehler KM, Pareo-Tubbeh SL, Romero LJ, Baumgartner RN, Garry PJ. Folate nutrition and older adults: challenges and opportunities. J Am Diet Assoc. 1997;97:167-173.

122 Althuis MD, Jordan NE, Ludington EA, Wittes JT. Glucose and insulin responses to dietary chromium supplements: a meta-analysis. Am J Clin Nutr. 2002;76:148-155.

123 Hasanain B, Mooradian AD. Antioxidant vitamins and their influence in diabetes mellitus. Current Diabetes Reports. 2002;2:448-456.

124 Waters DD, Alderman EI, Hsia J, et al. Effects of hormone replacement therapy and antioxidant vitamin supplements on coronary atherosclerosis in post-menopausal women. JAMA. 2002;288:2432-2440.

125 Lonn E, Yusuf S, Hoogwerf B, et al. On behalf of the Heart Outcomes Prevention Evaluation (HOPE) Investigators. Effects of vitamin E on cardiovascular and microvascular outcomes in high-risk patients with diabetes. Diabetes Care. 2002;25:1919-1927.

126 Franz MJ. Alcohol and diabetes. In: Franz MJ, Bantle JP, eds. American Diabetes Association Guide to Medical Nutrition Therapy for Diabetes. Alexandria, Va: American Diabetes Association; 1999:192-210.

127 Turner BC, Jenkins E, Kerr D, et al. The effect of evening alcohol consumption on next-morning glucose control in type 1 diabetes. Diabetes Care. 2001;24:1888-1893.

128 Koivisto VA, Tulokas S, Toivonen M, et al. Alcohol with the meal has no adverse effects on postprandial glucose homeostasis in diabetic patients. Diabetes Care. 1993;16:1612-1614.

129 Ben G, Gnidi L, Maran A, et al. Effects of chronic alcohol intake on carbohydrate and lipid metabolism in subjects with type II (non-insulin-dependent) diabetes. Am J Med. 1991;90:70-76.

130 Mukamal KJ, Conigrave KM, Mittleman MA, et al. Roles of drinking pattern and type of alcohol consumed in coronary heart disease in men. N Engl J Med. 2003;348:109-118.

131 Wei M, Gibbon LW, Mitchell TL, Kampert JB, Blair SN. Alcohol intake and incidence of type 2 diabetes in men. Diabetes Care. 2000;23:18-22.

132 Sacco RL, Elking M, Boden-Albala B, et al. The protective effect of moderate alcohol consumption on ischemic stroke. JAMA. 1999;281:53-60.

133 Bell RA, Mayer-Davis EJ, Martin MA, D'Agostino RB, Haffner SM. Association between alcohol consumption and insulin sensitivity and cardiovascular disease risk factors: the Insulin Resistance and Atherosclerosis Study. Diabetes Care. 2000;23:130-136.

134 Davis MJ, Baer DJ, Judd JT, Brown ED, Campbell WS, Taylor PR. Effects of moderate alcohol intake on fasting insulin and glucose concentrations and insulin sensitivity in postmenopausal women. JAMA. 2002;287:2559-2562.

135 Valmadrid CT, Klein R, Moss SE, Klein BK, Cruickshanks KJ. Alcohol intake and the risk of coronary heart disease mortality in persons with older-onset diabetes mellitus. JAMA. 1999;282:239-246.

136 Solomon CG, Hu FB, Stampfer MJ, et al. Moderate alcohol consumption and risk of coronary heart disease among women with type 2 diabetes. Circulation. 2000;102:494-499.

137 Ajani UA, Gaziano M, Lotufo PA, et al. Alcohol consumption and risk of coronary heart disease by diabetes status. Circulation. 2000;102:500-505.

138 Israelsson B. Role of alcohol, glucose intolerance and obesity in hypertriglyceridemia. Atherosclerosis. 1986;62:123-127.

139 Pownall HJ, Ballantyne CH, Kimball KT, Simpson SL, Yeshurum D, Grotto AM. Effect of moderate alcohol consumption on hypertriglyceridemia. Arch Intern Med. 1999;159:981-986.

140 Pastor JG, Franz MJ, Warshaw H, Daly A, Arnold M. How effective is medical nutrition therapy in diabetes care? J Am Diet Assoc. 2003; in press.

141 Yu-Poth S, Zhao G, Etherton T, Naglak M, Jonnalagadda S, Kris-Etherton PM. Effects of the National Cholesterol Education Program's Step I and Step II dietary intervention programs on cardiovascular disease risk factors: a meta-analysis. Am J Clin Nutr. 1999; 69:632-646.

142 Expert Panel on Detection, Evaluation, and Treatment of High Blood Cholesterol in Adults. Executive summary of the third report of the National Cholesterol Education Program (NCEP) expert panel on detection, evaluation, and treatment of high blood cholesterol in adults (Adult Treatment Panel III). JAMA. 2001; 285:2485-2497.

143 Cutler JA, Follmann D, Allender PS. Randomized trials of sodium restriction: an overview. Am J Clin Nutr. 1997;65(suppl 1):643S-651S.

144 Staessen J, Fagard R, Liunen P, Amery A. Body weight, sodium intake, and blood pressure. J Hypertens. 1989;7(suppl): S19-S23.

145 Appel LJ, Moore TJ, Obarzanek E, et al. A clinical trial of the effects of dietary patterns on blood pressure. N Engl J Med. 1997;336:1117-1124.

146 American Dietetic Association Medical Nutrition Therapy Evidence Based Guides for Practice. Nutrition Practice Guidelines for Type 1 and Type 2 Diabetes Mellitus [on CD-ROM]. Chicago: American Dictctic Association; 2001.

147 Franz MJ, Reader D, Monk A. Implementing Group and Individual Medical Nutrition Therapy for Diabetes. Alexandria, Va: American Diabetes Association; 2002.

148 Exchange Lists for Meal Planning. Alexandria, Va and Chicago: American Diabetes Association and American Dietetic Association; 2003.

149 Wheeler ML. Macronutrient and energy database for the 2003 exchange lists for meal planning. J Am Diet Assoc. 2003; in press.

150 Institute of Medicine of the National Academies. Dietary Reference Intakes: Energy, Carbohydrate, Fiber, Fat, Fatty Acids, Cholesterol, Protein, and Amino Acids. Washington, DC: Thc National Academies Press; 2002:5.1-5.114.

151 Maryniuk MD. Counseling and education strategies for improved adherence to nutrition therapy. In: Franz MJ, Bantle JP, eds. American Diabetes Association Guide to Medical Nutrition Therapy for Diabetes. Alexandria, Va: American Diabetes Association; 1999:369-386.

152 Kulkarni K, Castle G, Gregory R, et al. and the Diabetes Care and Education Practice Group of the American Dietetic Association. Nutrition practice guidelines for type 1 diabetes: an overview of the content and application. Diabetes Spectrum. 1997;10:248-256.

153 Basic Carbohydrate Counting. Alexandria, Va and Chicago: American Diabetes Association and American Dietetic Association; 2003.

154 Daly A, Franz M, Holzmeister LA, Kulkarni K, O'Connell B, Wheeler M. New diabetes resources. J Am Diet Assoc. 2003; in press.

155 US Department of Agriculture. The Food Guide Pyramid. Hyattsville, Md: USDA Human Nutrition Information Service; 1992.

156 Healthy Food Choices. Alexandria, Va and Chicago: American Diabetes Association and American Dietetic Association; 2003.

157 Eating Healthy with Diabetes: Easy Reading Guide. Alexandria, Va and Chicago: American Diabetes Association and American Dietetic Association; 2003.

158 Advanced Carbohydrate Counting. Alexandria, Va and Chicago: American Diabetes Association and American Dietetic Association; 2003.

159 My Food Plan and Mi Plan de Comidas. Minneapolis: IDC Publishing; 2000.

160 My Food Plan for Kids and Teens. Minneapolis: IDC Publishing; 1998.

161 My Food Plan for Early Kidney Disease. Minneapolis: IDC Publishing; 2000.

162 My Food Plan Made Easy. Minneapolis: IDC Publishing; 2000.

163 Being Healthy Rocks. Minneapolis: IDC Publishing; 2002.

164 Kittler PG, Sucher KP. Diet counseling in multicultural society. Diabetes Educ. 1990;16:127-134.

165 Cronin CC, Shanahan F. Insulin-dependent diabetes mellitus and celiac disease. Lancet. 1997;349:1096-1097.

166 Acerini CL, Ahmed ML, Ross KM, Sullivan PB, Bird G, Dunger DB. Celiac disease in children and adolescents with IDDM: clinical characteristics and response to gluten-free diet. Diabet Med. 1998;15:38-44.

167 Iafusco D, Rea F, Prisco F. Hypoglycemia and reduction of the insulin requirement as a sign of celiac disease in children with IDDM. Diabetes Care. 1998;21:1379-1381.

168 Andreeli F, Plotton I, Riou JP, Thivolet C. Diabetes instability and celiac disease. Diabetes Care. 1998;21:2192-2193.

169 Kaukinen K, Salmi J, Lahtela J, et al. No effect of gluten-free diet on the metabolic control of type 1 diabetes in patients with diabetes and celiac disease. Diabetes Care. 1999;22:1747-1748.

170 Thompson T. Oats and the gluten-free diet. J Am Diet Assoc. 2003;103:376-379.

171 Brunzell C, Schwarzenberg SA. Cystic fibrosis-related diabetes and abnormal glucose tolerance: overview and medical nutrition therapy. Diabetes Spectrum. 2002;15:124-127.

172 Rodman HM, Doershuk CF, Roland JM. The interaction of 2 diseases: diabetes mellitus and cystic fibrosis. Medicine. 1996;65:389-397.

173 Moran A, Hardin D, Rodman D, et al. Diagnosis, screening and management of cystic fibrosis related diabetes mellitus: a consensus conference. Diabetes Res Clin Pract. 1999;45:61-73.

174 Pencharz PB. Energy intakes and low-fat diets in children with cystic fibrosis. J Pediatr Gastroenterol Nutr. 1983;2:400-492.

175 American Diabetes Association. Translation of the diabetes nutrition recommendations for health care institutions (position statement). Diabetes Care. 2003;26(suppl 1):S70-S72.

176 Schafer RG, Bohannon B, Franz M, et al. Translation of the diabetes nutrition recommendations for health care institutions (technical review). Diabetes Care. 1997;20:96-105.

177 McMahon MM. Nutrition support and diabetes. In: Franz MJ, Bantle JP, eds. American Diabetes Association Guide to Medical Nutrition Therapy for Diabetes. Alexandria, Va: American Diabetes Association; 1999:335-348.

Resources

Annual Listing of Publications

American Diabetes Association. Diabetes Resource Catalog. Alexandria, Va: American Diabetes Association. Updated annually.

American Dietetic Association. Food & Nutrition Resources. Products and Services Catalog. Chicago: American Dietetic Association. Updated annually.

IDC Publishing. Making a Difference in Diabetes Education. Minneapolis: International Diabetes Center. Updated annually.

Other Resources

References 153 and 155 to 163 are valuable patient education tools.

Compu-Cal handheld computers. Olympia, Wash: Compu-Cal, Inc.

Foster-Powell K, Holt SHA, Miller JB. International table of glycemic index and glycemic load values: 2002. Am J Clin Nutr. 2002;78:5-56.

Franz MJ, Bantle JP, eds. American Diabetes Association Guide to Medical Nutrition Therapy for Diabetes. Alexandria, Va: American Diabetes Association; 1999.

Franz MJ, Reader D, Monk A. Implementing Group and Individual Medical Nutrition Therapy for Diabetes. Alexandria, Va: American Diabetes Association; 2002.

Ludwig DS, Eckel RH, eds. Is the Glycemic Index Important in Human Nutrition? Proceedings of a symposium held at Experimental Biology 2001. Am J Clin Nutr 2002:76(suppl):261S-298S.

Month of Meals: Classic Cooking, Meals in Minutes, Ethnic Delights, Old-Time Favorites, Vegetarian Pleasures. Alexandria, Va: American Diabetes Association.

Learning Assessment: Post-Test Questions

Medical Nutrition Therapy for Diabetes 1

1 Which of the following persons with type 2 diabetes would most benefit from food fat modifications?
   A 42-year-old female with a cholesterol of 205 mg/dL
   B 51-year-old male with low-density lipoproteins (LDL) of 124 mg/dL
   C 36-year-old female with triglycerides of 150 mg/dL
   D 60-year-old male with high-density lipoproteins (HDL) of 50 mg/dL

2 An effective strategy for achieving blood glucose goals in a person with type 1 diabetes is:
   A Moderate caloric restriction
   B Eating meals and snacks at specific times
   C Increasing NPH insulin if carbohydrate intake exceeds usual consumption
   D Integrating insulin regimen into usual eating habits

3 The macronutrient that exerts the greatest influence on postprandial blood glucose levels is:
   A Protein
   B Carbohydrate
   C Fat
   D Fiber

4 Insulin affects the use and storage of nutrients in each of the following ways except:
   A Facilitates cellular transport
   B Promotes lipogenesis by inactivating lipoprotein lipase
   C Stimulates glycogen synthesis
   D Suppresses gluconeogenesis (glucose production by the liver)

5 Which of the following intakes of the sugar substitute aspartame on a daily basis exceeds the acceptable daily intake (ADI) for a female who weighs 130 lb (59 kg)?
   A 14 cans (12 oz) of diet soft drinks
   B 18 cans (12 oz) of diet soft drinks
   C 45 packets of a tabletop sweetener
   D 75 packets of a tabletop sweetener

6 ML is a 39-year-old person with type 1 diabetes who weighs 121 lb (55 kg) and has overt nephropathy. Her protein requirement is:
   A 35 g
   B 44 g
   C 50 g
   D 55 g

7 If ML eats a meal that includes 1 serving from the starch group, 1 serving of meat (1 oz), 1 serving of fruit (1/2 c), and 1 serving of milk (8 oz), what will be her intake of protein?
   A 10 g
   B 14 g
   C 18 g
   D 20 g

8 Which of the following MNT strategies is consistent with the goal of attaining optimal lipid levels?
   A Limit fat consumption to 20% of daily calories in a person with normal lipid levels
   B Restrict dietary cholesterol to less than 200 mg/day if triglycerides are elevated
   C Limit saturated fatty acids to less than 7% of daily calories if LDL cholesterol is the primary concern
   D Increase polyunsaturated fat to 15% of total fat calories if VLDL levels are a primary concern

9 Assuming that blood glucose goals are being met, the guidelines for the use of alcohol in persons with diabetes include all of the following except:
   A Teach adult men with diabetes to limit consumption to 2 drinks with their regular meal plan
   B Eliminate 1 carbohydrate serving for each alcoholic beverage consumed
   C A 12-oz beer, 5-oz wine, or 1 oz of hard liquor (spirits) is considered 1 drink
   D Avoid consumption of alcoholic beverages during pregnancy

10 Persons with type 2 diabetes who are sodium sensitive and taking medications for hypertension should:

A Limit their intake of sodium to 3 000 mg daily

B Use no more than 2 tsp (5 g) of table salt as part of their total daily intake

C Be encouraged to choose entrees with 800 mg sodium or less per serving

D Limit their intake to low-sodium foods having 140 mg of sodium or less

11 Guidelines for the role of carbohydrate in meal planning include:

A The amount of carbohydrate to be included in the meal plan is determined before the protein and fat

B The amount of carbohydrate included will depend on the individual's current eating patterns and nutrition goals

C It is more important to count the carbohydrate from simple sugars than the total daily intake of carbohydrate

D The amount of fiber in the diet is important since it is not digested (available to the body)

12 Which of the following statements accurately describes the carbohydrate counting approach to meal planning?

A Individuals are ready to learn pattern management once they learn insulin-to-carbohydrate ratios

B Use of the basic diet planning guidelines is integral to a carbohydrate counting approach

C Carbohydrate counting can be used by persons with type 1 or type 2 diabetes to plan meals

D The carbohydrate counting approach restricts carbohydrate choices to starches and fruits

13 PS is a marketing director with type 1 diabetes who learned about insulin-to-carbohydrate ratios a month ago and has managed to reach her glucose goals since she implemented this approach. She now wants to adjust her insulin for a corporate dinner she will be attending and asks your assistance. Her usual insulin-to-carbohydrate ratio is 2:15 (2 lispro insulin units for each 1 carbohydrate choice), and she usually takes 8 units of lispro with her evening meal. She anticipates that she will select 6 carbohydrate choices at this dinner, which is more than her usual. How many additional units of insulin will she need to take?

A 1 unit

B 2 units

C 4 units

D 6 units

14 With her new flexibility in meal planning, she has also started to exercise. You advise her that:

A Her insulin-to-carbohydrate ratio will probably not change

B She'll need to recheck her insulin-to-carbohydrate ratios if she continues to exercise regularly

C She will need to add additional protein to her exercise snack

D She should eat high-carbohydrate snacks to cover for exercise

15 GH is an assembly line worker with type 2 diabetes and the equivalent of a fifth-grade education. She was referred to you by her employer for nutrition counseling because she has had to take more than the usual number of bathroom breaks while working. Which approach to meal planning is more likely to be appropriate for her?

A Carbohydrate counting

B Exchange system

C General diabetes nutrition guidelines

D Booklets featuring monthly menus

See next page for answer key.

Post-Test Answer Key

Medical Nutrition Therapy for Diabetes 1

1	B		**9**	B
2	D		**10**	C
3	B		**11**	B
4	B		**12**	C
5	B		**13**	C
6	B		**14**	B
7	C		**15**	C
8	C			

A Core Curriculum for Diabetes Education
Diabetes Management Therapies

Physical Activity/Exercise 2

Catherine A. Mullooly, MS, RCEP_SM_, CDE
Joslin Clinic
Boston, Massachusetts

Karen Hanson Chalmers, MS, RD, CDE
Joslin Clinic
Boston, Massachusetts

Introduction

1 The beneficial effects of exercise in treating diabetes were recognized as early as the ancient times.[1] Centuries later in the 1920s, exercise was first recommended as a therapeutic tool for lowering blood glucose levels.[2,3]

2 Today, implementing and maintaining an exercise program continues to be regarded as a primary component of diabetes management. However, not all persons with diabetes are capable or willing to participate in such programs. In these situations, other options can be explored to find alternatives to increase the amount of routine exercise for these individuals. One change has to do with the approach to exercise counseling. In this chapter the term "physical activity" will be used when discussing options that can lead to health and diabetes benefits. This broader term will include options that may have previously been overlooked. It will also do a better job in including options that can have an impact on blood glucose but are often overlooked.

3 Much of the morbidity and mortality among persons with diabetes is attributed to cardiovascular disease. Epidemiological evidence suggests that regular physical activity and physical fitness are associated with decreased cardiovascular disease in the general population as well as a decreased occurrence of type 2 diabetes.[4]

4 Because individuals, including people with diabetes, are living longer, the prevalence of diabetes in the elderly and the total number of people with diabetic complications are increasing. Consequently, the role of physical activity becomes even more significant.

5 This chapter focuses on the benefits, effects, risks, and precautions of physical activity for persons with diabetes. Also discussed are physical activity options for special populations, strategies for enhancing physical activity, guidelines for developing exercise prescriptions, and strategies for self-directed physical activity programs.

Objectives

Upon completion of this chapter, the learner will be able to
1 State the benefits of physical activity.
2 Describe the physiologic response to increased physical fitness in individuals with and without diabetes.
3 Identify the risks associated with physical activity and ways to minimize risks.
4 Explain the principles of increasing physical activity levels for people with diabetes.
5 Identify appropriate physical activity options for special populations.
6 Describe strategies for self-directed physical fitness programs.

Benefits of Physical Activity

1 Physical activity generally is regarded as having a salutary effect for everyone. The benefits are many and may be even more favorable for the person with diabetes.

2 Most of the benefits result from chronic (regular, long-term), aerobic (cardiovascular) exercise.

3 Resistance exercise to increase muscle strength is an important means of preserving and increasing muscular strength and endurance and of preventing falls and increasing mobility among the elderly. Resistance training also improves glycemic control and many of the abnormalities associated with the metabolic syndrome in older adults with diabetes.[5]

4 Because persons with diabetes have an increased risk of cardiovascular disease, the role of physical activity in reducing modifiable risks has primary importance. The potential benefits of improved physical fitness for persons with diabetes include the following:[6]

A Improved functioning of the cardiovascular system

B Improved strength and physical work capacity

C Decreased risk factors for coronary artery disease (CAD)
   - Reduction in plasma cholesterol, triglycerides, and LDL cholesterol (LDL)
   - Increase in high-density lipoproteins (HDL), particularly in the presence of weight loss

D Increased insulin sensitivity[7]

E Reduced hyperinsulinemia, a proposed risk factor for atherosclerosis[8-10]

F Enhanced fibrinolysis
   - Hypercoagulability frequently is present in persons with diabetes
   - Chronic physical activity can enhance fibrinolysis and affect other mechanisms responsible for this hypothesized risk factor for atherosclerosis[11,12]

G Favorable changes in body composition (reduction of body fat and weight; increase in muscle mass)

H Adjunct therapy for controlling hypertension

I Improved quality of life and self-esteem; reduced psychological stress[13]

5 In all persons, acute physical activity is associated with substantial improvement in insulin sensitivity, independent of any change in cardiorespiratory fitness or body composition. However, regular physical activity also improves insulin sensitivity independent of weight loss.[14] Because the beneficial effects of acute physical activity diminish quickly, the physical activity must be performed on a regular basis. Regular physical activity, therefore, improves insulin sensitivity, with or without weight loss, reducing the risk of cardiovascular disease and diabetes.

6 The chronic effects of increasing the physical activity level appear to benefit the person with type 2 diabetes by reducing the A1C level, improving insulin sensitivity, assisting in attainment and maintenance of desirable body weight, and decreasing CAD risk factors.[15]

A Several long-term studies[16-19] demonstrate a sustained improvement in glucose control while a regular physical activity program is maintained.

B Thus, remaining physically active is an essential component of diabetes self-management education for all individuals with type 2 diabetes.

7 Being physically active is also a critical part of the overall diabetes self-management education for type 1 diabetes, especially in light of the increased risk for macrovascular disease in this patient population.

A However, regular physical activity in type 1 diabetes has not been shown to consistently result in improved diabetes control as evidenced by A1C.[20-22] This finding may be due to the difficulty of balancing insulin adjustments with carbohydrate in concordance with physical activity.

B However, it may be possible for select patients with type 1 diabetes to obtain a sustained decrease in the A1C level.[23-26]

C Recommendations for the prevention of activity-induced hypoglycemia must be included in the physical activity plan and educational program.

8 Because of its effects on self-esteem and stress reduction, the addition of a regular physical activity program can serve as the first step in self-directed behavior change for many individuals with diabetes.

Physiology of Physical Activity/Exercise in Individuals Without Diabetes

1 Plasma glucose levels in individuals without diabetes who are physically active remain relatively stable due to an intricate regulation between the increase in glucose uptake by exercising muscles and increased hepatic glucose production.[27]

2 The contribution of carbohydrate (stored as glycogen in the liver and muscles) and fat (stored as triglyceride in adipose tissue) depends on the intensity and duration of the activity, the person's fitness level, and the time and content of the last meal.[6,28] This regulation involves a hormonal balance between decreased insulin secretion and increased action of catecholamines, glucagon, growth hormone, and cortisol (counterregulatory hormones).

A At the onset of exercise, fuel utilization by muscles progresses from fat (extracted from the bloodstream as free fatty acids [FFA] at rest) to high-energy phosphate compounds, such as adenosine triphosphate (ATP) and phosphocreatine (CP), to glucose utilization from intramuscular stores of glucose and triglycerides from adipose tissues.

- The immediate fuel sources available for muscle contraction are ATP and CP. The breakdown of these high-energy phosphate compounds contributes to the immediate resynthesis of ATP (the primary fuel source for muscle contraction).
- ATP and CP stores are limited and can only supply the energy needs of quick, powerful movements, such as sprinting for time periods of 8 to 12 seconds.
- As exercise moves from the quick, initial muscle action to an extended exercise session, the fuel supply for the contracting muscles shifts from the immediate high energy phosphate groups to the second system from which ATP is produced (glycolysis).[29]

B During the first few minutes of exercise, intramuscular glucose is broken down anaerobically (without oxygen present). Although this pathway does not provide an abundant quantity of ATP, this pathway is important at the onset of exercise when oxygen availability is limited. As exercise continues, an adequate supply of oxygen becomes available for the breakdown of carbohydrates, fats, and proteins, if necessary, for the resynthesis of ATP.

- During sustained exercise, carbohydrate, protein, and fat continually recharge the phosphate pool.
- After the first 5 to 10 minutes, muscle glycogen breakdown decreases, as circulating glucose from the liver becomes a major fuel source (hepatic glycogenolysis).[30]

C As exercise continues beyond 20 to 30 minutes, the muscle glycogen stores are depleted. Plasma glucose is maintained as glucose is broken down from the liver (hepatic glycogenolysis) and free fatty acids (FFA) (triglycerides mobilized from adipose tissue) are utilized.

- At the beginning of exercise, hepatic glucose production is mainly derived from glycogenolysis.
- As exercise continues, gluconeogenesis becomes increasingly important in providing glucose. The main substrates for hepatic gluconeogenesis during exercise are lactate, amino acids, and glycerol.

D As exercise duration increases, the contribution of FFA as a fuel increases relative to glucose. Exercise of low-to-moderate intensity relies primarily on FFA as the oxidative fuel for muscle.[6] The oxidation of fat-derived fuels cannot replace the utilization of glucose. When carbohydrate is limited, fat is not completely oxidized and ketone bodies are formed.

E Hormonal response to exercise determines substrate utilization during exercise (Table 2.1).

- Secretion of counterregulatory hormones increases and helps maintain glucose homeostasis.[26,31]
- Insulin secretion is decreased during exercise as a result of increased activity of the sympathetic nervous system.[31,32]
- The suppression of insulin secretion facilitates hepatic glucose production and lipolysis, which allows blood glucose to be maintained.[28,30,33]

F An ongoing increased uptake of glucose by muscle occurs during the postexercise period as one means of replenishing glycogen stores.

Table 2.1. Hormonal Response and Metabolic Effects During Exercise in Individuals Without Diabetes

Hormone	Response During Exercise	Metabolic Effect
Insulin	⬇	• Facilitates hepatic glucose and FFA production
Glucagon	⬆	• Increases hepatic glucose production, increases blood glucose
Epinephrine	⬆	• Stimulates FFA production, which provides glycerol as a substrate for gluconeogenesis
Norepinephrine	⬆	• Stimulates hepatic and muscle glycolysis, stimulates lipolysis
Growth hormone/Cortisol	⬆	• Increases lipolysis, decreases insulin-stimulated glucose uptake, increases gluconeogenic substrates

- Replenishment of glycogen stores may take 24 to 48 hours.[6,34]
- The postexercise recovery, particularly after exhaustive work, is characterized by enhanced insulin sensitivity.[35,36]
G Trained athletes demonstrate the following responses:
  - A reduction in fasting insulin secretion in response to a glucose load
  - An increase in muscle sensitivity to insulin despite reduced insulin secretion[28,37]
  - Less of a generalized secretion of counterregulatory hormones than sedentary individuals[32]
  - Less glucose utilization than sedentary individuals during exercise that is of similar intensity and duration. As a result, a slower rate and duration of glycogen usage as well as a greater reliance on fats for fuel, which are associated with greater endurance.[31,32]

Physiology of Physical Activity/Exercise in Individuals With Diabetes

1 A person with diabetes who increases his or her physical activity may have a decreased need for, or better utilization of, insulin; the result may be a decrease in diabetes medications needed to reach glucose goals.

A Acute effects of being physically active generally cause a reduction in plasma glucose.

B Chronically participating in a physically active lifestyle results in improved insulin sensitivity and glucose tolerance because of changes in body composition and the additive effects of daily physical exertion.

C The hormonal response to an episode of increased physical activity depends on the degree of diabetes control, medication, time and content of the last meal, fitness level, and type of activity performed.
  - Because the person with type 1 diabetes does not have a normal compensatory decrease in insulin secretion during physical activity, metabolic abnormalities may occur.[10,27,32,33,38]

2 Hypoglycemia is the most commonly encountered problem in individuals with diabetes when they are physically active and are treated with insulin or insulin secretagogues.

A Normally, plasma insulin decreases during the physical activity in individuals without diabetes. This decrease, along with increases in plasma counterregulatory hormones, allows hepatic glucose production and lipolysis to match glucose utilization.

B In persons with diabetes taking insulin, the plasma insulin concentration does not decrease. Because the insulin is exogenous in origin, the plasma insulin concentration actually may increase due to increased sensitivity or mobilization from subcutaneous depots (Table 2.2).
  - A high plasma insulin level during episodes of increased physical activity may enhance glucose uptake and further stimulate glucose oxidation in the exercising muscle.
  - A high plasma insulin level inhibits hepatic glucose production and FFA mobilization.[33] As a result, hepatic glucose production does not keep pace with peripheral glucose utilization and the blood glucose concentration falls.

Table 2.2. Factors That Contribute to Hypoglycemia in Type 1 Diabetes With Physical Activity

- Accelerated absorption of insulin
- Nonsuppressible plasma insulin levels
- Increased insulin sensitivity
- Possible impaired counterregulatory hormonal response

- Hypoglycemia also can result during physical activity in patients with type 2 diabetes treated with insulin secretagogues (sulfonylureas, meglitinide, and nateglinide) or insulin.[39] These individuals are less prone to activity-induced hypoglycemia, although it still can occur, and very rarely develop hyperglycemia with ketosis. Improvements in insulin sensitivity, insulin secretion, and glucose disposal rates have been well documented in type 2 diabetes as a result of regular physical activity, although the mechanisms underlying these improvements have not been clearly explained.[40] Changes in body composition (decrease in fat weight and increase in muscle mass) contribute to increasing sensitivity to endogenous and exogenous insulin. The potential result is a reduction in exogenous insulin and/or antihyperglycemic agents.[41]

3 A major concern for persons with diabetes who are taking insulin or insulin secretagogues, is post-activity, late-onset hypoglycemia (PAL) (that is, hypoglycemia occurring 4 or more hours following periods of increased physical activity). This is more frequently encountered in those individuals with type 1 diabetes.
   A PAL generally occurs following extended periods of increased physical activity of moderate to high intensity with a duration greater than 30 minutes.
   B PAL results from increased insulin sensitivity, ongoing glucose utilization, and repletion of glycogen stores.[42]

4 Physical activity of a high intensity can cause blood glucose levels to be higher after the activity is performed than before, even though blood glucose levels are in the normal range before beginning the activity. This hyperglycemia can also extend into the postactivity state and is mediated by the counterregulatory hormones. Hepatic glucose production no longer matches, but, in fact, exceeds the rise in glucose use.[43,44]

5 In type 1 individuals with hyperglycemia and/or ketosis, acute physical activity may result in a worsening of metabolic control.[38] A certain amount of insulin is required for glucose uptake. In the absence of adequate insulin, physical activity raises plasma glucose, FFA, and ketones (Table 2.3).

Special Considerations and Precautions for Physical Activity

1 The primary side effect of acute periods of physical activity is hypoglycemia. Occasionally, hyperglycemia and ketosis also occur in individuals with type 1 diabetes (Table 2.4).

Table 2.3. Consequences of Insufficient Insulin

- Impaired peripheral glucose utilization
- Excessive counterregulatory hormones
- Enhanced hepatic glucose production, lipolysis, and ketogenesis
- Rapid rise in already elevated blood glucose level and increased ketosis

Table 2.4. Exercise Considerations for People With Diabetes

Hypoglycemia (if diabetes is treated with insulin, sulfonylureas, or meglitinides)
- Exercise-induced hypoglycemia
- Postexercise, late-onset hypoglycemia (PAL)

Hyperglycemia after very strenuous (high-intensity) activity

Hyperglycemia and ketosis in insulin-deficient persons with type 1 diabetes

Precipitation or exacerbation of cardiovascular disease
- Presence of silent heart disease: arrhythmia, cardiac dysfunction
- Excessive increases in blood pressure with physical activity
- Angina pectoris
- Myocardial infarction
- Sudden death

Worsening of long-term complications with inappropriately prescribed physical activity program
- Proliferative retinopathy: vitreous hemorrhage, retinal detachment
- Nephropathy: increased proteinuria
- Peripheral neuropathy: soft tissue and joint injury, foot ulcers, orthopedic injury
- Autonomic neuropathy: decreased cardiovascular response during periods of physical activity, decreased maximum aerobic capacity, impaired response to dehydration, orthostatic hypotension, impaired counterregulatory response

Source: Adapted from Horton ES. Prescription for exercise. Diabetes Spectrum. 1991;4:250-257.[45]

A Blood glucose response to physical activity is affected by the type, amount, and intensity of the activity; the timing and type of previous meal and medication; the pre-activity blood glucose level; and the fitness level.[7,29,30]

B Hypoglycemia is a significant threat to persons who are physically active while taking insulin, sulfonylureas, or meglitinide; nateglinide, however, has a low potential for hypoglycemia. Persons who use biguanides, thiazolidinediones, alpha-glucosidases, or meal planning and physical activity alone to control type 2 diabetes are not at risk of hypoglycemia during physical exertion.

C General guidelines to either increase carbohydrate consumption or decrease medication(s) are based on planned versus unplanned physical activity. Initial guidelines should be provided and then adjusted based on the individual's response to the physical activity program.

2 Activity-induced hypoglycemia can be largely prevented by implementing certain guidelines.

    A During planned activity, the following self-management tasks can reduce the risk of hypoglycemia.

- Adjustments are needed to prevent hypoglycemia in the insulin-treated individual because hepatic glucose production is blocked or partially inhibited by exogenous insulin.[29,33] The physiological decrease in circulating insulin levels that occurs with physical activity cannot take place in patients treated with insulin.
- Reduction of the rapid-acting or short-acting insulin by 30% to 50% has been demonstrated to decrease the risk of hypoglycemia.[38,46]
- The recommendation to change the injection site to a part of the body not involved in the activity to prevent hypoglycemia was a recommendation based on published reports in the 1970s.[47] These studies demonstrated an increase in serum insulin levels in patients who are physically active shortly after an insulin injection. The recommendation to inject in the arm or abdomen instead of the leg if the activity was jogging or cycling emerged from these studies. Despite the increased absorption rate, subsequent research[48] demonstrated that simply changing the insulin injection site was not effective for preventing hypoglycemia. If the level of circulating insulin is elevated for any reason, hypoglycemia is likely to occur. Dose reductions should accompany any physical activity that is performed during the peak action of the insulin.[49]
- Proper administration of insulin requires injecting into the subcutaneous fat layer. Patients should be taught to avoid intramuscular injection of insulin because muscle contractions accelerate the absorption of insulin into the circulation.[49]
- Blood glucose monitoring before and after periods of physical activity provides needed feedback for the individual who is learning to adjust insulin and/or carbohydrate while active.
- Adjustments should be tailored to the specific response to physical activity of each individual (Table 2.5). The choice between decreasing medication or increasing carbohydrate will depend on the individual's goals.

    B During unplanned physical activity, carbohydrate replacement may be necessary to prevent hypoglycemia when insulin adjustments are not made or when the period of physical activity occurs several hours after a meal or when the activity is of a long duration.

Table 2.5. Physical Activity Adjustments

	Individual's Goals
Insulin Adjustment	• Weight loss • Improved control • Planned, regularly scheduled physical activity
Carbohydrate Replacement	• Long duration of physical activity • Unplanned physical activity

- The amount of additional carbohydrate needed depends on the time of the activity in relation to medication and previous meal; the type, intensity, and duration of the activity (Table 2.6); and the preactivity blood glucose level.
- Periods of physical activity performed 1 to 3 hours after a meal may not require any additional carbohydrate supplement.

Table 2.6. Carbohydrate Replacement During Exercise[50]

Intensity	Duration (minutes)	Carbohydrate Replacement	Frequency
Mild-to-moderate	<30	May not be needed	—
Moderate	30 to 60	15 g	Each hour
High	60+	30 to 50 g	Each hour

- Moderate-intensity activity increases glucose uptake by the muscle 2 to 3 mg/kg/body weight/min above resting levels.[38] For example, a 154 lb (70 kg) individual would require an additional 140 to 210 mg of glucose for every minute of moderate-intensity physical activity. This would mean an additional 8.4 to 12.6 g of glucose is required for every hour of the activity.
- High-intensity physical activity increases the rate of glucose utilization by the muscle to as much as 5 to 6 mg/kg/body weight/min or an additional 350 to 420 mg of glucose for every minute of the activity. Even though the rate of glucose utilization increases, the demand on glucose stores and risk of hypoglycemia is less because activity of this intensity cannot be sustained for long periods of time.[38]
- A snack is needed when the preactivity blood glucose level places the person at risk for hypoglycemia during or at the end of the physical activity session.
- Unfortunately, the starting blood glucose level that places an individual at risk for hypoglycemia is sometimes only defined after a period of trial and error. Blood glucose monitoring can help to determine the minimum level at which a carbohydrate snack is required. However, the blood glucose level before physical activity only reflects the glucose level at that time. It is unknown if the glucose level at this time is stable or dropping. If blood glucose has been elevated and the check before physical activity reflects a glucose level that is dropping, adding physical activity can contribute to hypoglycemia even if the glucose level was appropriate for activity.
- Preactivity snacks have been demonstrated to prevent postactivity hypoglycemia when taken 15 to 30 minutes before physical activity of short duration (less than 45 minutes).[51]
- Drinks containing less than 8% carbohydrate empty from the stomach more rapidly than drinks with a concentration of carbohydrate greater than 10%. Fruit juices and most regular soft drinks contain approximately 12% carbohydrate and lead to gastrointestinal upset, such as cramps, nausea, diarrhea, or bloating. For

the exerciser with diabetes, fruit juices diluted with water or fluid replacement beverages can provide both fluids and a source of carbohydrate.

C For individuals participating in extended periods of physical activity (longer than 2 hours), reducing insulin may be easier than continually supplementing with carbohydrate. It may be necessary to reduce the dose of both rapid-acting or short-acting and intermediate-acting or long-acting insulins depending on the time and type of physical activity.

3 Hypoglycemia remains a risk during periods of physical activity for persons using insulin pump therapy.

A The chances of developing hypoglycemia may be less for insulin pump users due to the steady infusion of insulin. Also, basal rates and boluses can be adjusted based on the timing, duration, and type of activity performed.

B The amount of insulin decrease or the amount of carbohydrate supplement depends on a person's fitness level and the duration and intensity of the activity.[46,52]

C Options for insulin pump users to maintain euglycemia during periods of physical activity include reducing the basal infusion rate, consuming additional carbohydrates, or temporarily suspending pump use.[46,51-53]

4 A link between the time of day when the activity is performed and the risk of activity-induced hypoglycemia has not been confirmed with research.

A The risk for hypoglycemia with physical activity may be lower when the level of circulating insulin is low. For example, physical activity performed prior to the morning insulin injection presents a lower risk of hypoglycemia.

B The risk for nocturnal hypoglycemia is increased when an activity is performed during the evening hours. However, decreasing the evening insulin dose can reduce this risk.

C The likelihood of activity-induced hypoglycemia can be decreased by avoiding activity during the time when the injected insulin is reaching the peak level. However, an insulin adjustment usually is required because it may be difficult to avoid physical exertion when medication is peaking.

5 Postactivity, late-onset hypoglycemia (PAL) occurs several hours following physical exertion and is a significant concern to persons treated with insulin; it also can occur in persons treated with insulin secretogogues.

A PAL can be the result of acutely increased insulin mobilization and sensitivity, increased glucose utilization, replenishment of glycogen stores, and defective counterregulatory mechanisms.[27,42]

B Options to minimize the occurrence of PAL include
• Providing patient education to increase awareness
• Reducing the insulin that peaks during the postactivity period
• Supplementing carbohydrate during the postactivity phase
• Avoiding physical activity prior to bedtime
• Monitoring blood glucose frequently during the postactivity period[41]

6 Activity-induced hyperglycemia can occur in individuals with type 1 diabetes.

A Hyperglycemia and worsening of ketosis can result if physical activity is initiated when fasting blood glucose levels are greater than 250 mg/dL (13.9 mmol/L) and ketones are present.[42]

- Patients should be taught to delay physical activity until blood glucose levels improve and ketones are negative.
- An insulin deficiency is not likely in persons with type 1 diabetes if a postmeal glucose level is greater than 250 to 300 mg/dL (13.9 to 16.7 mmol/L) due to excessive carbohydrate intake. Physical activity under this condition generally will cause a drop in glucose levels. Negative urine ketones confirm the absence of insulin deficiency.
- The American Diabetes Association position statement on physical activity and diabetes[42] provides the following guideline for metabolic control before physical activity. Avoid physical activity if FASTING glucose levels are >250 mg/dL (13.9 mmol/L) and ketosis is present, and use caution if glucose levels are >300 mg/dL (16.7 mmol/L).

B High-intensity, short-term, exhaustive physical activity causes an acute rise in blood glucose levels in persons with well-controlled diabetes.[43,44]

- Participation in highly competitive sports can sometimes result in postactivity hyperglycemia. This phenomenon may be due to excess sympathetic stimulation as a result of high-intensity activity; catecholamines are released that act on the liver to produce glucose. This has been observed to cause initial increases, followed by declines, in blood glucose levels. However, the existence of an undetected hypoglycemic reaction during physical exertion should not be overlooked as this sometimes can cause the same sympathetic response.
- An extra injection of insulin should not be administered in response to the hyperglycemia. The insulin action will coincide with the postactivity increase in insulin sensitivity and potentially result in severe hypoglycemia.

Other Safety Precautions

1 Teach all persons with diabetes who are treated with insulin, sulfonylureas, or meglitinides to carry some type of carbohydrate with them while performing physical activities.

2 Monitoring blood glucose, both pre- and postactivity, is the key to safety and understanding of how an activity affects blood glucose.

3 Advise persons with diabetes to wear some form of diabetes and personal identification.

4 Avoid vigorous physical exertion if the environment is extremely hot, humid, smoggy, or cold.

5 Wear proper equipment and exercise shoes appropriate for the activity to reduce the likelihood of injury.

6 Include warm-up and cool-down sessions with each workout. Stretching exercises performed following the cool-down enhance flexibility and prevent injury.

7 Certain medications can impair exercise tolerance. For example, beta-blockers alter the heart-rate response to physical activity as well as mask hypoglycemia and the body's counterregulatory response.

8 Maintain adequate hydration while exercising.

9 Stop the activity if pain, lightheadedness, or shortness of breath occurs.

10 Physical activity assessments for patients and educators are useful when planning to increase the level of physical activity. Direct special attention during assessments toward identifying a history of cardiac disease (including silent heart disease), the presence of complications, medications, medical and family history, and degree of diabetes control. The American Diabetes Association recognizes that an exercise tolerance test may be helpful if a patient is going to participate in a moderate- to high-intensity exercise program or for anyone at high risk for underlying cardiovascular disease.[42]

Exercise Programs

1 There are two types of exercise: aerobic and anaerobic.

   A Aerobic exercise is defined as an activity that involves repetitive, submaximal contraction of major muscle groups (eg, swimming, cycling, jogging) and requires oxygen to sustain muscular effort.[40,54] Aerobic exercise provides the greatest benefits for people with diabetes in terms of blood glucose control and cardiovascular status. The health-related benefits of improved physical fitness do not appear to be dependent on the type of aerobic exercise.

   B Anaerobic exercise is defined as an activity that does not require sustained oxygen to meet the energy demands and generally does not induce the same health benefits as an aerobic program.

   • Anaerobic exercise and certain types and intensity levels of aerobic exercise may cause excessive rises in blood pressure, cardiac workload, and intraocular pressure. These reactions could be potential problems in persons with diabetes and vascular disease or complications.

   • Studies[55,56] suggest that properly designed resistance programs may improve indices of cardiovascular function, glucose tolerance, strength, and body composition provided the person with diabetes does not have contraindications to weight training.

2 The duration of exercise is inversely related to the intensity of the exercise: lower intensity exercise needs to be conducted over a longer period of time than higher intensity exercise for maximum benefit. The duration of exercise to meet the required weekly energy expenditure is 20 to 60 minutes per session.[15]

   A All workouts should include a 5- to 10-minute warm-up and cool-down.

   • The warm-up increases core body temperature and prevents muscle injury; the cool-down prevents blood pooling in the extremities and facilitates removal of metabolic by-products.

   • All workout sessions should start with adequate warm-up and be concluded with the cool-down phase.[57]

   B Studies have shown similar cardiorespiratory gains to occur when physical activity is done in shorter bouts (~10 minutes) accumulated throughout the day, as when activity of similar duration and intensity occurs for 1 prolonged session (~30 minutes).[5,57] However, 30 minutes of continuous exercise seems to have a greater impact on weight loss.[58]

- These findings, although beneficial in terms of cardiorespiratory gains, have not been studied in the diabetes population.
- It may be necessary for severely deconditioned individuals to exercise in multiple sessions of short duration (~10 minutes).[57]

3 To achieve the desired fitness level, exercise needs to be done 5 times per week or 3 to 4 times per week for maintenance.[40]

A The duration of glycemic improvement after the last exercise session usually is greater than 12 hours but less than 72 hours.[18]

B Exercise needs to be done at least every other day to improve glycemic control, on at least 3 nonconsecutive days, and ideally 5 days per week.

C Obese individuals may need to exercise more frequently (5 to 7 days per week) to optimize weight loss or maintenance.

D Exercise that is limited to 2 days per week generally does not produce a meaningful change in maximal uptake.

E The minimum physical conditioning for health benefits requires expending at least 700 calories per week.

F For maximum health benefits, 2000 calories expended per week are required; there is limited substantial health benefit to expending greater than 2000 calories per week.[57]

4 According to the American College of Sports Medicine the intensity of exercise should be 55% to 90% of the maximal age-adjusted heart rate. This is comparable to 40% to 85% of maximal oxygen uptake reserve (VO_{2max}) or heart-rate reserve (HRR).

A Training intensity can be calculated accurately using the results of an exercise stress test.

B Based on the individual's maximum heart-rate response to the exercise stress test, the following HRR formula is commonly used to calculate target heart-rate zone: target heart-rate range = [($HR_{max} - HR_{rest}$) x 0.40 and 0.85] + HR_{rest}.

- Select a range between 55% to 90% based on the individual's fitness level, duration of diabetes, degree of complications, and patient's goals.

C Use the following equation to estimate the true maximal heart rate when the actual maximal exercise heart rate is unknown: HR_{max} = 220 – patient's age.

- This procedure may overestimate the maximal heart rate of some type 2 patients, particularly those with autonomic neuropathy.[40,57]
- Due to the high prevalence of occult cardiovascular disease, caution is required when applying standard heart-rate formulas to the diabetes population.

D Exercise performed at low levels (<50% HR_{max}) has less effect on glucose disposal than exercise performed at higher intensities. The effect on glucose disposal during high-intensity exercise is roughly proportional to the total work performed (time x intensity). However, high-intensity exercise may result in transient hyperglycemia and cause an excessive rise in blood pressure.

E When initiating an exercise program, it may be necessary to begin at low levels (50%) with brief rest intervals and progress weekly to higher intensity, continual exercise.[57]

5 Exercise components of duration, frequency, and intensity will help achieve aerobic training effects.

A Individual factors such as fitness level, age, and health status can affect the attainment of these goals.

B Medications (eg, ß-blockers) and the presence of secondary complications may affect the exercise plan and individual tolerance (Table 2.7).

Table 2.7. Summary of Physical Activity/Exercise Recommendations

Screening	• For patients intending on participating in moderate to high-intensity physical activity, a graded exercise test (GXT) may be helpful based on the following criteria:[42]
	 – Age >35
	 – Age >25 years and
	  Type 2 diabetes of >10 years duration
	  Type 1 diabetes of >15 years duration
	 – Presence of any additional risk factor for coronary artery disease
	 – Presence of microvascular disease (proliferative retinopathy or nephropathy, including microalbuminuria)
	 – Peripheral vascular disease
	 – Autonomic neuropathy

Exercise Prescription, Type 2 Diabetes[40]	• Aerobic preferred; anaerobic allowed if no secondary limitations (2 times/wk) *Intensity*[57] • 55% to 90% of age-adjusted maximal heart rate (equal to 40% to 85% of maximum oxygen uptake or heart rate reserve) *Duration*[40] • 30 to 60 min (can be divided into three 10-min sessions) *Frequency* • 3 nonconsecutive days up to 5 times per week; schedule every other day
Exercise Prescription, Type 1 Diabetes[42]	• All levels of exercise can be performed by those who do not have complications and are in good blood glucose control
Safety Precautions	• Warm up and cool down • Careful selection and progression of exercise program • Patient education • Monitor blood glucose pre-/postexercise • Adjust guidelines to prevent hypoglycemia • Management by healthcare personnel

Source: Adapted from the American Diabetes Association. Exercise and NIDDM: a technical review.[41]

6 It has been recommended that strength-developing exercises be included with cardiorespiratory endurance activities in order to improve musculoskeletal health, maintain independence in performing daily activities, and reduce the possibility of injury.[5,59] The acute components of a resistance-training program include the following:

A The choice of which physical activity to perform is based upon what the individual wants to achieve with the strengthening program.

   • Individuals who want to achieve specific strength gains should have a planned resistance program developed to target the particular action and muscular components that are essential in the desired activity.

   • Individuals who are interested in basic fitness can select exercises that use each of the major muscle groups of the body (shoulders, back, chest, abdomen, and legs).[60]

B Advise patients to exercise in a specific order to use the larger muscle groups first and then move to the smaller muscle groups.

   • By working the larger muscle groups and then proceeding to the smaller groups, the demanding exercises are performed early in the workout while the energy supply is the greatest and the individual has an abundance of energy.

   • By choosing to perform the exercises in an alternative manner, the exercises which have a small energy demand will start to deplete energy stores, leaving the individual with a reduced energy supply to complete more debilitative exercises (exercises including the larger muscle groups).[61]

C For individuals with diabetes and no known cardiac disease, it is important to find out what physical attributes are necessary to attain their goal before determining the appropriate resistance. Once these parameters have been identified, the resistance and repetition load can be determined.

   • The resistance used is determined through the individual's repetition maximum (RM), which is defined as the amount of weight that allows for successful completion of a specified number of repetitions (no more, no less).[61]

   • Studies have shown repetitions of 8 RM or less produce the greatest strength gains, and muscular endurance is maximized through the use of resistance that allows for the performance of more than 12 repetitions.

   • For an individual who wants to achieve both muscular strength and endurance, 8 to 12 repetitions would be the most appropriate range.

   • When working with individuals with cardiac disease, particular attention must be focused on blood pressure and heart-rate response to the resistance training. It is recommended that these individuals start at lighter resistance loads and perform exercises that utilize a smaller amount of muscle mass, which in turn will decrease the myocardial oxygen demand on the heart.[61] The heart rate and blood pressure need to remain within the limits established by the exercise tolerance test and, therefore, should be monitored throughout the training session.

D Performing 1 to 2 sets of each exercise has been proven to be beneficial to increase general muscle strength and endurance.

   • Instruct individuals with a low fitness level or little training experience to complete just 1 set of each exercise for the first 4 to 6 weeks. Once they are comfortable with the exercise and have demonstrated good technique, the number of sets can be increased.

E Rest for an adequate amount of time between sets to allow for successful completion of the next set.

- For individuals training at lower intensities, rest periods are short (15 seconds to 1 minute).
- Individuals training at higher intensities will take longer to recover and may take up 2 minutes to regain enough energy to successfully complete the next set.[60]

7 Special precautions need to be taken by patients with diabetes prior to starting a resistance-training program.

A Before starting the exercise sessions, the individual should be taught proper weight lifting technique:
- Keep the body properly aligned.
- Breathe properly, exhaling during the phase in which the muscle is exerting its force against the apparatus and inhaling while lowering the weight.
- Control the lifting movement.
- Obtain the adequate range of motion.
- Adjust the equipment to fit the body frame.

B Individuals with long-term microvascular or macrovascular complications will require program modifications to decrease the strain on their cardiovascular systems due to the resistive exercises.
- Patients with proliferative retinopathy or nephropathy should be taught to avoid resistive training as this may be harmful due to the excessive systolic pressure responses experienced.[61]
- Prior to beginning a resistance training program individuals with diabetes who also have cardiovascular disease should possess an ejection fraction of = 45% and a cardiorespiratory fitness level of = 7 metabolic equivalents (METs), without ischemic ST segment depression on their electrocardiogram, hypo- or hypertensive responses, serious ventricular arrhythmias, or symptoms of cardiovascular disease.[62]
- Patients with any complications that may be exacerbated by resistance training should always receive approval from their physician before starting a resistance program.

Physical Activity/Exercise Considerations for the Elderly

1 Age-associated changes in body composition in the elderly account for decreases in basal metabolic rate, muscle strength, activity levels, and a decreased energy expenditure.

A Reductions in lean body mass occur primarily as a result of loss of skeletal muscle mass and increase in body fat. This decrease in muscle mass is a direct cause of the decrease in muscle strength seen in older adults.

B Research has provided evidence that muscle mass, not muscular function, is the major determinant of age- and gender-related differences in strength.[63] As physical activity levels decline with advancing age, muscle power and strength become critical elements in walking ability.

C The capacity of the elderly to respond to increased activity levels is often underrated. Individuals over the age of 60 years have demonstrated greater benefits from aerobic and strength training in fitness capacity, strength, functional capacity, and glucose tolerance than comparable younger groups.

D Special attention needs to be directed toward potential hazards for the elderly population.[64,65]

- A thorough physical exam is required prior to initiation of a program to increase physical exertion. Emphasis is placed on detecting occult heart disease, cardiovascular and/or peripheral vascular disease, joint/bone disease, and secondary complications.
- Strength training improves performance activities of daily living and counteracts muscle weakness. Patients are given a regimen that includes exercises to train each major muscle group 2 to 3 times per week. Muscular toning can be accomplished via free weights, strap-on ankle/wrist weights, and traditional strengthening machines (eg, Nautilus®). The appropriate intensity is in the range of 1 set of 8 to 12 repetitions "somewhat hard" on the perceived exertion rating (12 to 13).[57]
- Aerobic fitness is beneficial for older persons (Table 2.8). Because of the progressive decline in oxygen transport and functional capacity, an effective training stimulus for this age group may be much less than is needed in a younger person.[64]

E Individuals with degenerative joint disease or osteoarthritis are taught to avoid orthopedic or musculoskeletal stress. Vary the activity options so that it is primarily weight-bearing one day and nonweightbearing on alternate days.[57]

F Sedentary individuals have an increased risk for cardiac arrest and cerebral vascular accidents if the physical exertion is too vigorous. Patients are educated to initiate the activity at lower levels, progress slower, and gradually increase in duration and frequency to reach their desired fitness level.

Table 2.8. Guidelines for Aerobic Exercise in the Elderly

- Beneficial aerobic activities include cycling, brisk walking, swimming, dancing, rowing.
- Intersperse initial activity sessions with brief rest periods until a continuous bout of activity is achieved over time.
- Adding 2 to 5 minutes per week to the workout usually is appropriate for achieving the following desired goals:[64]
  —Duration of 30 to 40 minutes
  —Frequency of 5 to 6 times per week
  —Intensity based on graded exercise test (GXT), risk factors, medical history (typical training heart rate in the elderly is 60% to 75% of maximal heart rate)
- Assess progress and reevaluate the fitness plan in about 4 to 6 weeks.

Physical Activity/Exercise Considerations for Obese Persons

1 Combined programs of physical activity, meal planning, and behavior change are effective for obese persons.

A The therapeutic approach that emphasizes increased levels of physical activity offers the advantage of enhancing caloric expenditure and providing the benefits of improved fitness in terms of influencing blood lipids, blood glucose control, blood pressure, mood, and attitude.[54]

B Often, the initial fitness goal of the obese person is to simply increase the amount of physical activity from an inactive state.

C A combination of meal planning plus increased physical activity has been shown to be more effective at long-term weight control than either meal planning or physical activity alone. The addition of physical activity to a weight-control program may facilitate more permanent weight loss than total reliance on caloric restriction.[7]

D Regular physical activity during a weight-control program helps to maintain muscle mass while promoting fat loss. Weight loss achieved by caloric restriction alone may lead to loss of lean muscle mass and less loss of fat.

E Continuous aerobic exercise has the greatest impact on weight loss because of enhanced caloric expenditure.
   • Walking is an effective choice for continuous aerobic exercise. Alternative types of exercise include cycling and water exercise.
   • Swimming (less likely to induce weight loss or provide aerobic effects) and running (too much knee stress for obese individuals) are less effective options.

F As the duration of physical activity increases, so does the utilization of fat as a fuel. A longer duration (eg, greater than 45 minutes) has been shown to have a greater calorie-burning and fat-mobilization effect than shorter activity periods.[6,57]

G Intensity should be at the low end of the target heart-rate range.
   • The duration of the activity should be sufficient to expend 200 to 300 kcal per session.
   • This calorie expenditure may be accomplished with low-intensity options of long duration (40 to 60 minutes) such as walking.[57]

H Frequency of exercise should be a minimum of 3 times per week. An exercise frequency of 5 times per week is recommended for increased weight loss and facilitation of blood glucose goal attainment.

Physical Activity/Exercise Considerations for Persons With Diabetes Complications

1 Persons with chronic complications of diabetes often do not take part in physical activity programs. Yet, it is useful for this group to increase their physical activity to improve or maintain their functional capacity, strength, and flexibility.[66] Since persons with diabetes have an increased risk of cardiovascular disease, comprehensive assessments may be necessary to determine the most appropriate physical activity options.

2 Patients with established cardiovascular disease usually require supervision in a cardiac rehabilitation program.
   A Hypertension and a hypertensive response to physical exertion (systolic blood pressure >260 mm Hg, diastolic blood pressure >125 mm Hg) are frequently seen in persons with diabetes.[57]
      • Activities should be performed at an intensity that avoids a hypertensive response.
      • Physical activities that involve heavy lifting, straining, and Valsalva-like maneuvers should be avoided.

- Physical activity that involves the upper body and arms generally induces larger increases in systolic blood pressure than similar workloads performed by the legs alone.

B Rhythmic activities using the lower extremities are recommended, such as walking, light jogging, and cycling. Weight training should involve low resistance with high repetitions.[57]

3 Patients with peripheral vascular disease will experience ischemic pain during physical activity as a result of insufficient oxygen supply and demand for the active muscles.

A A walking program for intermittent claudication may improve collateral circulation and muscle metabolism and, in turn, decrease pain.[67]

B An interval training program of walk/rest periods results in greater exercise tolerance of pain-limited work capacity.

- Determine the distance and duration of the patient's walk by a pain-limited threshold.
- Advise patients to keep the intensity low because higher intensity demands a greater blood supply and induces claudication pain.[65]
- Teach patients that conversation, music, and other elements can divert attention from the discomfort and pain.
- Discontinue the activity when the discomfort or pain accelerates from moderate to intense discomfort and the individual's attention cannot be diverted.[57]

C Weight-bearing activities are preferred, although activities that are not weight bearing may allow for longer duration and higher intensity workouts.

D Pain at rest and during the night are indications of severe peripheral vascular disease, which is an absolute contraindication for a walking program.[68]

E Daily activity sessions will maximize tolerable pain.[57]

4 Patients with advanced retinopathy have significant restrictions regarding the level of physical exertion and for their activity options.

A Provide physical activity recommendations based on the severity and stage of diabetic retinopathy. In general, physical activity has not been shown to accelerate retinopathy.

B In the early stages of retinopathy, there are limited restrictions on physical activity.

- Physical activity may actually reduce the risk of developing proliferative diabetic retinopathy (PDR) and diabetic macular edema by its positive effects on blood pressure and HDL cholesterol, which are associated with retinopathy.
- Strenuous activity may precipitate vitreous hemorrhage or traction retinal detachment for patients with active PDR; clearance for exercise must be provided by the patient's ophthalmologist.

C The level of retinopathy determines which activities are appropriate and which activities are to be avoided (Table 2.9).[69]

5 For persons with recent visual impairment, and for some with long-standing visual loss, aerobic capacity may be reduced due to loss of independent mobility.

A Suitable options for activity include swimming (using lane guides), stationary cycling, treadmill walking, tandem cycling, and folk dancing (using the sighted person as an anchor).

Table 2.9. Physical Activity/Exercise Guidelines for Persons With Diabetic Retinopathy

Level of Retinopathy	Physical Activity/Exercise Recommendation(s)
No diabetic retinopathy	• No physical activity/exercise limitations.
Mild nonproliferative	• No physical activity/exercise limitations.
Moderate nonproliferative	• Avoid activities that dramatically elevate blood pressure (eg, power lifting).
Severe to very severe nonproliferative	• Limit increase in systolic blood pressure (eg, Valsalva maneuvers), and avoid activities that jar the head. Heart rate should not exceed that which elicits a systolic blood pressure response greater than 180 mm Hg (eg, boxing and intense competitive sports).[66]
Proliferative	• Avoid strenuous activity, high-impact activities, Valsalva maneuvers, and activities that jar the head (eg, weight lifting, jogging, high-impact aerobic dance, racquet sports, strenuous trumpet playing, and competitive sports). • Encourage activities that are low-impact and aerobic and stress cardiovascular conditioning (eg, swimming without diving, walking, low-impact aerobic dance, stationary cycling, and endurance exercising).[69]

B Various teaching adaptations and organizations have broadened sports participation (snow skiing, track-and-field competition) for visually impaired individuals.[66]

6 Nearly all known risk factors for coronary artery disease are found in persons with end-stage renal disease, thus underscoring the need for a properly planned fitness program.

　　A Although aerobic activities are preferred, the ability to perform this type of activity depends on the degree of kidney impairment. These individuals usually have low functional and aerobic capacity.

　　B It is recommended that any aerobic activity begin at a low level, perhaps using interval work, followed by a gradual, progressive activity plan.[70] Brisk walking, swimming, and cycling are beneficial choices.

7 Peripheral neuropathy can result in sensory losses of pain, touch, and balance. For example, neuroarthropathy (Charcot's foot) can lead to disarticulations and injury in sensory-impaired individuals.

　　A Physical activity cannot reverse the symptoms of neuropathy, but it can prevent the further loss of muscle strength and flexibility commonly seen in patients with sensory polyneuropathy. Adaptive shortening of connective tissue can occur due to immobilization or limited awareness of how the body is moving through space. Thus, daily range-of-motion exercises are recommended.

B Extra care is needed to avoid injury and overstretching by sensory-impaired individuals.[66]

- Avoiding weight-bearing activities usually is recommended because of the increased likelihood of soft tissue and joint injury.
- Avoiding orthopedic stress is important; activity options such as cycling and swimming are beneficial choices.
- Brisk walking may be another alternative if balance is not impaired.[54]
- Jogging is contraindicated because it places a threefold increase on the foot compared with walking.

C Proper footwear and inspection of the feet after performing physical activity are strategies to prevent blisters and detect injuries. For persons with limited mobility, chair exercises may improve flexibility and strength.

8 Increases in the physical activity levels of people with autonomic neuropathy should be approached with caution because of the role of the autonomic nervous system in hormonal and cardiovascular regulation during exercise.

A Symptoms of angina are not reliable indicators of coronary artery disease due to the higher frequency of silent ischemia and myocardial infarction among people with diabetes.[27]

B Physical working capacity is reduced.

C High-intensity physical activities should be avoided.

D Dehydration may be a risk in individuals who have difficulty with hemoregulation; therefore, physical exertion in hot or cold environments should be avoided. Hypotension and hypertension following vigorous activities are possibilities.

E Recumbent cycling and water aerobics are options for persons with orthostatic hypotension.

F Frequent blood glucose monitoring is recommended during physical activity for people with defective counterregulatory mechanisms.[66]

Physical Activity/Exercise Participation

1 Little is known about how to increase and maintain participation in exercise programs.

A Only 22% of American adults perform the recommended amount of physical activity necessary for health benefits (light-to-moderate physical exertion sustained for at least 30 minutes). About 54% are somewhat active but do not meet this objective, and 24% or more are completely sedentary.[71-73]

B More is known about exercise relapse than effective interventions. Approximately 50% of people who join an exercise program drop out during the first 3 to 6 months.

2 The transtheoretical model for change has been applied to exercise participation, weight loss, smoking cessation, and mammography screening.[74,75]

A A perception of the pros (benefits) versus the cons (demands) of exercising determine the transition from consideration to participation to maintenance of a physical activity program.

B The stages of change can be used to tailor intervention strategies and exercise outcomes to include both readiness and behavioral changes (see Chapter 3, Behavior Change, in Diabetes Education and Program Management, for more information).

3 Stage-matched interventions are the most effective. These interventions provide strategies for overcoming barriers to participation at each stage.

A In the precontemplation stage, physical activity/exercise is not even a consideration. People in this stage lack confidence in their ability to begin or continue a fitness program and avoid reading, talking, and thinking about it.

- Asking that they begin to increase their physical activity level will have a negative effect.
- Building a trusting relationship and providing information are needed at this stage.

B Individuals in the contemplation stage think about physical activity/exercise and perceive the advantages and disadvantages to be equal, but they do not increase their physical activity level.

- Be supportive of these patients; they are looking for assistance and validation.
- It is important not to criticize any ambivalence about physical activity/exercise but rather to encourage discussion of concerns, questions, and personal reasons to increase their physical activity level.

C In the preparation stage, the individuals have thought about physical activity/exercise and are ready to begin.

- The patient is ready to set goals and develops a self-fitness plan.
- This stage is probably the most rewarding time for individuals.

D In the action stage, individuals are performing physical activity. They have achieved a regular level of physical activity/exercise of at least 20 minutes 3 times per week. There is a high risk of relapse because the behavior is new.

E In the maintenance stage, the rewards of physical activity/exercise are more subtle after 6 months. However, as the potential for relapse still exists, the educator's role is to keep activities interesting and assist the individuals in progressing with their program.

F Most people are not successful with their first try; they may need 3 or 4 attempts before an increase in their physical activity level becomes a long-term habit. When relapse does occur, feelings of failure, embarrassment, guilt, or shame may surface. Fifteen percent of people become demoralized and resist trying again, so support is important in all stages.

- Eighty-five percent will try again.
- Sixty percent of all New Year's resolutions are repledged the following year.
- People progress through the stages as they learn from their mistakes and try something different the next time.
- The more action taken, the better chance of progressing forward.

Self-Directed Physical Fitness Programs

1 Anecdotal reports suggest that personally designed programs enhance enjoyment and are more likely to be sustained. Persons who choose an activity that they enjoy are more likely to participate in it on a regular basis. Physical activity/exercise is more likely to occur when it is convenient (eg, close to home or work).

2 Asking individuals if they are thinking about increasing their physical activity level and their feelings about it provides cues for how to provide information.

3 It is important for individuals to establish realistic and practical goals at the beginning of a fitness program. Goals that are too vague, too ambitious, or too distant do not provide enough self-motivation to maintain long-term interest.

A The beginning of the fitness program is probably the most rewarding time for individuals.

B Ask individuals to identify barriers and develop strategies to overcome possible interruptions in their regular physical activity/exercise schedule (eg, inclement weather, seasonal change, vacations, and holidays).

C Individuals must learn strategies to optimize social support from the family, exercise class members, or a buddy system.

D Individuals should develop stimulus control strategies to initiate and continue physical activity/exercise participation (eg, write exercise in appointment books, set watch alarms for exercise time).

E Individuals should compare the time it takes to walk 2 miles at the beginning of their physical activity/exercise program with the time required to walk this distance after they have been active for a period of time.

F Individuals can obtain feedback by keeping a log of pre- and postactivity blood glucose levels or to chart A1C levels for the duration of the training program.

Key Educational Considerations

1 Assist individuals in designing a plan to increase their physical activity that will help them to safely achieve their goals. Reevaluate the fitness goals and plan between 5 and 7 weeks to establish new goals, as necessary, that reinforce the effects, benefits, and principles of the physical activity/exercise program.

2 Assist individuals in identifying barriers to the physical activity/exercise program and determine options for overcoming the barriers. For example, to overcome fear of hypoglycemia, discuss ways to make adjustments to prevent hypoglycemia.

3 Ask individuals to check blood glucose levels pre- and postactivity and record the results along with information about medication, food/carbohydrate intake, and the type and time of any symptoms that develop during or after physical exertion. By reviewing these records with the individuals, the educator can discuss the effects of physical activity/exercise and offer ideas about needed adjustments in management. Furthermore, record keeping may provide reinforcement for the fitness program.

4 Ask individuals to perform self-assessments to evaluate fitness results. Compare current level of physical activity to the amount of physical activity/exercise performed at the beginning of the program. Other parameters that can be monitored that reflect progress with the exercise program include weight, blood glucose, and lipid levels.

5 Assist individuals who may be self-conscious because of their weight or fitness level to find a group or class of similar status and with comparable goals. A significant deterrent for many overweight people is joining an exercise class that consists of people who are lean and relatively fit.

Self-Review Questions

1 What are the benefits of regular physical activity/exercise for individuals with diabetes?

2 Discuss the mechanisms for activity-induced hypoglycemia.

3 What precautions should be taken to help prevent activity-induced hypoglycemia, including postactivity, late-onset hypoglycemia?

4 For persons with type 1 diabetes, describe when and why physical exertion can result in a worsening of hyperglycemia and ketosis.

5 What are the components and examples of aerobic exercise?

6 What strategies can improve adherence to a fitness program?

7 What are the potential risks of physical activity/exercise for persons with type 1 and type 2 diabetes?

8 Briefly discuss and identify activity options that would be appropriate or contraindicated for persons with retinopathy and neuropathy.

9 Why are self-directed goals important for improving physical fitness?

Learning Assessment: Case Study

CD is a 64-year-old female with a 4-year history of type 2 diabetes. She has come to the diabetes center because she wants to start an exercise program to lose weight. She is very enthusiastic about her new health club membership, but she wants to know where to begin. During the assessment she tells you, "I have mild nonproliferative retinopathy and my feet are a little numb, but otherwise my diabetes is well controlled." AB is 5 ft 4 in tall, weighs 241 lb (108.1 kg), and her A1C level is >9.8% (normal = <6.2%). She is on a split dose of regular and NPH insulins at breakfast and dinner. She checks her blood glucose levels in the morning, and her results are around 180 mg/dL (10.8 mmol/L). She states that she has not seen her doctor in awhile.

Questions for Discussion

1 What questions would you ask CD about her diabetes management?

2 What does CD need to know before increasing her physical activity level?

3 What type of activity options are safe for CD (eg, exercise type, intensity, duration, restrictions)?

Discussion

1 Although CD states that her diabetes is fine, she has an elevated A1C level. This finding, together with her comments about her eyes and feet, indicate to the diabetes educator certain key facts about CD's diabetes.

  A Her diabetes is not adequately controlled.

  B Complications could be well established.

  C CD may not be adequately informed regarding diabetes and its management.

2 Since CD has not seen her physician for some time, she is encouraged to do so prior to increasing her physical activity level.

3 Based on the American Diabetes Association guidelines for her age and duration of diabetes, a graded exercise stress electrocardiogram test (GXT) is warranted prior to initiating an exercise program. The results of the GXT allow accurate and safe determinations of exercise tolerances and limitations.

4 A medical exam also is necessary and should include a plasma lipid profile and blood chemistries, kidney function tests, and a comprehensive eye exam. These assessments are important in view of CD's history and are necessary before she can safely begin her plans to increase her physical activity.

5 Results of the GXT show no cardiac dysfunction during exercise but reveal a poor tolerance for exercise, indicating a deconditioned state. Her resting HR was 77 bpm and her resting BP was 128/76. When CD walked on the treadmill, her exercise systolic blood pressure was 204 mm Hg when her heart rate was 136 beats per minute. Maximal exercise heart rate was 143 beats per minute.

6 Further assessments showed decreased sensation in the feet to stimuli, elevated lipids, and a low ratio of HDL:LDL cholesterol (risk factors for coronary artery disease), slight proteinuria, and stable nonproliferative retinopathy.

7 CD and her doctor decide that she will continue with the same insulin regimen, perform more frequent blood glucose monitoring, reevaluate her meal plan with the assistance of a dietitian, and incorporate her health club membership into a more physically active lifestyle. CD is referred to an exercise specialist.

8 The goals CD identifies for her fitness plan includes a weight loss of about 10 to 15 lb within 3 months (4.5 to 6.8 kg) (combined with a meal plan), improved lipid profile, improved aerobic capacity, improved overall diabetes control (combined with an education program), and increased feelings of control and self-worth.

9 A plan to increase CD's fitness level is established:
   A Treadmill walking at a heart rate of 131 beats per minute resulted in an elevated systolic blood pressure; therefore, CD's recommended intensity will be based on blood pressure response to exercise.
   B Physical activity will be performed at a workload that does not induce large systolic changes due to the cardiac concerns associated with elevated blood pressure response during activity.
   - CD's training intensity is 143 $[(HR_{max} - HR_{rest}) \times 0.60$ and $0.85] + HR_{rest} = [(143 - 77) \times 0.60$ and $0.85] + 77 = 116$ to 133 beats per minute.
   - At 130 beats per minute, CD's systolic blood pressure was 172 mm Hg, which is an appropriate training intensity.
   - CD has been inactive and is obese; therefore, she will need to initiate her fitness program at a lower training intensity (eg, 120 beats per minute).
   - CD may need some brief rest periods during the workout, initially performing only 10 to 15 minutes of activity at a time.
   - Alternating weekly additions of time and intensity to the workout will help accomplish the ultimate goal (within 6 to 8 weeks) of continual physical exertion for 45 to 60 minutes at a heart rate of 130 beats per minute.
   C CD decides to exercise 5 times per week. Focusing on increasing duration instead of only intensity will aid in fat mobilization and favorably alter the lipid profile.

D CD's blood glucose profile showed late-afternoon hyperglycemia prior to initiating the exercise prescription.

- A consistent physical activity program will eventually result in better blood glucose control 24 hours a day. An optimal time for CD to go to her health club is between 2 PM and 4 PM, when her blood glucose levels are elevated. This is also CD's preferred time because her workday is finished and her husband is not yet home.
- Exercising at this time will control CD's late-afternoon hyperglycemia.

E In addition to her health club activities, CD was instructed to identify some strategies to increase her usual daily physical activity level. She was able to list a few areas where she could become more active: spend less time in her car while running errands, stand while talking on the telephone, take short walks during her lunch break, and use the stairs at work instead of the elevator. CD agreed to find other strategies to add to this list.

10 CD's had noted her feet were a little numb, and she was found to have some decreased sensation during her medical exam; therefore, she should be instructed on proper foot care guidelines, proper shoe and sock selection and to choose her activities to decrease the risk of injury to her extremities. She should not begin with high-impact or heavy weight-bearing activities like step aerobics, prolonged walking, jogging or stair climbing. Cycling, Tai Chi, short bouts of walking, strength training, or water walking could be suggested as alternatives.

References

1 Sushruta SCS. Vaidya Jadavaji Trikamji Acharia. Bombay, India: Sagar; 1938.

2 Allen FM, Stillman E, Fitz R. Total Dietary Regulation in the Treatment of Diabetes. Exercise. 1919; Monograph 11.

3 Lawrence RH. The effects of exercise on insulin action in diabetes. Br Med J. 1926;1:648-652.

4 Helmrich SP, Ragland DR, Leung RW, Paffenbarger RS Jr. Physical activity and reduced occurrence of non-insulin-dependent diabetes mellitus. N Engl J Med. 1991;325:147-152.

5 Castaneda C, Layne JE, Munoz-Orians L, et al. A randomized controlled trial of resistance exercise training to improve glycemic control in older adults with type 2 diabetes. Diabetes Care. 2002;25:2335-2341.

6 McArdle WD, Katch FI, Katch VL. Essentials of Exercise Physiology. Philadelphia: Lippincott, Williams & Wilkins; 2000.

7 Bogardus C, Ravussin E, Robbins DC, Wolfe RR, Horton ES, Sims EAH. Effects of physical training with diet therapy on carbohydrate metabolism in patients with glucose intolerance and non-insulin-dependent diabetes mellitus. Diabetes. 1984;33:311-318.

8 Stout RW. Insulin and atheroma: 20 year perspective. Diabetes Care. 1990;13:631-654.

9 Fontbonne AM, Eschwege EM. Insulin and cardiovascular disease: Paris prospective study. Diabetes Care. 1991;14:461-469.

10 Schneider SH, Ruderman NB. Exercise and physical training in the treatment of diabetes mellitus. Compr Ther. 1986;12:49-56.

11 Colwell JA. Effects of exercise on platelet function, coagulation and fibrinolysis. Diabetes Metab Rev. 1986;1:501-512.

12 Hornsby WG, Boggess KA, Lyons TJ, Barnwell WH, Lazarchick J, Colwell JA. Hemostatic alterations with exercise conditioning in NIDDM. Diabetes Care. 1990;13:87-92.

13 Rodin J. Physiological effects of exercise. In: William RS, Wallace AG, eds. Biological Effects of Physical Activity. Champaign, Ill: Human Kinetics; 1990.

14 Duncan GE, Perri MG, Theriaque DW, Hutson AD, Eckel RW, Stacpoole PW. Exercise training, without weight loss, increases insulin sensitivity and postheparin plasma lipase activity in previously sedentary adults. Diabetes Care. 2003;26:557-562.

15 Schneider SH, Amorosa LF, Khachadurian AK, Ruderman NB. Studies on the mechanism of improved glycemic control during regular exercise in type II diabetes. Diabetologia. 1984;26:355-360.

16 Eriksson KF, Lindgarde F. Prevention of type II diabetes mellitus by diet and physical exercise. The 6-year Malmo Feasibility Study. Diabetologia. 1991;34:891-898.

17 Heath GW, Wilson RH, Smith J, Leonard BE. Community-based exercise and weight control: diabetes risk reduction and glycemic control in Zuni Indians. Am J Clin Nutr. 1991;53:S1642-S1646.

18 Schneider SH, Khachadurian AK, Amorosa LF, Clemow L, Ruderman NB. Ten-year experience with an exercise-based outpatient lifestyle modification program in the treatment of diabetes mellitus. Diabetes Care. 1992; 15(suppl 4):1800-1810.

19 Vanninen E, Uusitupa M, Siitonen O, Laitinen J, Lansimies E. Habitual physical activity, aerobic capacity, and metabolic control in patients with newly diagnosed type II diabetes mellitus: effect of a 1-year diet and exercise intervention. Diabetologia. 1992;35:340-346.

20 Stratton R, Wilson DP, Endres RK, Goldstein DE. Improved glycemic control after supervised 8-wk exercise program in insulin-dependent diabetic adolescents. Diabetes Care. 1987;10:589-593.

21 Landt KW, Campaigne BN, James FW, Sperling MA. Effects of exercise training on insulin sensitivity in adolescents with type 1 diabetes. Diabetes Care. 1985;8:461-465.

22 Wallberg-Henrikssonn H, Gunnarsson R, Henriksson J, et al. Increased peripheral insulin sensitivity and muscle mitochondrial enzymes but unchanged blood glucose control in type 2 diabetics after physical training. Diabetes. 1982;31:1044-1050.

23 Peterson CM, Jones RL, Dupuis A, Levine BS, Bernstein R, O'Shea M. Feasibility of improved blood glucose control in patients with insulin-dependent diabetes mellitus. Diabetes Care. 1979;2:329-335.

24 Wallberg-Henriksson H, Gunnarsson R, Henriksson J, Ostman J, Wahren J. Influence of training on formation of muscle capillaries in type 1 diabetes. Diabetes. 1984;33:851-857.

25 Zinman B, Zuniga-Guajardo S, Kelly D. Comparison of the acute and long-term effects of exercise on glucose control in type 1 diabetics. Diabetes Care. 1984;7:515-519.

26 Stratton R, Wilson DP, Endres RK. Acute glycemic effects of exercise in adolescents with insulin-dependent diabetes mellitus. Physician Sport Med. 1988;16:150-157.

27 Vitug A, Schneider SH, Ruderman NB. Exercise in type 1 diabetes. In: Terjung RL, ed. Exercise and Sport Sciences Reviews. New York: Macmillan; 1988:285-304.

28 Vranic M, Berger M. Exercise and diabetes. Diabetes. 1979;28:147-163.

29 Tzankoff SP, Norris AH. Longitudinal changes in basal metabolism in man. J Appl Physiol. 1978;45:536-593.

30 Franz MJ. Exercise and diabetes: fuel metabolism, benefits, risks and guidelines. Clin Diabetes. 1988;6:58-60.

31 Winder WW. Regulation of hepatic glucose regulation during exercise. In: Terjung RL, ed. Exercise and Sport Sciences Reviews. New York: Macmillan; 1985:1-32.

32 Hartley LH, Mason JW, Hogan RP, et al. Multiple hormonal responses to graded exercise in relation to physical training. J Appl Physiol. 1972;33:602-606.

33 Zinman B, Vranic M, Albisser AM, Leibel BS, Marliss ED. The role of insulin in the metabolic response to exercise in the diabetic man. Diabetes. 1979;28(suppl 1):76-81.

34 Wahren J. Glucose turnover during exercise in healthy men and in patients with diabetes mellitus. Diabetes. 1979;29(suppl 1):82-88.

35 Ahlborg G, Felig P. Lactate and glucose exchange across the forearm, legs and splanchnic bed during and after prolonged leg exercise. J Clin Invest. 1982;69:45-54.

36 Richter EA, Garetto LP, Goodman M, Ruderman N. Muscle glucose metabolism following exercise in the rat: increased sensitivity to insulin. J Clin Invest. 1982;69:785-793.

37 Mondon CE, Dolkas CB, Reaven GM. Site of enhanced insulin sensitivity in exercise-trained rats at rest. Am J Physiol 1980;239(Endocrinol Metab 2):E169-177.

38 Wasserman DH, Zinman B. Exercise in individuals with IDDM (technical review). Diabetes Care. 1994;17:924-937.

39 Kemmer FW, Tacken M, Berger M. Mechanism of exercise-induced hypoglycemia during sulfonylurea treatment. Diabetes. 1987;36:1178-1182.

40 Albright A, Franz M, Hornsby G, et al. for American College of Sports Medicine. Exercise and type 2 diabetes. Position stand. Med Sci Sports Exerc. 2000; 32:1345-1360.

41 Schneider, SH, Ruderman NB. Exercise and NIDDM (technical review). Diabetes Care. 1990;13:785-789.

42 American Diabetes Association. Physical Activity/Exercise and Diabetes Mellitus. Diabetes Care. 2003; 26(suppl 1):S73-77.

43 Mitchell TH, Abraham G, Schiffrin A, Leiter A, Marliss EB. Hyperglycemia after intense exercise in IDDM subjects during continuous subcutaneous insulin infusion. Diabetes Care. 1988;11:311-317.

44 Purdon C, Brousson M, Nyveen SL, et al. The roles of insulin and catecholamines in the glucoregulatory response during intense exercise and early recovery in insulin-dependent diabetic and control subjects. J Clin Endocrinol Metab. 1993;76:566-573.

45 Horton ES. Prescription for exercise. Diabetes Spectrum. 1991;4:250-257.

46 Schiffrin A, Parikh S. Accommodating planned exercise in type I diabetic patients on intensive treatment. Diabetes Care. 1985;8:337-342.

47 Koivisto VA, Felig P. Effects of leg exercise on insulin absorption in diabetic patients. N Engl J Med. 1978;298:79-83.

48 Kemmer FW, Berchtold P, Berger M, et al. Exercise-induced fall of blood glucose in insulin-treated diabetics unrelated to alteration in insulin mobilization. Diabetes. 1979;28:1131-1137.

49 Frid A, Ostman J, Linde B. Hypoglycemia risk during exercise after intramuscular injection of insulin in thigh in IDDM. Diabetes Care. 1990;13:473-477.

50 Franz MJ. Nutrition: can it give athletes with diabetes a boost? Diabetes Educ. 1991;17:163-172.

51 Nathan D, Madnek SF, Delahanty L. Programming preexercise snacks to prevent postexercise hypoglycemia in intensively treated insulin dependent diabetics. Ann Intern Med. 1985;102:483-486.

52 Sonnenberg GE, Kemmer FW, Berger M. Exercise in type I diabetic patients treated with continuous subcutaneous insulin infusion. Diabetologia. 1990;33:696-703.

53 Beaser RS. Outsmarting Diabetes. Minneapolis: Chronimed; 1994.

54 Roitman JL, Kelsey M, LaFontaine TP, Southard DR, Williams MA, York T, eds. American College of Sports Medicine. Resource Manual for Guidelines for Exercise Testing and Prescription. 3rd ed. Philadelphia: Lea & Febiger; 1998.

55 Durak EP, Jovanovic-Peterson L, Peterson CM. Randomized crossover study of effect of resistance training on glycemic control, muscular strength and cholesterol in type I diabetic men. Diabetes Care. 1990;13:1039-1043.

56 Goldberg AP. Aerobic and resistive exercise modify risk factors for coronary heart disease. Med Sci Sports Exer. 1989;21:669-674.

57 Franklin BA, Whaley MH, Howley ET, eds. American College of Sports Medicine. Guidelines for Exercise Testing and Prescription. 6th ed. Baltimore: Williams & Wilkins; 2000.

58 Fulton JE, Mâsse LC, Tortolero SR, et al. Field evaluation of energy expenditure from continuous and intermittent walking in women. Med Sci Sports Exerc. 2001;33:163-170.

59 National Institutes of Health. NIH Consensus Statement: Physical Activity and Cardiovascular Health. Bethesda, Md: Department of Health and Human Services, Public Health Service; 1995:13(3).

60 Kraemer WJ, Fleck SJ. Resistance training: exercise prescription. Physician Sport Med. 1988;16:69-81.

61 Soukup JT, Maynard TS, Kovaleski JE. Resistance training guidelines for individuals with diabetes mellitus. Diabetes Educ. 1994;20:129-137.

62 Franklin B, Bonzheim K, Gordon S, Timmis G. Resistance training in cardiac rehabilitation. J Cardiopulmonary Rehabil. 1991;11:99-107.

63 Frontera WR, Hughes VA, Lutz KJ, Evans WJ. A cross-sectional study of upper and lower extremity muscle strength in 45- to 78-year-old men and women. J Appl Physiol. 1991;71:644-650.

64 Graham C. Exercise and aging: implications for persons with diabetes. Diabetes Educ. 1991;17:189-195.

65 Schwartz RS. Exercise training in treatment of diabetes mellitus in elderly patients. Diabetes Care. 1990;13(suppl 2):77-85.

66 Graham C, Lasko-McCarthey P. Exercise options for persons with diabetic complications. Diabetes Educ. 1990;16:212-220.

67 Hiatt WR, Regensteiner JG, Hargarten ME, Wolfel EE, Brass EP. Benefit of exercise conditioning for patients with peripheral arterial disease. Circulation. 1990;81:602-609.

68 Levin, ME. The diabetic foot. In: Ruderman NB, Devlin JT, eds. The Health Professional's Guide to Diabetes and Exercise. Alexandria, Va: American Diabetes Association; 1995.

69 Aiello LM, Cavallerano J, Aiello LP, Bursell SE. Retinopathy. In: Ruderman NB, Devlin JT, eds. The Health Professional's Guide to Diabetes and Exercise. Alexandria, Va: American Diabetes Association; 1995.

70 Painter P. Exercise in end-stage renal disease. In: Terjung RL, ed. Exercise and Sport Sciences Reviews. New York: Macmillan; 1988:305-340.

71 Pate RR, Pratt M, Blair SN, et al. Physical activity and public health: a recommendation from the Centers for Disease Control and Prevention and the American College of Sports Medicine. JAMA. 1995;273:402-407.

72 Marcus BH, Rakowski W, Rossi JS. Assessing motivational readiness and decision making for exercise. Health Psychol. 1992;11:257-261.

73 Dishman RK, Sallis JF, Orenstein DR. The determinants of physical activity and exercise. Public Health Rep. 1985;100:158-171.

74 Marcus BH, Simkin LR. The transtheoretical model: applications to exercise behavior. Med Sci Sports Exerc. 1994;26:1400-1404.

75 Marcus BH, Selby VC, Niaura RS, Rossi JS. Self-efficacy and the stages of exercise behavior change. Res Q Exerc Sport. 1992;63:60-66.

Suggested Readings

General Exercise Physiology

American College of Sports Medicine. Exercise Management for Persons with Chronic Diseases and Disabilities. Champaign, Ill: Human Kinetics; 2003.

Franklin BA, ed. American College of Sports Medicine: ACSM's Guidelines for Exercise Testing and Prescription. 6th ed. Baltimore, Md: Lippincott, Williams & Wilkins; 2000.

McArdle WD, Katch FI, Katch VL. Essentials of Exercise Physiology: Diabetes Mellitus. Philadelphia: Lippincott, Williams & Wilkins; 2000.

Exercise and Diabetes

Albright A, Franz M, Hornsby G, et al. for American College of Sports Medicine. Exercise and type 2 diabetes. Position stand. Med Sci Sports Exerc. 2000;32:1345-1370.

American Diabetes Association. Handbook of Exercise in Diabetes. Alexandria, Va: American Diabetes Association; 2002.

American Diabetes Association. Physical activity/exercise and diabetes mellitus (technical review). Diabetes Care. 2003;26(suppl 1):S73-S77.

Franz M. Exercise and diabetes. In: Haire-Joshu D, ed. Management of Diabetes Mellitus: Perspectives of Care Across the Life Span. 2nd ed. St. Louis: Mosby Year Book; 1996:162-201.

Goodyear LJ. Exercise, glucose transport, and insulin sensitivity. Annu Rev Med. 1998;49:235-261.

Ivy JL. Role of exercise training in the prevention and treatment of insulin resistance and NIDDM. Sport Med. 1997;24:321-326.

Ivy JL, Aderic TW, Donovan FL. American College of Sports Medicine. Prevention and treatment of non-insulin-dependent diabetes mellitus. In: Exercise and Sport Sciences Reviews. Philadelphia: Lippincott, Williams & Wilkins; 1999:(27):1-35.

Mullooly C. Cardiovascular fitness and type 2 diabetes. Current Diabetes Reports. 2002, 2:441-447.

Wallberg-Henriksson H, Rincon J, Zierath JR. Exercise in the management of non-insulin-dependent diabetes mellitus. Sports Med. 1998;25:25-35.

Zinker BA. Nutrition and exercise in individuals with diabetes. Clin Sports Med. 1999;18:585-606,vii-viii.

Learning Assessment: Post-Test Questions

Physical Activity/Exercise 2

1 Which of the following are benefits of physical activity?
   A Reduced plasma cholesterol and triglycerides and enhanced fibrinolysis
   B Reduced body fat, muscle mass, and weight
   C Improved glucose tolerance and hypercoagulability
   D Increased insulin sensitivity and decreased high-density lipoproteins

2 In persons without diabetes, during the first 5 to 10 minutes of exercise, the major fuel for energy is:
   A Free fatty acids from adipose tissue
   B Intramuscular glucose from glycogen
   C Hepatic glucose from glycogenolysis
   D Hepatic glucose from gluconeogenesis

3 In persons without diabetes, during the postexercise recovery period, there is:
   A Replenishment of glycogen stores for 12 hours
   B Lessened insulin sensitivity
   C Increased uptake of glucose by muscle
   D Suppression of glucogenesis by the liver

4 After physical activity, which factor contributes to hypoglycemia in type 1 diabetes?
   A Mobilization of free fatty acids
   B Repletion of glycogen stores
   C Normal counterregulatory hormonal response
   D Decreased absorption of insulin

5 BD has type 1 diabetes and is on the high school track team. He runs the 4th leg of the 200-meter relay, which is a short, very intense workout. Ten minutes after the race, BD's blood glucose is 350 mg/dL. He should:
   A Inject himself with some regular insulin to cover the high blood glucose
   B Test his urine for ketones
   C Eat a snack of 1 bread exchange and 1 meat exchange
   D Run for about 40 more minutes to decrease his blood glucose

6 CN is age 55 years and has had type 2 diabetes for 10 years. He is 6 ft 1 in and weighs 300 lb. His fasting blood glucose is 145 mg/dL, and he is on metformin. He wants to start an exercise program. Which of the following would be the least important to teach him?
   A See his provider and have a stress test before beginning to increase his physical activity level
   B Wear properly fitting exercise shoes
   C Carry glucose tablets for hypoglycemia
   D Have an eye examination prior to his fitness program

7 What frequency of physical activity is optimal for weight loss for CN?
   A 2 to 3 days/week
   B 3 to 4 days/week
   C 4 to 5 days/week
   D 5 to 7 days/week

8 What maximum age-adjusted heart rate would provide an optimum aerobic workout for CN?
   A 50% to 70%
   B 55% to 75%
   C 60% to 85%
   D 65% to 90%

9 Which routine is most appropriate for an elderly patient with a degenerative joint disease?
   A No exercise at all
   B Aerobic exercise only
   C Anaerobic exercise only
   D Alternating aerobic and strength training exercise

10 Patients with moderate nonproliferative retinopathy should:
   A Avoid all strenuous activity
   B Avoid physical activity that dramatically increases their blood pressure
   C Limit physical activity to 2 days a week
   D Gradually incorporate resistance training into their normal physical activity routine

See next page for answer key.

Post-Test Answer Key

Physical Activity/Exercise

2

1	A		**6**	C
2	B		**7**	D
3	C		**8**	C
4	B		**9**	D
5	B		**10**	B

A Core Curriculum for Diabetes Education
Diabetes Management Therapies

Pharmacologic Therapies for Glucose Management

John R. White, Jr., RPh, PharmD, PA-C
Washington State University
Spokane, Washington

R. Keith Campbell, RPh, MBA, CDE
Washington State University
Pullman, Washington

Introduction

1 For some people with diabetes, nonpharmacologic interventions will suffice to attain an optimal level of blood glucose control:

A Medical nutrition therapy

B Regular physical activity

C Blood glucose monitoring

D Attention to relevant clinical educational and psychosocial needs

2 For the majority of people with diabetes, however, treatment will also require pharmacologic intervention. Approximately 90% of persons with diabetes require oral glucose-lowering medications, insulin injections, or both, to reach glucose goals.[1]

3 In addition to oral medications, the pharmacologic therapies for a person with diabetes often include other agents to treat the myriad of associated comorbid conditions or complications of diabetes. These pharmacologic therapies are considered part of standard diabetes care even though they are not used for the purpose of altering blood glucose levels. (For more information see Chapter 4, Pharmacotherapy for Dyslipidemia and Hypertension, in Diabetes Management Therapies.)

4 Diabetes educators must be cognizant of the total range of therapies that are available for comprehensive diabetes care, not just the therapies that are used for glycemic control. They also need to be able to advise patients about the effects of other drugs on blood glucose levels, diabetes complications, and other aspects of self-management.

5 This chapter will provide an update of the pharmacologic therapies for glycemic control and an overview of the impact of other drugs on diabetes management. The goal is for the educator to understand and be able to teach patients some of the intricacies of the pharmacologic interventions that are necessary for comprehensive diabetes self-management.

Objectives

Upon completion of this chapter, the learner will be able to

1 Explain the physiologic effects of insulin.

2 Differentiate insulin preparations based upon species/source, type, purity, and concentration.

3 Describe proper administration and storage guidelines for insulin.

4 Explain the limitations for insulin mixing.

5 Explain the similarities and differences of potential insulin therapy regimens, including the use of insulin pumps, and indications for specific insulin products.

6 Discuss the commonly encountered insulin regimens in persons with type 1 and type 2 diabetes.

7 Explain the differences between use of insulin in a person with type 1 and type 2 diabetes.

8 Explain the mechanism(s) of action of sulfonylureas, d-phenylalanine derivatives, meglitinides, biguanides, alpha-glucosidase inhibitors, and thiazolidinediones.

9 Describe the clinical use of the above-mentioned medications.

10 Explain the use of combination therapy in persons with type 2 diabetes.

11 Explain the clinical use of glucagon.

12 Describe potential drug-disease, drug-drug, or drug-food interactions.

Physiologic Effects of Insulin and Indications for Its Use

1 The following describes the physiologic actions and release of endogenous insulin:

  A Insulin is a hormone produced in the beta cells of the islets of Langerhans in the pancreas; it is formed from a substance called proinsulin (Figure 3.1).

- When the pancreas is stimulated, primarily by an elevated blood glucose level, the proinsulin is cleaved at 2 sections of the molecule—at the glycine position identified as the #1 amino acid of the "A" chain and at the alanine position identified as the #30 amino acid of the "B" chain (see Figure 3.1). When the proinsulin molecule is then broken apart, insulin and the connecting peptide (C-peptide) are both secreted and enter the bloodstream in equimolar amounts. Some uncleaved proinsulin also enters the blood.
- Once in the bloodstream, the half-life of free insulin has been reported to be on the order of 5.2 +/– 0.7 minutes but may be increased in persons with diabetes who have high insulin antibody titers.
- Normal daily insulin secretion in a healthy, nonpregnant, nonobese adult is approximately 0.5 to 0.7 unit insulin/kg/day.
- Since insulin and C-peptide are jointly secreted, a measurement of C-peptide level can be used as a clinical monitor of endogenous insulin production and to determine type of diabetes. Direct measurement of insulin secretion is difficult, except under controlled or research conditions, because insulin is rapidly removed from the blood as it exerts its pharmacologic action.
- Demonstration of measurable levels of C-peptide (normal fasting [0.78 to 1.89 ng/mL]) may also be used to rule out fictitious insulin administration as a cause of unexplained hypoglycemia in a person without insulin-requiring diabetes.
- Because insulin and C-peptide have different biologic durations, a measurement of C-peptide level may not accurately reflect the endogenous insulin level at that period of time.

  B Insulin exerts varied effects on body tissues. (See Chapter 1, Medical Nutrition Therapy for Diabetes, in Diabetes Management Therapies, for additional information.)

- Stimulates entry of amino acids into cells, enhancing protein synthesis.
- Enhances fat storage (lipogenesis) and prevents the mobilization of fat for energy (lipolysis and ketogenesis).
- Stimulates the entry of glucose into cells for utilization as an energy source and promotes the resultant storage of glucose as glycogen (glycogenesis) in muscle and liver cells.
- Inhibits production of glucose from liver or muscle glycogen (glycogenolysis).
- Inhibits formation of glucose from noncarbohydrates, such as amino acids (gluconeogenesis).

  C The major untoward effect of insulin therapy is hypoglycemia. Virtually all persons who inject insulin will experience hypoglycemia at some time.

- Frequent causes of hypoglycemia include too much (excessive dosage of) insulin; delayed, missed, or insufficient food intake; or too much (unplanned) exercise or physical activity.

Figure 3.1. Biochemical Formation of Human Insulin From Proinsulin

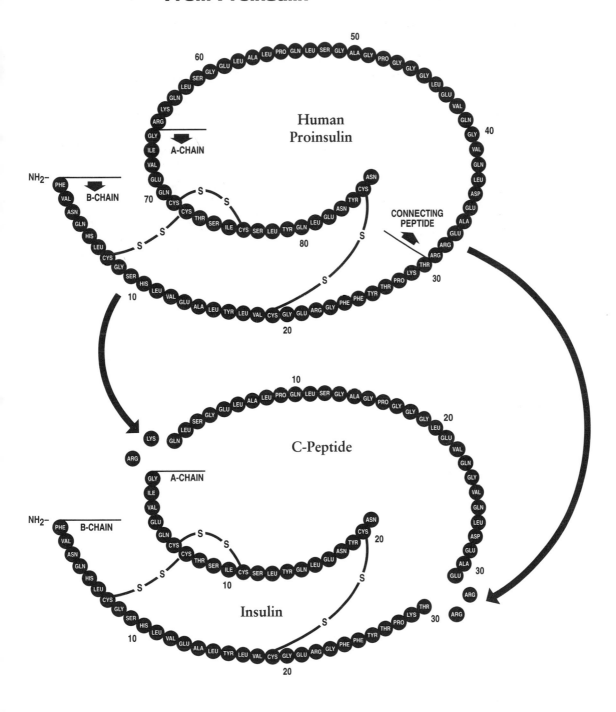

- Strategies to reduce the risk of hypoglycemia include routine self-monitoring of blood glucose levels; observing for and responding quickly to early symptoms of hypoglycemia; ingesting appropriate quantities and choices of a preexercise carbohydrate supplement; and using a consistent food/meal plan and pattern. (See Chapter 8, Hypoglycemia, in Diabetes Management Therapies, for additional information.)
- Instruct all insulin-using patients concerning the symptoms, prevention, and treatment of hypoglycemia. In addition, teaching patients to routinely carry a source of carbohydrate can help to prevent mild reactions from becoming severe.

D Endogenous insulin is defined as insulin that is supplied from the pancreas, while exogenous insulin is defined as injected pharmaceutical insulin.

2 There are several hormones in the body that exert antagonistic effects to the hypoglycemic actions of insulin. These hormones are collectively referred to as counterregulatory hormones. Blood glucose management in diabetes needs to take into account, and make compensation for, the release of 1 or more of these hormones throughout the day in response to a variety of stimuli. The primary counterregulatory hormones include

A Glucagon (produced in the alpha cells of the pancreas)

B Epinephrine

C Norepinephrine

D Growth hormone

E Cortisol

3 Insulin is indicated for specific persons with diabetes or in certain medical conditions.

A All individuals with type 1 diabetes require exogenous insulin to sustain life. In type 1 diabetes, production of insulin by beta cells is completely or largely lost.

B Individuals with type 2 diabetes may need insulin if other forms of therapy do not adequately control blood glucose levels or during periods of physiological stress such as surgery or infection.

C Women with gestational diabetes may need insulin if medical nutrition therapy alone does not adequately control blood glucose levels.

D Diabetic or nondiabetic patients receiving parenteral nutrition or high-caloric supplements to meet an increased energy need may require exogenous insulin to maintain normal glucose levels during periods of insulin resistance or increased insulin demand.

E Insulin is necessary in the treatment of diabetic ketoacidosis (DKA).

F Insulin is often needed in the treatment of hyperosmolar hyperglycemic state (HHS).

G Individuals with secondary diabetes, such as diabetes secondary to pancreatitis or other disease that severely diminishes beta cell production of insulin, may require insulin.

Insulin Species/Source, Type, Purity, and Concentration

1 Insulin preparations are differentiated by specific product characteristics (Table 3.1).

Table 3.

			Strength
Rapid-Acting			
			U-100
			U-100
Short-Acting			
			U-100, U-500
			U-100
			U-100
	Pork		
	Iletin® II regular	Lilly	U-100
	Purified Pork regular	Novo Nordisk	U-100
Intermediate-Acting	**Human**		
	Humulin® N (NPH)	Lilly	U-100
	Humulin® L (Lente)	Lilly	U-100
	Novolin® N (NPH)	Novo Nordisk	U-100
	Novolin® L (Lente)	Novo Nordisk	U-100
	Pork		
	Iletin® II NPH	Lilly	U-100
	Iletin® II Lente	Lilly	U-100
	Purified Pork NPH	Novo Nordisk	U-100
	Purified Pork Lente	Novo Nordisk	U-100
Long-Acting	**Human**		
	Humulin® U (Ultralente)	Lilly	U-100
	Human Insulin Analog		
	Lantus® (insulin glargine)	Aventis	U-100
Fixed Combination (all are U-100 insulins)			
	Human		
	Humulin® 70/30	Lilly	70/30 (NPH/reg ratio)
	Novolin® 70/30	Novo Nordisk	70/30 (NPH/reg ratio)
	Humulin® 50/50	Lilly	50/50 (NPH/reg ratio)
Fixed Combination Human Insulin Analog			
	Humalog® Mix 75/25 (neutral protamine lispro/lispro)	Lilly	75/25 (NPL/lispro ratio)
	Novolog® Mix 70/30 (neutral protamine aspart/aspart)	Novo Nordisk	70/30 (NPA/aspart ratio)

2 The species/sources for insulin are beef, pork, and human. The 4 product types include pork, which is isolated from animal pancreas glands; biosynthetic human insulin derived from bacteria (E coli), or fungal cells (Saccharomyces cerevisiae); and biosynthetic human insulin analog.

A Beef insulin differs from human insulin at 3 amino acid sites, while pork insulin differs at only 1 amino acid site (Table 3.2). Because of this difference, beef insulin induces more antigenic reactions than pork insulin. Beef-pork combination products were generally thought to induce the most antigenic reactions and were discontinued for this reason. Beef insulin is not available in the US.

Table 3.2. Amino Acid Sequence Differences Between Various Insulin Species

| Species | A Chain | | | B Chain | | | |
	A-8	A-10	A-21	B-30	B-29	B-28	B Chain Terminal
Human	Threonine	Isoleucine	Asparagine	Threonine	Lysine	Proline	
Lispro	Threonine	Isoleucine	Asparagine	Threonine	**Proline**	**Lysine**	
Aspart	Threonine	Isoleucine	Asparagine	Threonine	Lysine	**Aspartate**	
Glargine	Threonine	Isoleucine	**Glycine**	Threonine	Lysine	Proline	2 Arginines added
Bovine	**Alanine**	**Valine**	Asparagine	**Alanine**	Lysine	Proline	
Porcine	Threonine	Isoleucine	Asparagine	**Alanine**	Lysine	Proline	

B Human insulin, the human insulin analog lispro, the human insulin analog aspart, and the human insulin analog glargine are manufactured by using recombinant-DNA technology (biosynthetic). Human insulin and rapid-acting insulins are less antigenic than beef insulin and slightly less antigenic than pork insulin.

C Human biosynthetic NPH, Lente, and Ultralente insulins appear to be absorbed faster and therefore act more quickly than animal-derived insulins, even though they have similar pharmacologic effects. Commercially prepared human insulins are effective and chemically identical to endogenous human insulin.

D There are virtually no contraindications to human insulin, although there are rare instances of hypersensitivity.

E Human insulin has provided an option for vegetarians, Muslims, Orthodox Jews, or Hindus who prefer not to use pork or beef insulins.

F Animal-derived insulins induced insulin antibody formation to a greater degree than human insulins or rapid-acting insulins. When insulin is bound to insulin antibodies, the predictability of the insulin's peak effect and duration of action will be altered.

3 Insulin is generally classified according to onset, peak effect, and duration of action (Table 3.3).[2] The currently available rapid-acting insulins are lispro and aspart, the short-acting insulin is regular, the intermediate-acting insulins are NPH and Lente, and the long-acting insulin is Ultralente. Additionally, a true "peakless" long-acting insulin analog Lantus® (insulin glargine) is now available.

A Regular insulin, lispro and aspart, and glargine are the clear insulins or solution of insulin; all of the others are suspensions. Regular insulin is the only insulin product routinely used for intravenous administration, although lispro may be given intravenously.

Table 3.3. Comparison of Human Insulins and Analogs

Insulin Preparations	Onset of Action	Peak	Duration of Action
Lispro/Aspart	5-15 minutes	1-2 hours	4-6 hours
Human Regular	30-60 minutes	2-4 hours	6-10 hours
Human NPH/Lente	1-2 hours	4-8 hours	10-20 hours
Human Ultralente	2-4 hours	Unpredictable	16-20 hours
Glargine	1-2 hours	Flat	~24 hours

Note: The time course of action of any insulin may vary in the same individual. Because of this variation, time periods indicated here should be considered general guidelines only.

Source: Adapted from White JR Jr, et al.[2]

B Insulin lispro is an insulin analog identical to human insulin in its structure with the exception of the juxtaposition of lysine and proline in positions 28 and 29 on the B chain (see Figure 3.1). This molecular alteration yields insulin with a faster rate of absorption than regular human insulin.[3]

- A dose of lispro insulin peaks in half the time and in double the concentration of a comparable subcutaneous injection of regular insulin.
- Lispro insulin can generally be used in place of regular insulin to provide better coverage of postprandial glycemic excursions.[4]
- Lispro insulin can be injected immediately prior to eating (generally less than 15 minutes preprandially); injecting lispro insulin 30 to 60 minutes prior to meals may result in profound hypoglycemia.
- Several studies show reduced hypoglycemia in patients with type 1 diabetes treated with lispro insulin compared with those treated with regular human insulin.[5-7]
- Insulin lispro has also been shown to be a suitable pump insulin.[8,9] Insulin lispro insulin pump therapy compared to regular insulin reduced A1C levels; however, both reduced the incidence of hypoglycemia compared to injected insulin.[9]
- Lispro insulin is available in the US only by prescription.

C Insulin aspart is an insulin analog in which aspartic acid has been substituted for the amino acid proline at the B28 position (see Figure 3.1). In comparison to human short-acting insulin, insulin aspart can improve postprandial glycemic control by reducing hyperglycemic and hypoglycemic excursions.[10,11]

- Insulin aspart has a glucose-lowering response similar to insulin lispro and its duration of action is shortest after abdominal subcutaneous injection.[12]
- Compared to regular human insulin, insulin aspart is associated with a lower number of hypoglycemic episodes.[10]
- Insulin aspart is also reported to be effective when used in insulin pump therapy.[13]

D NPH is an abbreviation for neutral protamine Hagedorn. It is neutral in pH, contains the protein protamine (as well as zinc), and was named for the chemist who derived the formulation. The zinc/protamine complex prolongs the duration of action. Lente and Ultralente insulins are formulations with varying amounts of zinc, which prolongs the duration of action.

- Both protamine and zinc have occasionally been implicated as the causative agents of immunologic reactions such as urticaria at the injection site. Since protamine is the antidote for heparin toxicity, some have expressed concerns about sensitizing patients to protamine with NPH insulin, but these concerns have not been proved to be warranted.

E Insulin glargine (Lantus) is a long-acting human insulin analog which differs from human insulin in that asparagine at position A-21 is replaced by glycine and 2 arginines are added to the C terminus of the B chain.[14]

- Insulin glargine is a long-acting, "peakless" insulin which provides insulin in a basal pattern for up to 24 hours (see Figure 3.2).[15] It is a clear and colorless.

- Studies in persons with type 1 and type 2 diabetes have shown that insulin glargine when administered once daily provides similar control to NPH insulin administered once or twice daily.[16,17] In addition, in individuals with type 2 diabetes treated with insulin glargine, the risk of nocturnal hypoglycemia was lower and there was less weight gain compared with NPH.[17]

- Insulin glargine should be administered once daily. It is usually given at bedtime but can be given at any time of the day.[18]

- Insulin glargine must not be mixed in the same syringe with other insulins. Mixing glargine with other insulins alters its pharmacokinetic characteristics. The syringe must not contain any other medicine or residue.[18]

- The most common adverse event reported in phase III trials with glargine use was pain of mild intensity at the injection site.[18]

- Insulin glargine provides only basal insulin coverage and in many cases will be used in combination with other insulin preparations, with oral agents, or possibly in the future with inhaled insulin.

F Insulin detemir (NN304) is a soluble basal insulin analog also being developed to provide exogenous basal insulin. It has been shown to be as effective as NPH in maintaining glycemic control, with reduced risk of hypoglycemia, but has a higher mean dose requirement compared to NPH.[19]

4 Purity of animal-source insulin is expressed as parts per million (ppm) of proinsulin, the primary contaminant after extraction from the pancreas. Concern about purity is a less significant issue in insulin therapy today than previously, as all insulins are now highly purified.

5 The concentrations of insulin currently available in the US are U-100 and U-500, indicating 100 units/mL or 500 units/mL, respectively.[20] U-100 insulin is the insulin of choice for nearly all patients. U-100 insulin is not always available worldwide; instruct patients to take extra supplies when traveling to foreign countries as some countries may still use U-40 insulins.

A Patients requiring large doses of insulin may benefit by using U-500 regular insulin. The onset and duration of action of U-500 is not the same as U-100 regular. It may have a slower onset and slightly longer duration of activity.

B U-500 regular (Humulin R, Eli Lilly) is available in the US only by prescription.

Figure 3.2. Time Action Profiles of Glargine vs NPH Insulin in Type 1 Diabetes

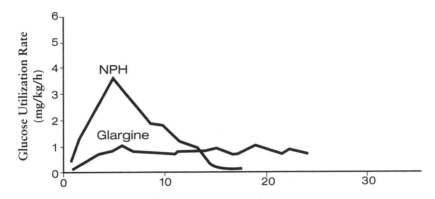

Source: Reprinted with permission from Lepore.[15]

Administration and Storage Guidelines

1 Effective use of insulin requires the correct equipment, insulin preparation, and consistent use of proper technique.

2 Teach patients to store insulin according to the manufacturer's recommendations.

A Generally, insulin should be refrigerated at 36°F to 46°F (2C° to 8°C).
  • Unopened insulin products may be stored under refrigeration until the expiration date noted on the product label.

B To reduce local irritation at the injection site that may occur when injecting cold insulin, advise patients to roll the prepared syringe between the palms, bring the bottle of insulin to room temperature before withdrawing the dose, or store the insulin at room temperature. Opened or unopened vials of insulin may be stored at a controlled room temperature of 59°F to 86°F (15°C to 30°C) for a period of 1 month; unused insulin should be discarded after that time.[20]

C Storage guidelines differ for use and storage of used (punctured) or unused cartridge insulin (Penfill®) and disposable prefilled insulin pens.
  • Insulin cartridges or regular prefilled insulin pens may be kept unrefrigerated for 28 days (1.5-mL or 3.0-mL cartridges).
  • Humalog Mix 75/25 may be used for 10 days capped at room temperature (72°F) and out of direct sunlight; unused can be stored without refrigeration for 28 days, but should be stored in the refrigerator.
  • 70/30 insulin cartridges or prefilled insulin pens may be kept unrefrigerated for 10 days.
  • NPH insulin cartridges or prefilled insulin pens may be kept unrefrigerated for 14 days.

D Keep extemporaneously prepared, prefilled syringes of either single formulations or mixtures of insulins refrigerated and use within 21 to 30 days.[20]

E Availability of insulin and supplies may vary; teach patients to carry insulin and supplies when traveling. Due to variance of temperature, insulin should not be left in a car or checked through in airline baggage.

F Instruct patients to examine vials of insulin for sediment or other visible changes before withdrawing the insulin into the syringe. Cloudiness or discoloration of clear insulin, clumping of insulin suspensions, or flocculation (frosting) of insulin suspensions indicates that the insulin has lost potency and should not be used but returned to the pharmacy for exchange. The incidence of frosting may be minimized if temperature is stabilized through refrigeration and if agitation or shaking of the vial is minimized.

3 Insulin administration equipment includes the following and requires consistent use of proper technique.
  A Disposable insulin syringes with attached needles for U-100 insulin are available in different syringe sizes, chosen according to the dose of insulin to be injected:
  - 0.25 cc (for doses <25 units), 0.3 cc (for doses <30 units), 0.5 cc (for doses <50 units), or 1 cc (for doses 50 to 100 units).
  - Needle length may be 5/16-inch or 1/2-inch. The "short needle" (5/16-inch length) is appropriate only for individuals with normal or near-normal body mass index (BMI <27 kg/m²).
  B In most circumstances, and with proper training, syringes and needles may be safely reused; however, reuse may carry an increased risk of infection for some individuals.[20] Advise patients who choose to reuse syringes that the markings on the syringe may rub off and that the needle becomes dull with repeated use. Instruct patients to safely recap the needle and store at room temperature.
  C Alternative equipment to the traditional syringe-needle unit is available. The variety of injection devices includes automatic needle injectors, automatic needle and insulin injectors, pen injectors, and needle-free jet injectors.
  - The first major alternative device, the continuous subcutaneous insulin infusion pump became available in 1974. An insulin pump consists of a reservoir filled with insulin, a small battery-operated pump and a computer chip that allows the user to control the insulin delivery.[21] (For more information see Chapter 7, Insulin Pump Therapy, in Diabetes Management Therapies.)
  - Jet injectors are a novel, needle-free system that delivers insulin transcutaneously. Jet injectors release a fine stream of insulin at high-speed and under high-pressure to penetrate the skin.
  - Pen devices have been a popular insulin delivery option in Europe for years. They were introduced in the United States in 1987. They combine the insulin container and the syringe into a single modular unit which allows for convenient insulin delivery. Insulin pens are available in a variety of types and styles. Pens may be reusable or a prefilled device. Reusable pens and prefilled pens both hold cartridges of insulin. With the reusable pen, the patient must first load an insulin cartridge. This step is eliminated with prefilled pen devices.
  - In the future, insulin may be delivered by implantable insulin pumps or transdermal systems. Two types of implantable pumps exist: a closed-loop system and an open-looped system. Transdermal insulin technologies use a process called iontophoresis (electrical currents move large, charged molecules, like insulin, across the skin).
  - Pulmonary delivery of insulin is also under development and is discussed later.

4 Teach patients to follow a specific routine for insulin injections, including consistent technique, accurate dosage, and site rotation.

A Injections are given into the subcutaneous tissue. Most individuals are able to lightly grasp a fold of skin and inject at a 90° angle. Thin individuals or children may need to pinch the skin and inject at a 45° angle to avoid intramuscular injection.[20]

B Insulin may be injected into the subcutaneous tissue of the upper arm, the anterior and lateral aspects of the thigh, the buttocks, and the abdomen (with the exception of a circle with a 2-inch radius around the navel).[20] These sites are chosen because of general patient acceptability and accessibility (see Chapter 5, Monitoring, in Diabetes Management Therapies).

- Areas for injection must be determined individually, allowing for scar tissue, areas with less subcutaneous fat, and patient preference.

- Both the patient and the health professional need to examine injection areas at regular intervals to detect bruising, redness, infection, lipoatrophy, or lipohypertrophy.

- Teach patients to rotate injection sites to prevent local irritation. Rotating within one area is recommended (eg, rotating injections systematically within the abdomen) rather than rotating to a different area with each injection. This practice may decrease variability in absorption from day to day.[20]

C Insulin absorption may vary depending upon several parameters.

- Abdominal injection provides the most rapid absorption followed by the arms, thighs, and buttocks.[20] However, note that insulin glargine does not display this difference of absorption rates at different sites.[18] Deeper intramuscular injections induce faster absorption and shorter duration of action. High levels of insulin antibodies can also inhibit insulin action following injection.

- Exercise or massage of the injection site may induce more rapid absorption and action from a dose of insulin probably by increasing the rate of blood flow through the tissue around the site.[20]

5 Various problems or complications may arise from insulin impurity, species/source, and improper injection technique.

A Insulin impurity can cause lipodystrophies (atrophy and hypertrophy).

- Atrophy, which is a concavity or pitting of the fatty tissue, is an immune phenomenon that occurs in a small number of patients and is related to species/source or purity. Use of highly purified insulins such as human insulin or purified pork reduces the occurrence of atrophy. Patients who develop this problem may benefit from injecting human or highly purified insulin around the periphery of the atrophied areas.[22]

- Hypertrophy, which is a fatty thickening of the lipid tissue, is best prevented by rotation of injection sites.

B Allergies to insulin are rare. Insulin allergy may occur as local reactions (rash, urticarial cutaneous reaction) or systemic reactions (serum sickness, anaphylaxis).

- Prior to insulin purification, local cutaneous reactions were more common.

- Zinc or protamine in the insulin, preservatives, and rubber or latex stoppers have all been implicated in inducing allergic reactions.

- Both local and systemic reactions appear to be immunologically mediated through induction of high titers of IgG and IgE antibodies.

- If systemic reaction occurs, desensitization to the insulin will be necessary. If desensitization is needed, the attending physician should be encouraged to contact the insulin manufacturer for the desensitization kit and the procedure to follow.

Mixing Insulins

1 Organizing the necessary materials prior to insulin injection will limit errors.

2 Guidelines for extemporaneous insulin mixtures are listed in Table 3.4. These standards are based on published data.[23]

   A Varying the time delay for injecting after mixing may result in a different insulin action.

   B As a general rule, the 2 insulins being mixed should be of the same brand.

   C Rapid-acting or regular insulin is usually drawn up first, followed by the intermediate-acting insulin. This practice limits the potential for contamination, which may result in dose variance.

Table 3.4. Guidelines for Mixing Insulin and/or Prefilling Syringes

Regular and NPH	• Mixture stable in any ratio • Mixture of choice, if regular and intermediate combination is needed • Extemporaneously prepared syringes that are refrigerated are stable for at least 1 month • Prefilling is acceptable
Regular and Lente	• Binding of regular begins immediately • Binding continues for 24 hours • Activity of regular is blunted • Velosulin should not be mixed with Lente insulins • If mixed or prefilled, the interval between mixing the insulins and administering the insulin should be standardized
Commercially Prepared Premixed Insulins	• Prefilling is acceptable
Lente and Ultralente	• Mixture stable in any ratio • Mixture stable for 18 months • Prefilling is acceptable
Lispro Insulin With NPH or Ultralente	• Mixture stable in any ratio • Administer immediately after mixing
Glargine Lantus	• Should not be mixed with other insulins

Source: From American Diabetes Association.[20]

3 Commercially available premixed insulins (70/30, 50/50, 75/25) are manufactured and stabilized by altered buffering. These products may be advantageous for individuals unable to mix insulins accurately or reliably. All insulin mixtures must be thoroughly resuspended immediately prior to an injection or after storage for any time period.

Patients should be instructed to gently roll the vial or prefilled syringe or pen device between the palms several times to thoroughly mix the component insulins.

Insulin Therapy Programs

1 Insulin dosing schedules vary among individuals (see Chapter 6, Pattern Management of Blood Glucose, in Diabetes Management Therapies).

   A Physiologically, insulin is released throughout the day in dynamic fashion. Insulin is secreted in response to a variety of stimuli such as the glycemic rise from ingestion of carbohydrate or the release of counterregulatory hormones. Insulin release in response to carbohydrate intake is referred to as a bolus secretion; insulin release to counteract ongoing hormonal or other glycemic influences is referred to as basal secretion. Basal insulin secretion typically occurs at a rate of 0.5 to 1 unit per hour. The metabolic balance between basal insulin, the counterregulatory hormones, hepatic glucose production, and circulating glucose normally provides the body with sufficient glucose to function between meals. Bolus insulin is rapidly released in response to nutrient intake and under normal circumstances reduces postprandial glycemic excursions back to baseline in 60 to 90 minutes. Thus, the physiologic insulin profile is one of peaks (bolus) superimposed on a baseline (basal) amount of insulin throughout the day (Figure 3.3).

   B A goal of insulin therapy is to mimic, as nearly as possible, the physiologic profile of insulin secretion (basal/bolus). Such a pattern was difficult to achieve prior to the era of the insulin analogs.

Figure 3.3. Time Action of Physiologic (Endogenous) Insulin*

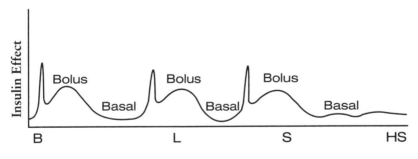

B = breakfast, L = lunch, S = supper, HS = bedtime.

"Bolus" secretion: The biphasic release of insulin in response to food intake.
"Basal" secretion: The release of insulin to counteract ongoing hormonal or other glycemic influences.

*Schematic representation only

C To optimize glycemic control, the pharmacology and pharmacokinetics of insulin require that a person receive insulin continuously (basal, also referred to as background insulin), with boluses of insulin before meals and snacks (often called mealtime insulin).

D The evolution of insulin management in the US is clearly moving from single injection therapy with intermediate-acting insulin to multiple injection therapy with human insulins.

E The time action profiles of various insulin products are shown in Table 3.3.

2 The starting dose and schedule of insulin administration is based on the type of diabetes the patient has and on the clinical assessment of insulin deficiency and suspected insulin resistance and on the patient's preferences for eating times and amounts of carbohydrate, physical activity, and waking/sleeping patterns.[24]

A Insulin requirements for individuals with type 1 diabetes or who are within 20% of ideal body weight are usually 0.5 to 1.0 unit/kg body weight/day.

  • Insulin requirements will be higher (even double) in the presence of intercurrent illness or other metabolic instability.

  • Insulin requirements will be less (0.2 to 0.6 unit/kg body weight/day) during the honeymoon phase, the period of relative remission early in the course of the disease.

B Insulin requirements for individuals with type 2 diabetes vary considerably and may range from as little as 5 to 10 units/day to as much as several hundred units per day.[25] This variability may be attributed to interpatient variability of insulin deficiency and insulin resistance.

C Insulin requirements for women with preexisting diabetes during the second and third trimesters of pregnancy gradually increase and are usually 0.9 to 1.2 units/kg body weight/day (as much as twice the total daily dosage of insulin needed before pregnancy).[26] These increases in plasma insulin are opposed by diminished responsiveness to insulin action due to placental production of contrainsulin hormones. Women with preexisting diabetes should be treated with an intensive insulin regimen. (See Chapter 4, Pregnancy With Preexisting Diabetes, in Diabetes in the Life Cycle and Research, for additional information on the use of insulin during pregnancy with preexisting diabetes.)

D Approaches to insulin therapy for gestational diabetes differ greatly. A total dose of 20 to 30 units given before breakfast is commonly used to initiate therapy.[26] The total dose is usually divided into two-thirds intermediate-acting insulin and one-third rapid-acting or short-acting insulin. For obese women, a higher starting dosage of insulin is usually necessary. The total initial dosage may be as high as 0.8 to 1.0 units/kg body weight/day.[26] (See Chapter 5, Gestational Diabetes, in Diabetes in the Life Cycle and Research, for additional information on the use of insulin in gestational diabetes.)

E Target blood glucose levels for before meals, after meals, and during sleep should be established. Setting targets with the patient (rather than for the patient) enhances patient understanding and decision-making as the person observes changes in blood glucose levels in relation to changes in food, exercise, stress, or illness.

F Subsequent adjustments in dose or timing of the insulin are based on self-monitoring of blood glucose (SMBG) and clinical signs and symptoms of hypoglycemia or hyperglycemia.

G Other parameters used to refine the insulin dose and schedule include glycosylated hemoglobin levels, achievement of weight or lipid goals, and variability of lifestyle or activities from day to day.

3 Regimens for insulin monotherapy vary as needed, to meet the needs of the individual's daily habits with regard to meals, exercise, medications, work or activity schedule, and emotional factors. Note: The following regimens assume that the patient's lifestyle includes a waking time in the morning, meals spaced consistently during the day and waking hours, with a late evening bedtime. Appropriate alterations can be made in the insulin program to accommodate a midnight or rotating work schedule or other lifestyle preferences. Combination therapy using insulin with oral glucose-lowering medications is discussed later.

A In a single daily injection regimen, insulin is administered in the morning or at bedtime in patients with type 2 diabetes (Figure 3.4A).

- **This regimen is not indicated for type 1 diabetes.**
- An intermediate-acting or a long-acting insulin is usually utilized, but could include a combined dose of a rapid-acting or short-acting and intermediate-acting insulin product.
- Bedtime administration may offer the advantage of improved fasting blood glucose control by suppressing nocturnal hepatic glucose production or increasing the basal-metabolic clearance of glucose.[27] Bedtime administration of insulin has also sometimes been associated with less weight gain.
- Single daily injections of conventional intermediate-acting or long-acting insulins may be used when doses are <30 units/day; however, for larger daily insulin doses, 2 or more doses may be needed due to an enhanced peak effect with larger doses.
- Higher single daily doses of insulin glargine may be used.
- This regimen is commonly used in type 2 patients who are also being treated with 1 or more oral agents.

B In 2-injection regimens, insulin is administered in the morning before breakfast and before the evening meal or at bedtime.

- This regimen may include only intermediate-acting insulin (Figure 3.4B), or doses of regular or rapid-acting insulins mixed with intermediate-acting insulin, or pre-mixed formulations (ie, mixtures such as Humalog Mix 75/25[28] or Novolog Mix 70/30) at 1 or both injection times. Mixed doses in the morning and before the evening meal is often called a split-mixed regimen and is considered fixed or conventional insulin therapy.
- Two-injection regimens which utilize only intermediate-acting insulins are sometimes useful in patients with type 2 diabetes but not in patients with type 1 diabetes.
- Usually two thirds of the total daily dose of insulin is given before breakfast (using a ratio of 1 part rapid-acting or short-acting insulin to 2 parts intermediate-acting insulin) and one third is given before the evening meal (using a ratio of 1:1 or 1:2, rapid-acting or short-acting to intermediate insulin) (Figure 3.5A and B).
- Daily 2-injection regimens are commonly used in patients with type 2 diabetes who are also being treated with 1 or more oral agents.

Figure 3.4. Time Action of Insulin,*
One or Two Daily Injections

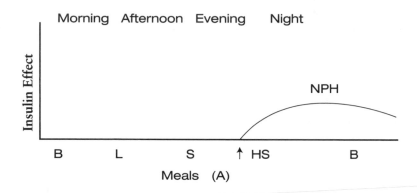

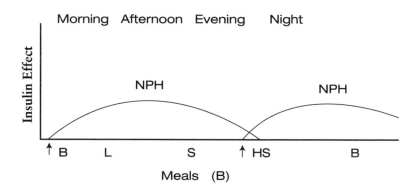

A: Idealized insulin effect provided by insulin regimen consisting of a bedtime (HS) injection of intermediate-acting insulin (NPH).

B: Idealized insulin effect provided by insulin regimen consisting of 2 daily injections of intermediate-acting insulin.

B = breakfast; L = lunch; S = supper; HS = bedtime snack; arrow = time of insulin injection, 30 minutes before meals
*Schematic representation only

Source: Reprinted with permission from Skyler.[24]

c Multiple injections of insulin (3 or more) are components of the system called flexible or intensive insulin therapy. In 3-injection regimens, insulin is administered in the morning before breakfast, before the evening meal, and at bedtime, or before each meal.

Figure 3.5. Time Action of Insulin,*
Two Split-Mixed Daily Injections

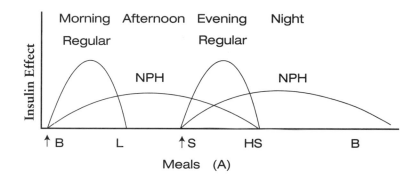

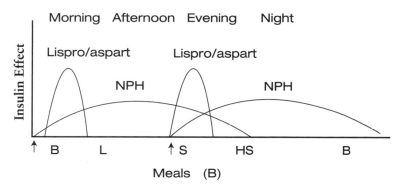

A: Idealized insulin effect provided by split-mixed insulin regimens consisting of 2 daily injections of short-acting (regular) and intermediate-acting insulin (NPH). B: Idealized insulin effect provided by insulin regimen consisting of rapid-acting insulin (lispro or aspart) and intermediate-acting insulin.

B = breakfast; L = lunch; S = supper; HS = bedtime snack; arrow = time of insulin injection, 30 minutes before meals
*Schematic representation only

Source: Reprinted with permission from Skyler.[24]

- Combination of rapid-acting or short-acting and intermediate-acting insulin before breakfast, rapid-acting or short-acting insulin alone before the evening meal, and intermediate-acting insulin at bedtime is illustrated in Figure 3.6A and B. This type of therapy reduces the risk of nocturnal (2 to 4 AM) hypoglycemia, allows better insulin coverage for early morning (5 to 10 AM) hyperglycemia from the release of cortisol and growth hormone (the dawn phenomenon), and, in some cases, may accommodate "sleeping in."

Figure 3.6. Time Action of Insulin,*
Three Multiple-Dose Daily Injections

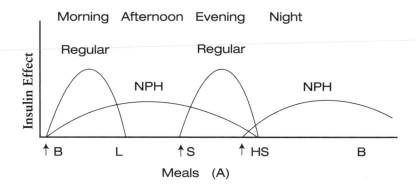

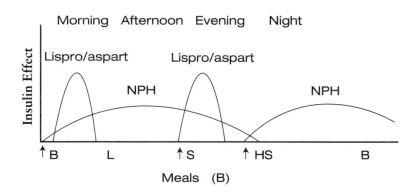

Idealized insulin effect provided by insulin regimen consisting of a morning injection of short-acting insulin and intermediate-acting insulin (NPH), a presupper injection of short-acting insulin, and a bedtime (HS) injection of intermediate-acting insulin.

A: Regular insulin

B: Rapid-acting insulin (lispro or aspart)

B = breakfast; L = lunch; S = supper; HS = bedtime snack; arrow = time of insulin injection, 30 minutes before meals
*Schematic representation only

Source: Reprinted with permission from Skyler.[24]

D In 4-injection regimens, a long-acting insulin such as insulin glargine is administered once a day and at mealtimes a rapid-acting or short-acting insulin is administered. If snacks contain more than 15 grams of carbohydrate, an injection of rapid-acting insulin may be needed before a snack. This regimen is illustrated in Figure 3.7A and B.

• The rapid-acting or short-acting insulin provides postmeal glycemic control, while the long-acting insulin dose ensures a low, steady rate of insulin throughout the day.

• This type of regimen can best duplicate normal physiologic insulin action. In patients with type 1 diabetes, physiologic replacement using basal insulin and a mealtime rapid-acting insulin, improves A1C levels and results in fewer episodes of hypoglycemia than conventional regimens.[29] This regimen can provide individuals with diabetes the flexibility in insulin doses necessary for busy and active lifestyles.

Figure 3.7. Time Action of Insulin*, Four Multiple-Dose Daily Injections

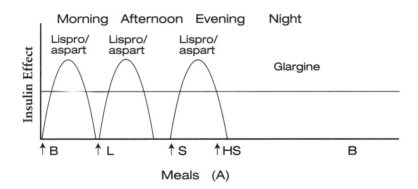

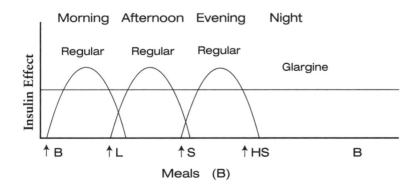

Idealized insulin effect provided by multiple-dose regimen providing basal long-acting (Glargine) insulin and preprandial injections of rapid-acting or short-acting insulin
A: Rapid-acting insulin (lispro or aspart)
B: Regular insulin

B = breakfast; L = lunch; S = supper; HS = bedtime snack; arrow = time of insulin injection, 30 minutes before meals
*Schematic representation only

Source: Reprinted with permission from Skyler.[24]

E Pump therapy is a continuous basal amount of insulin (0.5 to 1.0 U/hour) that is usually administered in addition to bolus doses given prior to meals (Figure 3.8)

Figure 3.8. Time Action of Insulin,* Pump Therapy

Pump Therapy With Regular Insulin

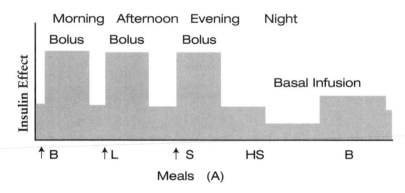

Meals   (A)

Pump Therapy With Lispro or Aspart Insulin

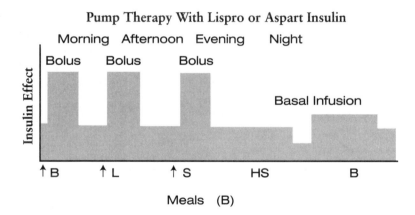

Meals   (B)

Schematic representation of idealized insulin effect provided by pump therapy with either regular insulin (A) or lispro or aspart insulin (B). The insulin pump is programmed to deliver a determined rate of insulin throughout the day; prior to each meal, the patient activates the pump to deliver a bolus of insulin to control the glycemic response to food intake.

B = breakfast; L = lunch; S = supper; HS = bedtime snack; arrow = time of insulin injection, 30 minutes before meals
*Schematic representation only

Source: Reprinted with permission from Skyler.[24]

F Insulin in persons with type 1 and type 2 diabetes
  • Larger daily doses of insulin (up to several hundred units per day) may be needed in the person with type 2 diabetes.
  • Persons with type 2 diabetes may progress from regimens requiring daily injection to more complex regimens as their disease progresses.

- Oral agents are commonly used in combination with insulin in persons with type 2 diabetes.
- Persons with type 2 diabetes may be back-titrated off of oral agents when their insulin regimens are intensified.
- Persons with type 1 diabetes will need a minimum of a 2-injection regimen (split/mixed) but will have much more flexibility if they are on a 4-injection regimen.
- Fixed-ratio premixed insulins are suboptimal in the person with type 1 diabetes.
- Thin persons with type 2 diabetes may have insulin requirements which are significantly lower than those of the obese person with type 2 diabetes.

Pulmonary Insulin

1 Recent technological advances have made it feasible to deliver insulin to the alveolar space where it is rapidly absorbed into the alveolar capillaries and disbursed throughout the systemic circulation.[30]

    A Insulin administered via the pulmonary route in human studies has a soluble, rapid-acting formulation. However, in the future a pulmonary administration of longer acting insulin may also be possible.

    B Two inhalation systems use different technology to deliver insulin via the pulmonary route.

- One system uses a fine-powdered formulation of insulin. The particle size is less than 5 μm in diameter. Particles of this size are able to reach the deep lung with slow, deep inhalation, and they then pass a single cellular layer into the circulation. Insulin from this system will be available in "blister packs" and will remain stable at room temperature for up to 2 years. The device used to deliver the insulin is the size of a mechanical flashlight.
- The other system being evaluated in the US uses a handheld inhalation device that is regulated with microprocessors to produce a consistent dose using commercially available liquid insulins. Liquid insulin is inserted into the device and the aerosol delivers particles 2 to 3 μm in size directly to the alveoli.

2 Clinical trials have demonstrated the effectiveness, safety, and acceptability of inhaled insulin in persons with type 2 and type 1 diabetes.[31,32] At this time, inhaled insulin is not yet clinically available.

Oral Glucose-Lowering Medications in the Management of Diabetes

1 Currently, there are 6 chemical classes of oral agents available in the US for the management of diabetes.

    A Sulfonylureas: first- and second-generation (insulin secretagogues)

    B Benzoic acid derivative: repaglinide (insulin secretagogue)

    C D-Phenylalanine derivative: nateglinide (insulin secretagogue)

    D Biguanide: metformin (insulin sensitizer)

    E Thiazolidinediones (glitazones): rosiglitazone and pioglitazone (insulin sensitizer)

    F Alpha-glucosidase inhibitors: acarbose, miglitol (delay glucose absorption)

2 These agents may be used as monotherapy for the treatment of type 2 diabetes, for treatment of secondary diabetes in individuals with substantial capacity for insulin production, or in combination with each other or with insulin.[33,34]

3 Oral glucose-lowering agents may be used in type 1 diabetes only as an adjunct to insulin therapy.

4 These agents are not advised for use during preconception care or pregnancy (pregestational diabetes or gestational diabetes). Only metformin has been approved for use in children.

5 Generally, monotherapy with any of these agents is associated with a reduction in A1C levels of approximately 0.5% to 1.5%.[35] This does not mean, however, that any agent will be equally efficacious for all patients; matching the pharmacologic action of a given agent with the patient's pathophysiologic basis(es) of hyperglycemia is a major determinant in therapeutic efficacy.

6 When combination therapy is utilized (2 or more oral agents or an oral agent combined with insulin), an additive effect is observed, as demonstrated by a further decrease in the A1C level.[33,34]

   A Frequently used and/or well-studied combination therapies:
- Sulfonylurea with metformin
- Sulfonylurea with insulin
- Sulfonylurea with alpha-glucosidase inhibitor
- Glitazone with insulin
- Glitazone with sulfonylurea
- Glitazone with metformin
- Nateglinide with metformin
- Metformin with insulin

   B Less frequently used and/or less well-studied or not-studied combination therapies:
- Triple combination therapy
- Metformin with alpha-glucosidase inhibitor
- Alpha-glucosidase inhibitor with insulin
- Repaglinide with metformin

Sulfonylureas

1 Available agents: Sulfonylureas can be classified as first- and second-generation oral hypoglycemic agents as shown in Table 3.5.[36] The first-generation agents are further divided into rapid-acting, intermediate-acting, and long-acting products.

2 The pharmacologic actions of sulfonylureas include

   A Hypoglycemic agent: The major pharmacologic action has the potential to reduce the blood glucose level below normal (ie, cause hypoglycemia).

   B Primary effect: Increases release of insulin from the pancreas, especially at the onset of therapy.

3 They have the following pharmacokinetics:

   A Absorption is generally rapid, fairly complete, and unaffected by food except for short-acting glipizide, which is most effective when taken on an empty stomach.

   B Metabolism and excretion of these agents varies greatly. Most sulfonylureas are metabolized in the liver to active or inactive metabolites except for chlorpropamide,

Table 3.5. Oral Glucose-Lowering Agents

Second-Generation Sulfonylureas

Drug	Glyburide (DiaBeta®, Micronase®, Glynase Prestabs®)	Glipizide (Glucotrol®/Glucotrol XL®)	Glimepiride (Amaryl®)
Recommended dose	1.25 to 10 mg single or divided dose; 0.75 to 12 mg (Glynase)	2.5 to 20 mg single or divided dose; single dose for extended release (XL)	1 to 4 mg single dose
Maximum dose	20 mg; 12 mg (Glynase)	40 mg; 20 mg (XL)	8 mg
Half-life, h	Biphasic 3.2 + 10	3.5 to 6	2.5 ± 1.2
Onset, h	1.5	1	2 to 3
Duration, h	24	12 to 16	24
Metabolism/excretion	24% absorbed; completely metabolized in liver to nonactive derivatives; excreted in urine and bile 1:1	Metabolized in liver to inactive metabolites; excreted primarily in urine	Completely metabolized via oxidative biotransformation to 2 major metabolites; metabolites excreted 60% renal and 40% hepatic elimination
Comments	50 to 200 times more potent than first generation agents; no disulfiram-like reaction; caution in elderly	Glucotrol needs to be taken on an empty stomach; no disulfiram-like reaction; caution in elderly	Take with first main meal, once-daily dosing; no disulfiram-like reaction

First-Generation Sulfonylureas

Drug	Tolbutamide (Orinase®)	Tolazamide (Tolinase®)	Chlorpropamide (Diabinese®)
Recommended dose	0.25 to 3.0 g divided doses	0.1 to 1.0 g single or divided doses	0.1 to 0.5 g single dose
Maximum dose	2 to 3 g	0.75 to 1.0 g	0.5 g
Half-life, h	5 to 7	7	24 to 48
Onset, h	1	4 to 6	1
Duration, h	6 to 12	10 to 14	72
Metabolism/excretion	Totally metabolized to inactive form; inactive metabolite excreted via kidney	Absorbed slowly; metabolite active but less potent than parent compound; excreted via kidney	Previously thought not to be metabolized, but recently found that metabolism may be quite extensive; significant percentage excreted unchanged via kidney
Comments	Most benign; least potent; short half-life; especially useful in kidney disease	Essentially no advantage over tolbutamide; said to be equally effective with less severe side effects	Longest duration; caution in elderly patients and those with kidney disease; disulfiram-like reactions may occur with alcohol; hyponatremia may be a problem

Table 3.5. Oral Glucose-Lowering Agents (cont.)

Nonsulfonylureas

Drug	Repaglinide (Prandin®)	Nateglinide (Starlix®)	Metformin (Glucophage®)	Metformin Extended Release (Glucophage XR®)
Recommended dose	0.5 to 4.0 before meals	120 mg before meals	500 to 850 mg tid or 1000 mg bid	500 to 2000 mg once daily with evening meal
Maximum dose	16 mg/day	120 mg before meals	2550 mg/day	2000 mg/day
Half-life, h	1	1.5	6	1.5 to 4.9
Onset, h	0.25 to 0.5	Within 20 minutes	Not related to dose	Not related to dose
Duration, h	2 to 3	2 to 3 hours	~6	Up to 24 h
Metabolism/excretion	Hepatic metabolism to inactive metabolites: <1% of parent drug excreted via kidney	Hepatic metabolism with approximately 16% of the parent compound excreted via the kidneys	Excreted unchanged in the urine	Excreted unchanged via the kidneys
Comments	Short duration; potential for accumulation is minimal; frequency of dosing dependent upon frequency of meals	Shortest duration; effect dependent on glucose levels; potential for accumulation is minimal; frequency of dosing dependent on frequency of meals	Do not use in patients with renal or active liver disease	Same precautions as metformin

Drug	Pioglitazone (Actos®)	Rosiglitazone (Avandia®)	Acarbose (Precose®)	Miglitol (Glyset®)
Recommended dose	15 to 45 mg daily	2 to 8 mg daily	25 to 100 mg tid	25 to 100 mg tid
Maximum dose	45 mg daily	8 mg daily	300 mg/day	100 mg tid
Half-life, h	16 to 24	103 to 158	2	2 to 3
Onset, h	Days	Days	Immediate	Rapid
Duration, h	n/a	n/a	~6	Short
Metabolism/excretion	Primarily hepatic metabolism	Extensive hepatic metabolism	<2% absorbed, metabolized in GI tract	Unchanged via kidney and feces
Comments	Monitor liver function tests every 2 months for first year, then periodically thereafter	4 mg bid more effective than 8 mg daily; monitor liver function tests every 2 months for first year, then periodically thereafter	Take with first bite of meal for maximum effectiveness	

Source: Adapted from Campbell and White.[36]

which is partially excreted unchanged in the urine. Biliary excretion is significant with glyburide and to a lesser extent with glipizide.[37]

4 Significant contraindications or precautions to sulfonylurea therapy:

A Not recommended for use during pregnancy, for breastfeeding women, or for children

B Sulfonylurea hypersensitivity

C Diabetic ketoacidosis

D Severe infection

E Surgery, trauma, or other severe metabolic stressor

F Elderly, debilitated, or malnourished patients and patients with adrenal, pituitary, or hepatic insufficiency who are particularly susceptible to the hypoglycemic effects of glucose-lowering agents

G Refer to package labeling for specific agents for additional contraindications and precautions

5 Adverse effects associated with sulfonylurea agents:

A Hypoglycemia is the most serious complication of sulfonylurea therapy. An age-related decline in renal function can contribute to susceptibility to hypoglycemia in the elderly.[38]

B Weight gain, probably secondary to increased insulin secretion

C Skin rashes in approximately 2% of users

D Gastrointestinal disturbances in approximately 5% of users

E Metabolic disorders such as a renal syndrome of inappropriate antidiuretic hormone (SIADH) can occur with the use of chlorpropamide. SIADH (ADH=vasopressin), manifested by hyponatremia and hypervolemia, occurs in about 4% of patients treated with chlorpropamide.

F Hepatic changes—abnormal hepatic function tests and icterus—are rare.

G Hematologic changes—thrombocytopenia, agranulocytosis, and hemolytic anemia—have been described with tolbutamide and chlorpropamide but appear to be very rare with second-generation sulfonylureas.

6 Treatment failure occurs when an individual is insensitive to the effects of sulfonylureas.

A Primary failure: No response to the initial sulfonylurea therapy; occurs in 20% of patients.

B Secondary failure: No or diminished response to the sulfonylurea, after an initial therapeutic response; occurs in 5% to 10% of those individuals whose blood glucose initially responded to a given agent.

7 Clinically important drug interactions with sulfonylurea agents are listed in Table 3.6.

8 The role of sulfonylurea agents in the treatment of diabetes include

A Use as monotherapy only in type 2 diabetes or secondary diabetes with substantial capacity for insulin production.

  • Typical candidate for initial sulfonylurea monotherapy: Has type 2 diabetes, without dyslipidemia, not overweight, and a fasting plasma glucose level >20 mg/dL above the target concentration.[39]

Table 3.6. Drug-Disease and Drug-Drug Interactions

Interacting Drug	Drug-Disease (Intrinsic Effect)	Drug-Drug Interaction*	Net Effect on Blood Glucose	Notes
Allopurinol	No	Sulfonylureas and Meglitinide	↓	• Decreased renal tubular secretion of chlorpropamide
Androgens/anabolic steroids	Yes	—	↓	• Mechanism unknown
Anticoagulants, oral (Dicumarol)	No	Sulfonylureas and Meglitinide	↓	• Interfere with metabolism of tolbutamide, chlorpropamide
Asparaginase I	Yes	—	↑[1] ↓[2]	1. Hyperglycemia associated with inhibition of insulin synthesis 2. Hypoglycemia reported occasionally
Aspirin	Yes[3]	Sulfonylureas[4] and Meglitinide	↓	3. Large daily doses (~4 gm/d): Increased basal and stimulated release of insulin 4. Displace sulfonylurea from protein binding; decrease urinary excretion of sulfonylurea
Beta-adrenergic antagonists	Yes	—	↑↓	• Both hypoglycemic and hyperglycemic response has been reported; may alter physiologic response to, and subjective symptoms of, hypoglycemia; may reduce hyperglycemia-induced insulin release or decrease tissue sensitivity to insulin
Calcium channel blockers	Yes	—	↑	• Hypoglycemia reported with verapamil • Hyperglycemia reported with diltiazem, nifedipine
Cholestyramine	No	TZD[5] and Acarbose[6]	↓[5] ↑[6]	5. Cholestyramine reduces absorption of coadministered drugs 6. Cholestyramine may enhance effects of acarbose; interactions may be avoided by administering cholestyramine 2 hours apart from other medications
Chloramphenicol	No	Sulfonylureas and Meglitinide	↓	• Decreased hepatic metabolism and/or protein-binding displacement of tolbutamide, chlorpropamide
Chloroquine	Yes	—	↓	• Mechanism unknown

Table 3.6. Drug-Disease and Drug-Drug Interactions (cont.)

Interacting Drug	Drug-Disease (Intrinsic Effect)	Drug-Drug Interaction*	Net Effect on Blood Glucose	Notes
Cimetidine/possible other H₂ antagonists	No	Sulfonylureas,[7] Meglitinide and Metformin[8]	↑	7. Increased absorption and/or decreased clearance of glipizide, glyburide, tolbutamide 8. Decreased renal tubular secretion of metformin; other drugs excreted via renal tubular transport *may* similarly interfere with metformin clearance
Clofibrate	Yes[9]	Sulfonylureas[10] and Meglitinide	↑	9. Intrinsic hypoglycemic effect: Mechanism unknown 10. Displace certain sulfonylureas from protein binding
Corticosteroid	Yes		↓	• Increased gluconeogenesis; transient insulin resistance
Cyclosporine	Yes		↓	—
Diazoxide	Yes		↓	• Inhibition of insulin secretion
Dicumarol	No	Sulfonylureas and Meglitinide	↑	• Inhibits hepatic metabolism of tolbutamide, chlorpropamide
Disopyramide	Yes		↓	• Most susceptible: Elderly or patients with renal or liver impairment
Diuretics	Yes		↓	—
Estrogen products	Yes		↓	• Mechanism unknown
Ethanol	Yes	Sulfonylureas[11] and Meglitinide	↓[12] ↑[13]	11. Disulfiram-like reaction may also occur, especially with chlorpropamide; not noted with second-generation sulfonylureas 12. Chronic alcohol ingestion may increase metabolism of sulfonylurea; alcohol ingestion, especially with carbohydrate-based drink (beer, mixed drink), has caloric effect. 13. Intrinsic hypoglycemic effect; impairs gluconeogenesis and increases insulin secretion; effect is potentiated if alcohol consumed without food or in fasting state

Table 3.6. Drug-Disease and Drug-Drug Interactions (cont.)

Interacting Drug	Drug-Disease (Intrinsic Effect)	Drug-Drug Interaction*	Net Effect on Blood Glucose	Notes
Fluoxetine	Yes	—	↓ ↑	• Hypoglycemia and hyperglycemia have been reported
Fluconazole	No	Sulfonylureas and Meglitinide	↓	• Reported interaction with glipizide
Gemfibrozil	Yes	—	↑	—
Glyburide	Yes	Acarbose and Miglitol[14]	↑	14. Miglitol reduces the area under the curve (AUC) and peak concentration of glyburide
Guanethidine	Yes	Sulfonylureas[15] and Meglitinide	↓ ↑[16]	15. Protein-binding displacement of certain sulfonylureas 16. Intrinsic glycemic effect
NSAID (nonsteroidal anti-inflammatory drugs)	Yes[17]	Sulfonylureas[18] and Meglitinide	↓	17. Possible intrinsic hypoglycemic effect 18. Protein-binding displacement (tolbutamide, tolazamide)
Isoniazid	Yes	—	↓	• Increases glycogenolysis
Ketoconozol	Yes	Pioglitazone	↓	• In vitro studies suggest that ketoconozal inhibits the metabolism of pioglitazone
Metformin	No	Alpha-glucosidase inhibitors	↓	• Acarbose reduces metformin bioavailability by ~35% when coadministered; separate doses to avoid
Monoamine oxidase inhibitors	Yes[19]	Sulfonylureas[20] and Meglitinide	↓	19. May stimulate insulin secretion (beta-adrenergic stimulation) or may be secondary to hepatotoxicity 20. May interfere with metabolism of sulfonylurea
Nicotinic acid (niacin)	Yes	—	↑	• Dose dependent, when lipid-lowering doses are used • Insignificant effect at vitamin supplement dose
Octreotide	Yes	—	↓ ↑	• Hypoglycemia and hyperglycemia have been reported
Oral contraceptives	Yes	Pioglitazone[21] and Rosiglitazone[22]	↓ ↑	21. Pioglitazone has not been evaluated; however, caution should be used 22. No clinically significant effect on ethinyl estradiol or norethindrone
Pancrelipase/pancreatic enzymes	Yes	—	↓	• Do not administer these agents concurrently with acarbose
Pentamidine	Yes	—	↓ ↑	• Initially, hypoglycemia; hyperglycemia may occur days or even months after initiation of therapy

Table 3.6. Drug-Disease and Drug-Drug Interactions (cont.)

Interacting Drug	Drug-Disease (Intrinsic Effect)	Drug-Drug Interaction*	Net Effect on Blood Glucose	Notes
Phenothiazines	Yes	—	↓ ↑	• Hypoglycemia observed with some phenothiazines, hyperglycemia with others
Phenytoin	Yes	—	↑	• Decreased insulin secretion
Probenecid	Yes[23]	Sulfonylureas[24] and Meglitinide	↓	23. Intrinsic glycemic effect 24. Decrease urinary excretion of chlorpropamide
Protease inhibitors	Yes	—	↑	—
Rifampin	Yes[25]	Sulfonylureas[26] and Meglitinide	↑[26] ↓[25]	25. Possible intrinsic hypoglycemic effect 26. Increased metabolism of chlorpropamide, glyburide, tolbutamide
Salicylates	Yes[27]	Sulfonylureas[28] and Meglitinide	↓	27. Large daily doses (~4 gm/d): Increase basal and stimulated release of insulin 28. Displace sulfonylurea from protein binding; decrease urinary excretion of sulfonylurea
Sulfonamides, highly protein-bound	No	Sulfonylureas and Meglitinide	↓	• Various effects upon chlorpropamide, tolbutamide kinetics: displacement from protein binding, decreased urinary excretion, and/or altered metabolism
Tacrolimus	Yes	—	↑	—
Thyroid products	Yes	—	↑	• Once euthyroid status is achieved, diabetes medications may need to be adjusted to compensate for glycemic effect of thyroid product
Urinary acidifiers	No	Sulfonylureas and Meglitinide	↓	• Interfere with chlorpropamide excretion

This listing is not intended to be inclusive. Before any new medication is initiated, consult the package labeling (insert) or other reference. In general, these interactions are based on moderate to severe clinical significance and/or possible or established documentation.

• Interactions with sulfonylureas, meglitinide, metformin, pioglitazone and rosiglitazone (both thiazolidinediones), alpha-glucosidase inhibitors, and insulin are listed.

B Therapy initiated at a low, single daily dose, with gradual increases to reach glucose goals.

- Doses of the sulfonylurea preparations are listed in Table 3.5. Although there is noticeable variance in the relative weight potency between first- and second-generation agents, the maximum hypoglycemic effect between these agents is similar.[40]
- Initial dosage may need to be adjusted for patients with hepatic or renal dysfunction.
- Use chlorpropamide with caution in patients who are elderly or have renal insufficiency because of the potential for accumulation.

C Combination therapy, or transition to insulin monotherapy, is considered when sulfonylurea therapy approaches the maximum dose. In most cases at one half the maximum dose, additional increases in dosage will not yield additional increases in therapeutic effect; this phenomenon is referred to as the "ceiling effect."

- In many patients, half the recommended maximum dose of sulfonylureas may be as effective as maximum doses.[41]

D Compared with the first-generation agents, the second-generation sulfonylureas generally interact less frequently with other agents, elicit fewer significant adverse effects, and have alternate routes of excretion.

Meglitinide Analogs

1 Available agents are

A Benzoic acid derivative: Repaglinide (Prandin®)

B D-Phenylalanine derivative: Nateglinide (Starlix®)

2 Meglitinides are hypoglycemic agents whose major pharmacologic action has the potential to reduce the blood glucose level to below normal.

Repaglinide   *Prandin*

1 Repaglinide is a nonsulfonylurea agent, but shares many of the pharmacologic actions and adverse effects of sulfonylureas. It increases release of insulin from the pancreas; the effect is glucose-dependent and diminishes at low blood glucose concentrations.

A Treatment with repaglinide is effective in well-controlled patients with type 2 diabetes[42] or in patients whose control is suboptimal.[43] Patients treated with repaglinide who missed or delayed a meal had less risk of hypoglycemia compared to treatment with longer acting sulfonylurea drugs.[42]

B Repaglinide also resulted in better glycemic control when combined with a glitazone than monotherapy with either agent alone.[44] However, addition of repaglinide to a sulfonylurea results in no additional glycemic benefit and is a therapeutic duplication.

C Repaglinide (Prandin) is available in 0.5-mg, 1-mg, and 2-mg tablets.

2 Pharmacokinetics include

A Absorption from the GI tract is rapid and complete; food slightly decreases absorption.[45]

B Protein binding and binding to serum albumin: >95%.

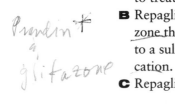
Prandin + a glitazone

C Rapid hepatic metabolism to inactive metabolites; half-life of the drug is approximately 1 hour. Less than 1% of the parent drug is excreted by the kidneys. Because of the short half-life, the potential for accumulation is minimal with normal dosing regimens.[45]

3 Significant contraindications or precautions to repaglinide therapy:
  A Not recommended for use during pregnancy, for breastfeeding women, or for children
  B Diabetic ketoacidosis
  C Severe infection
  D Surgery, trauma, or other severe metabolic stressor
  E Impaired hepatic function: Use cautiously. Titrate doses upward very gradually, with careful monitoring of blood glucose concentrations, to detect accumulation of parent drug and/or metabolites.
  F Elderly, debilitated, or malnourished patients and those with adrenal, pituitary, or hepatic insufficiency who are particularly susceptible to the hypoglycemic effects of glucose-lowering agents
  G Refer to package labeling for additional contraindications and precautions

4 Adverse effects associated with repaglinide therapy:
  A Gastrointestinal disturbances in approximately 4% of users
  B Upper respiratory infection or problems
  C Arthralgia or back pain ✳
  D Headache
  E Hypoglycemia (16% to 31%)

[handwritten margin note: Arthralgia = Joint pain]

5 Treatment failure occurs when an individual is insensitive to the effects of repaglinide.
  A Primary failure: No response to the initial repaglinide therapy.
  B Secondary failure: No or diminished response to repaglinide, after an initial therapeutic response.

6 Clinically important drug interactions with repaglinide are listed in Table 3.6.

7 Role of repaglinide in the treatment of diabetes mellitus:
  A Use as monotherapy only in type 2 diabetes or secondary diabetes in individuals with substantial capacity for insulin production.
    • Typical candidate for initial repaglinide monotherapy: Type 2 diabetes, without dyslipidemia, with or without renal failure, not overweight, and fasting plasma glucose level >20 mg/dL above the target concentration.
  C Therapy initiated at a low, single daily dose, with gradual increases to reach glucose goals.
    • Instruct patients to take 15 minutes (0 to 30 minutes) before each meal. The number of daily doses taken is determined by the number of meals eaten. The "meal-based" dosing frequency may offer advantages for patients who vary frequency of daily meals or for those who choose to eat only 2 meals a day and need to avoid persisting hypoglycemic activity between the meals.
    • Initial dose for patients not treated previously with glucose-lowering drugs or with an A1C level <8%: 0.5 mg with each meal.[43]

- Initial dosage does not need to be adjusted for patients with renal dysfunction; however, upward titration should proceed cautiously.
- Initial dose for patients previously treated with glucose-lowering drugs and with an A1C level >8%: 1 or 2 mg with each meal.
- At 1-week intervals, each preprandial dose may be doubled, up to 4 mg, until desired effect is attained.
- Maximum dose: 16 mg daily.

C Combination therapy, or transition to insulin monotherapy, is considered when repaglinide therapy approaches the maximum dose. Repaglinide is not effective in patients who have experienced primary or secondary failure on a sulfonylurea.

Nateglinide   *Starlix*

1 The major pharmacologic action of nateglinide is its potential to reduce the blood glucose level to below normal; however, its effects are linked to ambient glucose levels.[46,47] In combination with metformin, nateglinide decreased mealtime glucose excursions, whereas metformin affected fasting glucose concentrations.[48]

  A Nateglinide is a D-phenylalanine (amino acid) derivative and is a very rapid-acting oral insulin secretagogue which stimulates insulin secretion when needed (postprandial) and then allows insulin concentrations to return to normal basal concentrations.[46,47]

  B Nateglinide (Starlix®) is available in 60-mg and 120-mg tablets.

2 Pharmacokinetics include

  A The mean time to reach maximum concentrations of nateglinide after oral administration is 0.82 hours. High-fat meals reportedly result in a 12% increase in maximum concentration and a 52% reduction in the time to reach that concentration.[49]

  B Metabolism is by extensive hepatic metabolism via cytochrome P450 enzymes, primarily by CYP3A4 and CYP2C9.[50]

  C It is eliminated predominately by the kidneys (80% of the parent compound and metabolites). The average terminal half-life is an average of 1.5 hours.[50]

3 Significant contraindications or precautions to D-phenylalanine derivatives are

  A Not recommended for use during pregnancy, for breastfeeding women, or for children

  B Diabetic ketoacidosis

4 Adverse effects associated with nateglinide include

  A Mild hypoglycemia in approximately 2.4% of patients in clinical trials. There were no reports of hypoglycemia requiring third-party assistance or nocturnal hypoglycemia in the phase III trials (2400 patients).

  B Dizziness in approximately 3.6% of users.

  C Weight gain of <1 kg from baseline; this is attenuated with the concomitant use of metformin.[48]

5 No clinically important drug interactions with nateglinide have been identified to date.

6 Role of nateglinide in the treatment of diabetes mellitus:

A To be used as monotherapy in patients with type 2 diabetes with a capacity for insulin production whose hyperglycemia cannot be adequately controlled by nutrition therapy and physical activity and who have not been treated long-term with other oral glucose-lowering agents. The usual initial and maintenance dose of nateglinide is 120 mg taken just before (1 to 30 minutes) meals. Titration of dose is not usually necessary. The 60-mg dose may be used in patients who are near their A1C goal.

B Combination oral therapy, or transition to insulin monotherapy, may be considered when nateglinide therapy is ineffective as monotherapy. The addition of nateglinide to a sulfonylurea results in no additional benefit and is therefore not recommended. Nateglinide is efficacious when used in combination with metformin. The usual initial and maintenance dose of nateglinide when used in combination with metformin is 120 mg taken just before (1 to 30 minutes) meals. Titration of dose is not usually necessary. The 60-mg dose may be used in patients who are near their A1C goal.

C Nateglinide is not effective in patients who have experienced primary or secondary failure on a sulfonylurea.

D Dose adjustment is not needed in the elderly, in patients with mild to severe renal insufficiency, or in patients with mild hepatic insufficiency.

Biguanides

1 Available agents include

A Metformin (Glucophage®) in 500-mg, 850-mg, and 1000-mg dosage units

B Metformin (Glucophage XR®) in 500-mg dosage unit

C Glyburide/metformin (Glucovance®) in 1.25/250-mg, 2.5/500-mg, and 5/500-mg dosage units.

D Metformin/glipizide (Metaglip®) in 2.5 mg of glipizide combined with 250 mg of metformin; 2.5 mg/500 mg and 5 mg glipizide with 500 mg metformin.

E Metformin/rosiglitazone (Avandamet®) in 1 mg rosiglitazone with 500 mg of metformin; 2 mg/500 mg and 4 mg rosiglitazone with 500-mg of metformin.

F Fixed-dose combinations may not match with the specific dose needs of an individual patient. For example, most patients using metformin require 2 000 mg total daily dose.

2 Biguanides have the following pharmacologic actions:

A They are not a hypoglycemic agent because their major pharmacologic action does not increase insulin secretion and thus does not increase the risk of hypoglycemia. These agents have proven to be an effective antihyperglycemic agent or an insulin sensitizer.[51-55]

- Frequently, there is a slight (2-kg to 5-kg) weight loss seen with metformin therapy; however, the actual cause of weight loss is not known.

B Primary effects include

- Reduces hepatic glucose production primarily by reduction in glycogenolysis.[56]
- Enhances insulin-stimulated glucose transport in adipose tissue and skeletal muscle, thus reversing or partially reversing insulin resistance.[51]

C Decreases intestinal absorption of glucose (minor effect).

D Causes a reduction in triglyceride concentrations of approximately 16%, in LDL cholesterol by approximately 8%, and in total cholesterol by approximately 5% and is associated with an increase in HDL cholesterol by approximately 2%.[51,53]

3 Pharmacokinetics include

  A The oral bioavailability is 50% to 60%. Food decreases the extent of bioavailability and slightly delays the absorption of metformin.

  B Does not bind to liver or plasma proteins.

  C Major excretion is by the kidneys, largely unchanged, through an active tubular process.

4 Significant contraindications or precautions to metformin therapy:

  A Generally not indicated during pregnancy or for breastfeeding women

  B Renal dysfunction with serum creatinine levels >1.5 mg/dL in males or >1.4 mg/dL in females. Because metformin is excreted renally by the kidneys, it can accumulate in patients with renal dysfunction.

  C Hepatic dysfunction (lactate metabolism is carried out in the liver)

  D Acute or chronic lactic acidosis

  E History of alcoholism or binge ingestion of alcohol

  F Metformin should be temporarily withheld in any situation which would predispose the individual to acute renal dysfunction or tissue hypoperfusion, including

  • Cardiovascular collapse

  • Acute myocardial infarction

  • Acute exacerbation of congestive heart failure

  • Use of iodinated contrast media

  • Major surgical procedure

  G Refer to package labeling for additional contraindications and precautions[57,58]

5 Adverse effects associated with metformin therapy:

  A Metformin monotherapy is not associated with hypoglycemia.

  • Patients using combination therapy (metformin with insulin or metformin with sulfonylureas [eg, Glucovance or Metaglip]) may experience hypoglycemia secondary to the hypoglycemic agent.

  B Gastrointestinal effects in up to 30% of users: Abdominal bloating, nausea, cramping, feeling of fullness, diarrhea.[59]

  • Usually self-limiting, transient (7 to 14 days), and can be minimized by taking the medication with food, starting with a low dose, and slow upward titration of dosage.

  C Miscellaneous: Agitation, sweating, headache, and metallic taste.

  D Associated with a reduction in vitamin B_{12} levels, although no cases of anemia have been reported in the US.

  E Lactic acidosis can occur with the administration of metformin but is rare (0.03 cases per 1000 patient years). Lactic acidosis is primarily associated with its use in patients who have contraindications to the drug or in cases of overdose.[60]

6 Clinically important drug interactions with metformin are listed in Table 3.6.

7 Role of metformin in the treatment of diabetes mellitus:

  A Use as monotherapy only in type 2 diabetes or secondary diabetes with substantial capacity for insulin production.

  • Typical candidate for initial metformin monotherapy: Type 2 diabetes, with dyslipidemia, with obesity or genetic factors favoring insulin resistance, and fasting plasma glucose level >20 mg/dL above the target concentration.[23]

B Therapy initiated at a low dose, with gradual increases to obtain desired control.
- Usual initial dose: Standard formulation—500 mg or 850 mg qd or 500 mg bid, with doses taken prior to a meal. Glucophage XR formulation—500 mg with the evening meal.[57]
- Titrate dose upward as tolerated (to GI effects) to reach glucose goals. Increases usually occur at 14-day intervals for the standard formulation and at 7-day intervals for the XR formulation.[57]
- Maximum daily dose: Standard formulation—2550 mg daily (850 mg tid) (note, however, that the greatest reduction in fasting plasma glucose is seen at 2000 mg/day (1000 mg bid). XR formulation—2000 mg daily in 1 or 2 doses.
- In children, start with 250 mg twice daily and titrate the dose slowly until treatment objectives are achieved.

C Combination therapy, or transition to insulin monotherapy, is considered when metformin therapy approaches the maximum dose.[61]

Thiazolidinediones (TZDs)

1 Available agents are
- **A** Pioglitazone (Actos) available in 15-mg, 30-mg, and 45-mg tablets
- **B** Rosiglitazone (Avandia) available in 2-mg, 4-mg, and 8-mg tablets
- **C** Fixed-dose combination (Avandamet®) available in 1 mg/500 mg, 2 mg/500 mg and 4 mg/500 mg. Pioglitazone can be given with either metformin or with sulfonylureas.

2 TZDs have the following pharmacologic actions:
- **A** TZDs are not hypoglycemic agents; the major pharmacologic action does not increase insulin secretion and thus does not increase the risk of hypoglycemia. These agents may best be described as antihyperglycemic agents or insulin sensitizers. These drugs probably reduce insulin resistance and improve blood glucose levels via the stimulation of peroxisome-proliferator-activated receptor-gamma (PPAR-y).[62,63]

- **B** They enhance insulin action at the receptor and postreceptor level in hepatic and peripheral tissues, thus reversing or partially reversing insulin resistance.

3 Pharmacokinetics are
- **A** Both of these medications are well absorbed without regard to meals. Pioglitazone is always given once daily whereas rosiglitazone may need to be given twice daily in many persons with type 2 diabetes.
- **B** Both medications are extensively bound (>99%) to serum albumin.
- **C** Both drugs are extensively metabolized in the liver.
- **D** Metabolites and parent compounds are eliminated primarily in the feces with minor amounts in the urine.

4 Significant contraindications or precautions to thiazolidinedione therapy include
- **A** Generally not indicated during pregnancy, for breastfeeding women, or for children.
- **B** TZDs may cause fluid retention, which can exacerbate or lead to heart failure. Patients should be observed for signs and symptoms of heart failure.
- **C** TZDs should be used with caution in patients with hepatic dysfunction. Rare cases of severe idiosyncratic hepatocellular injury have occurred with troglitazone. Serum transaminase levels should be monitored every 2 months during the first year of therapy and then periodically thereafter.

D In premenopausal anovulatory women with insulin resistance, thiazolidinedione therapy may result in resumption of ovulation, with a subsequent risk of pregnancy.

E TZDs are contraindicated in patients with NYHA class III and IV failure since their safety in this population has not been studied.

F Refer to package labeling for additional contraindications and precautions.[64,65]

5 Adverse effects associated with thiazolidinedione therapy are

A Elevated hepatic enzymes. Rare cases of severe idiosyncratic hepatocellular injury occurred with troglitazone. It is not clear if this effect is a class effect or if it was specific to troglitazone. While the hepatic injury associated with troglitazone was generally reversible, rare cases of hepatic failure, including death, were reported, which prompted removal of this drug from the market.[63]

B Plasma volume expansion, resulting in small reductions in hemoglobin, hematocrit, and neutrophil counts.

C Weight gain is probably a class effect of the TZDs.

D Both TZDs have been associated with mild to moderate edema.[63]

E Other considerations include incidences similar to that of placebo: GI discomfort, headache, pharyngitis.

F Small increases in HDL and LDL cholesterol may occur with rosiglitazone while reductions in triglycerides and elevations of HDL have been reported with pioglitazone. The clinical significance of the lipid effects of this class or drugs is unclear at this time.

6 Clinically important drug interactions with thiazolidinediones are listed in Table 3.6

A Rosiglitazone is metabolized by CYP2C9 and CYP2C8. In vitro studies have suggested that inhibition of these isoenzymes by rosiglitazone does not occur at concentrations usually encountered clinically. The isoenzyme CYP3A4, which is responsible for the metabolism of several drugs including erythromycin, calcium channel blockers, corticosteroids, and HMG-CoA reductase inhibitors, is also partially responsible for the metabolism of pioglitazone. However, specific studies evaluating these agents have not been carried out. Therefore, the possibility of altered safety or efficacy should be considered when using these agents with pioglitazone.

7 Role of TZDs in the treatment of diabetes mellitus:

A Use as monotherapy only in type 2 diabetes or secondary diabetes with substantial capacity for insulin production.[66,67]

- Typical candidate for initial TZD monotherapy: Type 2 diabetes, obesity or genetic factors favoring insulin resistance, and fasting plasma glucose level >20 mg/dL above the target concentration.

B Therapy initiated at a low dose, with gradual increases to reach plasma glucose goals. Instruct patients to take with main meal of day for maximum absorption.

- Usual initial dose: Rosiglitazone—2 mg bid or 4 mg qd; pioglitazone—15 to 30 mg qd.
- Titrate dose upward until desired therapeutic effect is reached. Dose increases should not occur less often than 4 weeks.
- Maximum recommended daily dose for rosiglitazone is 4 mg bid or 8 mg qd and for pioglitazone, 45 mg qd.

C Combination therapy is considered when TZDs are ineffective at maximum dose.

Alpha-Glucosidase Inhibitors

1 Available agents are

  A Acarbose (Precose®) available in 25-mg, 50-mg, and 100-mg tablets

  B Miglitol (Glyset®) available in 25-mg, 50-mg, and 100-mg tablets

2 Pharmacologic actions include

  A They are not hypoglycemic agents; the major pharmacologic action does not increase insulin secretion and thus does not increase the risk of hypoglycemia. This agent may best be described as an antihyperglycemic agent.

  B They inhibit alpha-glucosidase enzymes in the brush border of the small intestine[68] and pancreatic alpha-amylase,[69] leading to a reduction in carbohydrate-mediated postprandial blood glucose elevation.

  • Alpha-glucosidase enzymes (maltase, isomaltase, glucoamylase, and sucrase) hydrolyze oligosaccharides, trisaccharides, and disaccharides to glucose and other monosaccharides in the brush border of the small intestine.

  • Alpha-amylase enzymes hydrolyze complex starches to oligosaccharides in the lumen of the small intestine.

  • Inhibition of these enzyme systems reduces the rate of digestion of starches and the subsequent absorption of glucose.

3 Pharmacokinetics are

  A Oral bioavailability: Acarbose has a negligible absorption of unchanged drug, about 35% of the intestinal metabolites of acarbose are absorbed. Miglitol is almost completely absorbed.

  B Acarbose is metabolized within the GI tract by intestinal bacteria and by digestive enzymes. Excretion of absorbed acarbose and its metabolites is by the kidneys, Miglitol is excreted unchanged in the urine with any unabsorbed drug being eliminated in the feces.

  C Acarbose plasma levels are elevated in patients with creatinine clearance (CrCl) <25 mL/min, suggesting accumulation of acarbose. However, dosage adjustment in this setting is not feasible because acarbose acts locally.

4 Significant contraindications or precautions to alpha-glucosidase inhibitor therapy:

  A Generally not indicated during pregnancy, for breastfeeding women, or for children

  B Inflammatory bowel disease, colonic ulceration, or obstructive bowel disorders; chronic intestinal disorders of digestion or absorption; or any medical condition that might deteriorate with increased intestinal gas formation[69]

  C Acarbose is contraindicated in patients with cirrhosis of the liver

  D Acarbose is not recommended in patients with serum creatinine levels >2.0 mg/dL since studies have suggested increases in drug or metabolite plasma concentrations with renal dysfunction, and long-term studies have not been carried out in this population.[35] Neither agent is recommended in patients with creatinine clearances of <25 mL/min.[69]

5 Adverse effects associated with alpha-glucosidase inhibitor therapy:

  A Alpha-glucosidase inhibitor monotherapy is not associated with hypoglycemia.[69]

- Patients using combination therapy (alpha-glucosidase inhibitor with insulin or alpha-glucosidase inhibitor with sulfonylureas) may experience hypoglycemia secondary to the insulin or sulfonylurea.
- Hypoglycemia in this situation can be managed with oral glucose (if the patient is conscious) or intravenous glucose or glucagon (if the patient is unconscious). Because these drugs blunt the digestion of complex sugars to glucose, oral sugar sources other than glucose or lactose (eg, glucose tablets, milk) are unsuitable for rapid correction of hypoglycemia.[69]

B Gastrointestinal effects, occurring primarily at initiation of therapy or when dosage is increased, are diarrhea, abdominal pain, and flatulence (in one third to two thirds of patients).
- Usually self-limiting, transient, and can be minimized by starting with a low dose and slow upward titration of dosage. Redistribution of the inhibited enzymes usually occurs after several weeks of therapy resulting in a mitigation of adverse effects.[69]

C Elevation of serum transaminases (AST or ALT) has been observed in clinical trials in patients taking acarbose at a dose of 200 to 300 mg tid. Elevations in hepatic enzymes have only been observed in patients taking greater than 100 mg tid.[35]

6 Clinically important drug interactions with alpha-glucosidase inhibitors are listed in Table 3.6.

7 Role of alpha-glucosidase inhibitors in the treatment of diabetes mellitus:
  A Use as monotherapy only in type 2 diabetes or secondary diabetes with substantial capacity for insulin production.[70]
  - Typical candidate for initial alpha-glucosidase inhibitor monotherapy: Type 2 diabetes, with dyslipidemia or obesity, and symptoms suggesting—or blood glucose profile demonstrating—significant postprandial hyperglycemia.
  - Individuals demonstrating significant premeal hyperglycemia without a significant premeal-to-postmeal glucose rise would not be expected to respond optimally to alpha-glucosidase inhibitor monotherapy.
  B Therapy initiated at a low dose to minimize GI adverse effects, with gradual increases to reach glucose goals.
  - The usual initial dose is 25 mg qd. Instruct patients to take with the first bite of the meal for the drug to be effective.
  - Titrate dose upward as patient tolerance (to GI effects) allows, until desired therapeutic effect is reached.[71] The following titrated doses can be used:
  Acarbose
    — 25 mg qd for 2 weeks
    — 25 mg bid for 1 to 2 weeks
    — 25 mg tid for 4 to 8 weeks
    — Increase to 50 mg tid for 4 to 8 weeks
    — Maintenance dose: 50 or 100 mg tid (50 mg tid if patient <60 kg)
    — Maximum daily dose: 50 mg tid if patient <60 kg; 100 mg tid if patient >60 kg
  Miglitol
    — 25 mg tid initially for 4 to 8 weeks
    — 50 mg tid for 3 months
    — Increase to 100 mg tid, if tolerated and if needed

C Combination therapy, or transition to insulin, should be considered when the maximum dose is reached.

Amylin Agonists

1 Amylin is a hormone secreted by the pancreatic beta cells in response to hyperglycemia; its secretion parallels that of insulin. The main mechanism of amylin is to inhibit gastric emptying and, to a lesser extent, suppression of glucagon secretion.[72]

2 Pramlintide acetate (SYMLIN™) is a synthetic version of human amylin. Amylin Pharmaceuticals has submitted the drug to the FDA for approval to market SYMLIN as an adjunctive therapy to insulin. It must be injected and currently can not be combined with insulin.

3 Clinical trials in patients with type 1 and type 2 diabetes indicate that pramlintide improves postprandial hyperglycemia and modestly improves A1C levels.[73,74] It is expected that Symlin will be FDA approved to be given by injection in individuals who also use insulin to assist in decreasing A1C levels.

Use of Glucagon Injection for Severe Hypoglycemia

1 The available agent is glucagon, which must be given by injection: 1 mg lyophilized powder in a single-dose vial with 1 ml diluent contained in a disposable syringe/needle to allow rapid reconstitution of the powder and administration of the dissolved drug. This is the Glucagon Emergency Kit.
  A The dose is mixed by adding the diluent from the prefilled syringe in the emergency kit to the contents of the vial.
  B A 10-mg glucagon injection is commercially available, but is not intended for use as a glucose elevating agent; this product is used as a diagnostic aid in gastrointestinal examinations.

2 Pharmacologic actions are
  A The primary effects are to raise blood glucose levels by accelerating hepatic glycogenolysis and stimulating hepatic gluconeogenesis.
  B Other effects are to stimulate catecholamine and insulin release.
  C Glucagon is effective if adequate hepatic glycogen (stored glucose) is available, but may not be beneficial in patients with inadequate glycogen stores (eg, patients with alcoholic hepatic disease, starvation, adrenal insufficiency, or chronic hypoglycemia).

3 Pharmacokinetics include
  A The bioavailability is 100% and it may be injected intramuscularly, intravenously, or subcutaneously.
  B It is degraded in the liver, kidney, and plasma. The plasma half-life is 3 to 6 minutes.

4 Significant contraindications or precautions for glucagon:
  A Insulinoma: Marked hypoglycemia may occur following the initial increase in blood glucose

B Pheochromocytoma: Marked hypertension may occur

C Safety during pregnancy or for breastfeeding women is not known

D Refer to package labeling for additional contraindications and precautions

5 Adverse effects associated with glucagon use include

A Nausea, vomiting (most common adverse effect)

B Generalized allergic reactions including urticaria, respiratory distress, and hypotension

6 Clinically important drug interactions with glucagon:

A Oral anticoagulants: Hypoprothrombinemic effects may be increased, possibly with bleeding, which may occur after several days. Appears to be dose-related, and occurs minimally with a single 1-mg dose for hypoglycemia.

7 Role of glucagon injection in diabetes mellitus:

A Indicated for the treatment of severe hypoglycemia, in situations when the individual requires assistance from another person (see Chapter 8, Hypoglycemia, in Diabetes Management Therapies, for more information). Situations in which glucagon is indicated:

- Patient is unconscious or uncooperative
- Patient cannot take oral fluids
- Emergency staff are not available to treat the hypoglycemia with an injection of 50% dextrose; patients with a significant component of hypoglycemic unawareness.
- If a hospitalized patient develops severe hypoglycemia, is unconscious, and an intravenous line is not running, glucagon may be administered until intravenous access can be obtained

B Dosage is based upon patient's age and clinical condition:

- Adults and children over 5 or 6 years of age (>20 kg): 1 mg SC or IM
- Children under 5 years of age (<20 kg): 0.5 mg SC or IM
- Infants: Should probably be given 0.25 mg SC or IM

C Blood glucose response usually occurs in 5 to 20 minutes. If response is insufficient, an additional dose may be needed.

- Liquids containing glucose are needed when the patient becomes conscious to restore hepatic glycogen stores and to prevent secondary hypoglycemia.
- Instruct patients to eat a snack containing carbohydrate when nausea subsides. The snack may need to be repeated because glycogen reserves can take 8 to 12 hours to be replenished.

D Protect patients from injury or aspiration if convulsions occur. A common adverse effect of glucagon is nausea and possibly vomiting as the patient returns to consciousness.

Use of Other Drugs in Diabetes Care

1 A variety of drugs other than antihyperglycemic agents are commonly used in the care of people with diabetes (see Chapter 4, Pharmacotherapy for Hypertension and Dyslipidemia, in Diabetes Management Therapies).

A Medications are used for the treatment or prevention of the following complications of diabetes:

- Autonomic neuropathy
- Cardiovascular disease
- Problems of peripheral circulation
- Distal symmetric polyneuropathy
- Hyperlipidemia
- Nephropathy
- Periodontal disease
- Circulation abnormalities

B Medications are used for the treatment of the following conditions or diseases that occur frequently in people with diabetes:
- Hypertension
- Glaucoma
- Cataracts
- Hypothyroidism
- Infections (eg, vaginitis)
- Certain forms of joint disease

C Medications are used for the treatment of the following conditions or diseases that are unrelated to the diabetes:
- Colds
- Coughs
- Birth control/hormone replacement therapy
- Smoking cessation
- Arthritis
- Depression/anxiety
- Sunburn
- Acid indigestion
- Allergies
- Contact dermatitis
- Others

2 Because of the number of drugs that may be used for various concurrent problems, it is important to examine the overall potential consequences when 1 or more drugs are added to or removed from the drug regimen for a person with diabetes (for more information, see chapters on complications in Diabetes and Complications).

Potential Effects of Other Drugs

1 Certain drugs have an effect on blood glucose levels. The following types of interactions can occur.

A A drug-disease or pharmacodynamic interaction is defined as a desirable or undesirable alteration of blood glucose level by a drug prescribed for a purpose other than its glycemic effect (Table 3.6). This interaction has an intrinsic physiologic effect.

B A drug-drug interaction is defined as a desirable or undesirable effect of a drug on the efficacy or toxicity of the oral glucose-lowering drug(s) (Table 3.6).

c A drug-food interaction is defined as a desirable or undesirable effect of food on the efficacy or toxicity of the hypoglycemic or oral glucose-lowering drugs(s) (Table 3.7).

Table 3.7. Drug-Food Interactions of Diabetes Medications

Sulfonylurea Agents	• Administration of most sulfonylurea agents with food only slightly alters absorption characteristics. • Patients are often advised to take these agents ½ to 1 hour prior to eating to allow the onset of action to occur more closely with the postprandial glucose rise. • When sulfonylurea-induced gastric distress occurs, patients may be advised to take these agents with food to minimize stomach upset. • Glipizide (short-acting) is the only sulfonylurea specifically recommended to be taken on an empty stomach.
Repaglinide *Nateglinide*	• Food only slightly affects absorption; however, patients are advised to take repaglinide 15 minutes before eating so that the rapid action of the drug matches the timing of glucose rise following the meal.
Metformin	• Food decreases the extent of and slightly delays the absorption of metformin. • Taking metformin with or after food is usually advised to reduce stomach upset.
Thiazolidinediones	• No significant interaction.
Acarbose *Miglitol*	• No reported food interactions. • Must be taken with the meal ("first bite of the meal") to attain optimal therapeutic effect.
Insulin	• Not applicable because insulin must be taken by injection. • Timing of injection prior to eating may be an important factor in postprandial glycemic control. • Lispro or aspart insulin is injected no more than 5 to 15 minutes prior to eating to avoid preprandial hypoglycemia.

2 Certain drugs have an effect on the complications of diabetes (Table 3.8).

Table 3.8. Adverse Drug Effects Related to Diabetes

Specific Drugs or Drug Classes (see Table 3.6 for blood glucose effects)

Drugs within a drug class often share adverse effects, although to varying degrees. Certain drug classes warrant particular attention to effects that may have an impact upon complications or comorbidity conditions for specific patients.

Alpha-1 antagonists (prazosin, terazosin, doxazosin)	Impotence; constipation (aggravates chronic constipation from autonomic neuropathy); diarrhea (aggravates diarrhea from autonomic neuropathy); dizziness, headache, weakness (may be confused for signs of hypoglycemia); blurred vision, drowsiness, xerostomia (may be confused for signs of hyperglycemia)
Antihistamines, anticholinergic	Contraindicated in neurogenic bladder (may occur in diabetic autonomic neuropathy); blurred vision; constipation, abdominal pain
Antihypertensives in general	Impaired sexual function; constipation (selected agents); orthostatic hypotension may occur in diabetic autonomic neuropathy
Anti-inflammatory agents	Nonsteroidal: Renal effects; hypertensive effects Steroidal: Osteoporosis; hypertension; weight gain/increase in appetite may worsen diabetes control; diminished wound healing; thin fragile skin; glaucoma
ß-blockers	Mask signs/symptoms of hypoglycemia; impaired sexual function; reduced peripheral circulation and cold extremities
Calcium channel blockers	Constipation (selected agents aggravate chronic constipation from autonomic neuropathy); orthostatic hypotension (aggravate diabetes-related orthostatic hypotension); glycemic effects (selected agents)
Chemotherapeutic agents	Nausea, vomiting, stomatitis, anorexia, alterations in taste (makes diabetes nutrition therapy difficult or inconsistent); diarrhea
Clonidine	Urinary retention; constipation; diminished sexual function; orthostatic hypotension; nocturia, lethargy, xerostomia, drowsiness (may be confused for signs of hyperglycemia)
Codeine (as cough suppressant) or opiate analgesics	Constipation (aggravate chronic constipation from autonomic neuropathy)
Diuretics	Changes in lipid profile; total body potassium loss (unless potassium-sparing diuretic or formulation); diuresis mimics polyuria/nocturia which may interfere with use of these signs as a warning sign of hyperglycemia; diminished effectiveness in decreasing renal function; aggravate diabetes-related orthostatic hypotension
Sorbitol, as compounding ingredient and/or sweetening agent	Loose stools, diarrhea, flatulence (aggravate diarrhea from autonomic neuropathy)
Sympathomimetics	Hypertension; peripheral vasoconstriction

A A complication or comorbid condition may be worsened when certain drugs are added to or removed from the overall diabetes treatment program.

B Potential effects can be best anticipated by carefully examining the pharmacologic action or adverse effects of a drug that are described in the package labeling (insert) or other therapeutic reference.

C The following are examples of drugs that have an effect on the complications of diabetes.

- An antacid with an adverse effect of constipation may aggravate constipation associated with diabetic autonomic neuropathy.
- An oral decongestant with vasoconstriction adverse effects may aggravate peripheral vascular problems such as intermittent claudication.
- An antihypertension medication with an adverse effect of impotence may worsen diabetes-related sexual dysfunction.

3 Certain drug adverse effects have an impact on diabetes self-management.

A Patients are taught to be attentive to particular signs and symptoms that may indicate impending hypoglycemia or hyperglycemia. In addition, certain procedures and aspects of diabetes care require the patient to be alert, coordinated, and capable of making self-management decisions. A drug that mimics a patient's usual warning signs of hypoglycemia or hyperglycemia, or one that impairs a patient's ability to perform necessary self-care tasks, may adversely affect glycemic control.

- Frequent urination or nocturia from initiation of diuretic therapy may be mistakenly interpreted as a symptom of hyperglycemia.
- Central nervous system adverse effects such as dizziness, headache, fatigue, weakness, loss of energy, or tingling of extremities may be mistaken for symptoms of hypoglycemia.
- Adverse effects of drowsiness, tiredness, lethargy, or depression could be mistaken for symptoms of hyperglycemia or may affect diabetes control by interfering with the patient's ability or desire to exercise or carry out other self-management activities.
- Blurred vision as an adverse effect of another agent may lead to a dosing error in insulin administration.
- Drug-induced night blindness may aggravate night blindness from previous retinal photocoagulation or autonomic neuropathy.

4 The package labeling (insert) or product information usually provides a list of adverse effects by body system affected and in the order of frequency of occurrence. Certain adverse effects should arouse suspicions or raise questions about the potential for drug-related problems in patients with diabetes (Table 3.9).

Significance of Drug-Related Effects

1 Some problems have major clinical significance, which means an event is relatively well-documented (established documentation) and has the potential of being harmful to the patient.

2 Some problems have moderate clinical significance, which means more documentation is needed (possible documentation) and/or the potential harm to the patient is less.

3 Some problems have minor clinical significance, which means an event may occur but may be less significant because of poor documentation, minimal potential harm to the patient, or low incidence of the interaction.

Table 3.9. Adverse Effects of Drugs on Body Systems

Gastrointestinal (GI)	• Nausea, vomiting, constipation, diarrhea, bloating, gas: Additive problem with various forms of autonomic neuropathy • Dry mouth: Could be mistakenly interpreted as a symptom of hyperglycemia
Genitourinary (GU)	• Impotence, failure to ejaculate, reduced libido: Additive problem with diabetes-related impotence
Renal	• Glycosuria listed as an adverse effect: Carefully read the package insert to ascertain if this adverse effect refers to a lowered threshold for glucose or an indication of hyperglycemia • Frequent urination, nocturia, polyuria: Could be mistakenly interpreted as a symptom of hyperglycemia; could lead to hypovolemia and problems with orthostatic hypotension • Elevations of creatinine or BUN: May pose problems in patient predisposed to renal dysfunction
Central nervous system (CNS)	• Dizziness: Additive problem with orthostatic hypotension, hypoglycemia • Headache, fatigue, weakness, loss of energy, blurred vision, tingling of extremities: Could be mistakenly interpreted as symptom of hypoglycemia • Drowsiness, tiredness, lethargy, depression: Could be mistaken for symptom of hyperglycemia; could affect diabetes control by interfering with ability and desire to exercise • Numbness/tingling of extremities, paresthesias, neuropathy: Additive problem with diabetes-related neuropathy
Dermatologic	• Pruritus, rash, dry skin: Aggravate the dry skin and itching associated with peripheral neuropathy and venostasis
Ophthalmic	• Night blindness: May aggravate night blindness resulting from retinal photocoagulation
General	• Elevated cholesterol or triglyceride levels: May pose problems in patient predisposed to lipid disorders • Hypoglycemia, hyperglycemia: May require adjustment of diabetes treatment plan • Peripheral edema: Aggravate problems in patient with impaired peripheral circulation and venous return

4 It is important to note that the classification of "major" versus "minor" significance is not solely a matter of the degree of documentation. The individual patient characteristics must be considered in making this determination. For example, in the following situations the first would represent a problem of minor significance whereas the second could be major.

  A A 37-year-old man with type 2 diabetes, who is relatively healthy otherwise, has been taking an oral hypoglycemic agent for the past 2 years. Today his provider has added a diuretic. If this individual experiences hypoglycemia during the first few days of diuretic therapy, it is unlikely that the potential diuresis, hypovolemia, or dizziness from the diuretic would exaggerate the dizziness/weakness of hypoglycemia to a dangerous state.

  B An 87-year-old widow with type 2 diabetes, osteoporosis, sporadic nutrition and fluid ingestion, and occasional disequilibrium has been taking an oral hypoglycemic agent for the past 2 years. She lives alone. Today her provider has added a diuretic. If this patient experiences hypoglycemia at the same time she experiences dizziness from the diuretic, the drug-related problem may have major significance: a fall, broken hip, and no one in the house to render assistance.

Caveats to Drug Interactions and Drug-Related Problems

1 Drug interactions may be beneficial or detrimental. For example, using a drug with intrinsic hypoglycemic activity may be detrimental for a patient with hypoglycemia unawareness (drug-disease interaction and an effect on a diabetes complication).

2 Drug interactions are not necessarily predictable because they do not always happen to all people.

3 Drug interactions are usually dose dependent.

4 A specific combination of interacting drugs can have a different interaction profile depending on the order in which the drugs are initiated.

  A Adding a diuretic to an established dose of sulfonylurea can reasonably be expected to raise the blood glucose level, thus lessening the apparent effectiveness of the sulfonylurea.

  B When a sulfonylurea is added to an established dose of a diuretic, the blood glucose would not be expected to rise further.

5 The severity of an interaction is different for different people (variable responses) depending on the following individual variables:

  A Current metabolic control

  B Self-monitoring practices

  C Lability/stability of complications and concurrent conditions

  D Duration/dosage of proposed therapy

  E Potential for administration error

Ways to Help Prevent, Minimize, or Prepare for Potential Drug-Related Problems

1 Inform the patient if a drug-related problem is likely to occur and the usual signs and symptoms to watch for.

2 If possible, inform the patient as to when the interaction/drug problem would be expected to occur. Some interactions may occur after the first dose while others may not occur until the problem drug has reached steady state or has accumulated in the body.

3 Devise a strategy by which the patient can determine if the anticipated problem has occurred.

A Recommend blood glucose monitoring at specific times of day or at more frequent intervals until the patient's response to the drug is established.

B Stress the importance of additional monitoring or observation.

4 Provide an action plan for the patient to use if the suspected drug-related problem has occurred. This action plan is based on the drug and the severity of the interaction/problem.

A For problems of major clinical significance, instruct the patient to notify the provider as soon as possible. Specify whether the drug should be stopped or continued while attempting to reach the health professional.

B For problems of moderate clinical significance, the problem may be resolved by making appropriate compensations. A member of the healthcare team may need to be contacted for assistance.

C For problems of minor clinical significance, the problem is primarily an inconvenience or is self-limiting and does not generally require any specific action.

5 Prepare a backup plan should problems arise. Determine alternatives the patient might use if the drug problem occurs.

Self-Review Questions

1 What are the effects of insulin on fat, protein, and glucose utilization.

2 List 4 categories of patients who are candidates for insulin therapy.

3 What concentrations of insulin are available and which concentration is most commonly used in the United States?

4 Describe the guidelines for insulin storage.

5 Compare and contrast the sulfonylureas, meglitinides, biguanides, thiazolidinediones, alpha-glucosidase inhibitors, and D-phenylalanine derivatives as to adverse effects and contraindications.

6 How should metformin therapy be initiated and titrated?

7 How should acarbose therapy be initiated and titrated?

8 Which oral glucose-lowering medications must be taken with a meal ("first bite of the meal") to attain their therapeutic effect?

9 Which oral glucose-lowering medication is specifically recommended to be taken on an empty stomach?

10 List the indications for use of glucagon.

11 What are 3 drugs with intrinsic hyperglycemic activity?

12 What are 3 drugs with intrinsic hypoglycemic activity?

13 What are 3 adverse effects of various drugs which may mimic symptoms of hypoglycemia and cause confusion in the perception of hypoglycemia?

14 What are 2 adverse effects of various drugs which may mimic symptoms of hyperglycemia and cause confusion in the perception of hyperglycemia?

15 Define the following terms: (a) major clinically significant problem, (b) moderate clinically significant problem, (c) minor problem.

Key Educational Considerations

1 Oral glucose-lowering agents are not a substitute for meal planning and physical activity, but will work best when all aspects of therapy are combined.

2 Many patients assume that sulfonylureas are "oral insulin" and become confused by what they hear about insulin.

3 It is common for patients who take oral agents to believe that they have a "touch of sugar" or "mild diabetes." If this information is obtained as part of the educational assessment, it can prompt the educator to ask additional questions about the patient's perceptions and beliefs about diabetes and then to provide relevant content.

4 The recognition and treatment of hypoglycemia is essential information for all patients taking insulin or insulin secretagogues.

5 Teach patients to inform all healthcare providers about their diabetes and their medications so that the potential for drug interactions will be recognized.

6 The dosage of metformin or acarbose may be titrated over weeks in order to minimize adverse effects. Written dosage instruction handouts may help patients minimize adverse effects.

7 Persons with type 2 diabetes taking oral agents often assume that when they must start insulin, it is a signal that they are "getting worse" or that it is because they have not "followed the diet right." Explain that over time, the oral agents do not lower the blood glucose as well as they did originally.

8 Persons with type 2 diabetes who change from oral agents to insulin sometimes assume that they no longer have to be concerned about the amounts of food eaten because the insulin will regulate the blood glucose. It should be explained that the insulin is being started to meet the patient's physiologic insulin requirement, not to replace meal planning related to amounts, timing, and consistency of eating.

9 Most insulin-requiring individuals will need 2 or more daily insulin injections, often using 2 types of insulin in each injection to provide insulin in a more physiologic manner.

Learning Assessment: Case Study 1

LR is a 22-year-old woman with type 1 diabetes that was diagnosed 5 years ago. She has cared for her diabetes with 2 insulin injections daily for the past 15 months as follows:

AM: 20 units NPH insulin and 8 units regular insulin

PM: 10 units NPH insulin and 4 units regular insulin

She has hypertension, for which she is taking 50 mg hydrochlorothiazide daily. She has also been taking an oral contraceptive for 3 months. Today she comes to the clinic expressing concern about her glucose levels. Her SMBG record averages for the past 3 weeks are as follows:

SMBG Levels	7 AM mg/dL (mmol/L)	11 AM mg/dL (mmol/L)	4 PM mg/dL (mmol/L)	9 PM mg/dL (mmol/L)
Previous month	107 (6.0)	112 (6.2)	129 (7.1)	120 (6.6)
Week 1	151 (8.3)	168 (9.2)	112 (6.3)	176 (9.7)
Week 2	158 (8.7)	167 (9.2)	142 (7.9)	168 (9.2)
Week 3	167 (9.2)	172 (9.5)	141 (7.8)	171 (9.4)

She reports that her activity, weight, and dietary intake are unchanged.

Questions for Discussion

1 What other information do you need?

2 What possible explanations could be given for her blood glucose levels?

3 What therapeutic options are available for LR?

Discussion

1 An initial review of these data suggests that further information is needed.

    A Your assessment reveals that LR's insulin administration routine is accurate, including storage of insulin, injection sites, timing, and technique.

    B She reports no significant change in her food intake or the introduction of new food products.

    C There has been no change in her activity level, daily habits, level of stress, or coping methods.

2 Potential explanations are either the hydrochlorothiazide or the estrogen-containing contraceptive is causing a drug interaction that is inducing an increase in blood glucose level. LR has been taking hydrochlorothiazide for 3 years with no previous problem. The contraceptive has produced no problem thus far.

3 A trial period of other medications for hypertension and/or contraception might be indicated.

    A Unless the HCTZ was specifically chosen for diuresis as well as antihypertensive effects (ie, the patient has problems with peripheral edema or other fluid accumulation) an angiotensin-converting-enzyme inhibitor (ACE inhibitor) is the drug of choice for hypertension in diabetes. Unlike HCTZ, an ACE inhibitor does not have a potential for causing hyperglycemia or lipid abnormalities.

B A "low dose" contraceptive agent may be considered.

4 Adjustments in insulin are also an option, such as

A The evening dose of intermediate-acting insulin could be increased by 1 to 2 units, or LR could eat less carbohydrates for supper or exercise in the evening to reduce her 7 AM glucose concentration.

B The AM regular insulin could be increased by 1 or 2 units, or LR could eat less carbohydrates for breakfast to reduce her 11 AM glucose concentration.

C Evaluate the 9 PM level based on when LR eats her evening meal.

D Her 4 PM level may be improved by reducing the morning glucose levels.

E If LR is open to the idea of 3 daily injections, the evening dose could be changed to rapid-acting insulin or regular insulin at the evening meal and NPH at bedtime. Administering her NPH at bedtime would help to lower her fasting glucose.

5 Suggest to LR an alternative insulin regimen such as glargine at bedtime and rapid-acting insulin at mealtimes. This type of regimen would provide her with more flexibility in lifestyle, and insulins can be adjusted for improved glycemic control.

Learning Assessment: Case Study 2

AH is a 57-year-old male referred to the diabetes clinic for evaluation of his glycemic control. He was diagnosed with type 2 diabetes about 15 months ago. He remains overweight in spite of numerous attempts to lose weight. His fasting blood glucose concentrations have risen lately and range from 170 to 185 mg/dL (9.4 to 10.3 mmol/L) over the last few weeks. He complains of weakness, fatigue, increased urination, and increased thirst.

Past Medical History
Hypertension x 10 y
Type 2 diabetes mellitus

Family History
(+) Diabetes
(+) Hypertension

Social History
Smokes, ½ to 1 pack per day
Alcohol, none

Current Medications
Hydrochlorothiazide (HCTZ) 50 mg qd
KCl 40 mEq q AM
Propranolol 40 mg qid

Physical Examination
Weight 198 lb (90 kg), increase of 3 kg
Height 5 ft 8 in
BP 154/94 (previous BP ranged from 150/92 to 160/96)
Pulse 88 regular
RR 14

Questions for Discussion

1 How do the antihypertensive agents affect AH's blood glucose level?
2 Which class of oral agent might be appropriate for AH?

Discussion

1 It would be appropriate to begin by substituting different drugs for those that worsen glucose tolerance (HCTZ and propranolol).

A This patient's hypertension might be better treated with an ACE inhibitor or a calcium channel blocker.

B If the HCTZ is discontinued or an ACE inhibitor is initiated the potassium supplement should probably be discontinued as well.

2 The effects of HCTZ and propranolol on glucose tolerance may take a number of weeks to resolve. In the interim, his hyperglycemia should be treated with oral agents or low-dose insulin in order to relieve his symptoms. Metformin may be a good choice for AH because he is overweight and probably insulin resistant. Metformin could lower his blood glucose levels, weight, and lipid levels (if elevated).

3 Prior to initiation of any new therapy, evaluation for potential contraindications (particularly hepatic or renal dysfunction) or drug allergies is needed.

4 Other considerations include cost, patient convenience, patient preference, and lifestyle concerns.

A Many of the sulfonylurea agents are available generically, which are generally less expensive than the brand or newer products.

B A once-a-day agent such as glyburide, glipizide long-acting, glimepiride, or pioglitazone may offer the advantage of being easier to take correctly and consistently.

C If hypoglycemia poses a particular risk for AH (eg, due to work or living situation), a nonhypoglycemic agent such as acarbose, metformin, or a thiazolidinedione may offer an advantage.

D The patient's willingness or ability to self-monitor blood glucose levels may influence the type of agent chosen or blood glucose goals.

5 As the effects of the propranolol and HCTZ wane following their discontinuance, AH may no longer need an oral glucose-lowering medication.

6 Assess the patient's level of interest in meal planning for glucose control and referral to a dietitian.

Learning Assessment: Case Study 3

MC is a 79-year-old female with type 2 diabetes who resides in a nursing home. You are the nursing home consultant. You notice that 10 days ago MC developed a urinary tract infection (UTI), which was initially treated with co-trimoxazole (Septra DS®). After the second dose of Septra DS, intense pruritus and a rash appeared on her arms and upper chest. The Septra was discontinued and ampicillin was prescribed. Diphenhydramine (Benadryl®) and a methylprednisolone dose pack (Medrol®) were given for the sulfonamide reaction.

Over the next several days, you notice that symptoms of increased urination, incontinence, and mental confusion are documented in the nursing notes. After reading the notes and talking with the staff, you learn that these observations were attributed to her advancing age and deteriorating mental status, so no action was taken.

You suspect that the changes observed are related to drug problems rather than changes in patient's mental status.

Questions for Discussion

1 What information would you need to help determine if this reaction is a drug-related problem?
2 What possible explanations could be given for what has happened to MC?
3 Assuming your suspicions are correct and MC has experienced a drug-related reaction, what recommendations could you make to resolve MC's problem?
4 What could be done to prevent this from occurring in the future?

Discussion

1 The following information is needed to help determine the causes of MC's problem:
   A Current drug profile (Is she taking oral agents? Insulin? Have other drugs been recently initiated that would cause symptoms of polyuria or mental confusion?)
   B Recent blood glucose results (Have her blood glucose levels been increasing recently, and did the increase coincide with the onset of UTI symptoms? Did the blood glucose levels increase further when the steroid was initiated?)
   C Ongoing blood glucose patterns and A1C test results (Has chronic hyperglycemia predisposed this patient to infection?)
   D Description of MC's mental status during the period of the UTI and treatment
   E Lab results and vital signs to assess if the UTI is responding to therapy
   F Blood chemistries to assess for possible hyperglycemic hyperosmolar state (HHS)

2 A urinary tract infection is an example of physical stress that can raise blood glucose concentrations (release of counterregulatory hormones). If MC's diabetes was previously poorly controlled or "brittle" (blood glucose fluctuating dramatically with changes in her meal plan, exercise, illness, stress), the hyperglycemic effect of illness would be more exaggerated.

3 Subsequent hyperglycemic factors include the allergic reaction (causing endogenous release of corticosteroid) and the initiation of methylprednisolone (intrinsic hyperglycemic activity).

4 The increased urination, incontinence, and mental confusion may be symptoms of the resulting hyperglycemia; depending upon severity of neurologic symptoms and blood chemistries, HHS may be developing.

5 Diphenhydramine in an elderly person may substantially alter mental alertness or cause urinary retention resulting in overflow incontinence.

6 The following measures can be taken to resolve MC's symptoms:
A Assure adequate hydration.
B Insulin may be needed temporarily in place of oral agents; if MC is already on insulin, doses need to be increased temporarily.
C Monitor blood glucose more frequently until control is reestablished.
D Continue to follow signs and symptoms of UTI to assure resolution of infection.
E Discontinue diphenhydramine. Institute shorteracting or nonsedating antihistamine if antipruritic agent still needed. Topical steroid creams may provide relief.
F Discontinue methylprednisolone as soon as feasible. A slow taper is not necessary.

7 The following preventive recommendations could be instituted:
A The nursing home could establish standard policies regarding detection and management of acute loss of glycemic control in residents with diabetes.
• Blood glucose testing is essential even for residents with well-controlled diabetes. An increase in blood glucose levels often precedes the clinical manifestations of infection and may thus serve as a warning that illness may be developing.
B Blood glucose testing (at least qd or bid) is performed under the following conditions:
• When infection is suspected or confirmed, more frequent testing is needed until blood glucose results return to preinfection levels.
• Upon initiation of drugs with intrinsic hyperglycemic or hypoglycemic activity, more frequent testing is needed until the drug interaction is resolved.
• Upon initiation of drugs with potential adverse effects that mimic hyperglycemia or hypoglycemia, more frequent testing is needed until the patient's response to the drug is determined.

References

1 Fertig BJ, Simmons DA, Martin DB. Therapy for diabetes. In: National Diabetes Data Group. Diabetes in America. 2nd ed. Bethesda, Md: National Institute of Diabetes and Digestive and Kidney Diseases; 1995. NIH Publication 95-1468:519-540.

2 White JR, Davis SN, Cooppan R, Davidson MB, Mulcahy K, Manko GA, Nelinson D, and the Diabetes Consortium Medical Advisory Board. Clarifying the role of insulin in type 2 diabetes management. Clinical Diabetes. 2003;21:14-21.

3 Howey DC, Bowsher RR, Brunelle RL, Woodworth JR. [Lys(B28), Pro(B29)]-human insulin, a rapidly absorbed analogue of human insulin. Diabetes. 1994;43:396-402.

4 Ciofetta M, Lalli C, Del Sindaco P, et al. Contribution of postprandial versus interprandial blood glucose to HbA1c in type 1 diabetes on physiologic intensive therapy with lispro insulin at mealtime. Diabetes Care. 1999;22:795-800.

5 Lalli C, Ciofetta M, Del Sindaco P, et al. Long-term intensive treatment of type 1 diabetes with the short-acting insulin analogue lispro in variable combination with NPH insulin at mealtime. Diabetes Care. 1999;22:468-477.

6 Holleman F, Schmitt H, Rottiers R, Rees A, Symanowski S, Anderson JH Jr. Reduced frequency of severe hypoglycemia and coma in well-controlled IDDM patients treated with insulin lispro. The Benelux-UK Insulin Lispro Study Group. Diabetes Care. 1997;20:1827-1832.

7 Brunelle BL, Llewelyn J, Anderson JH Jr, Gale EA, Koivisto VA. Meta-analysis of the effect of insulin lispro on severe hypoglycemia in patients with type 1 diabetes. Diabetes Care. 1998;21:1726-1731.

8 Renner R, Pfutzner A, Trautmann M, Harzer O, Sauter K, Landgraf R, on behalf of the German Humalog–Pump Therapy Study Group. Use of insulin lispro in continuous subcutaneous insulin infusion treatment. Diabetes Care. 1999;22:784-788.

9 Zinman B, Tildesley H, Chiasson JL, Tsui E, Strack T. Insulin lispro in pump therapy: results of a double blind crossover study. Diabetes. 1997:46:440-443.

10 Home PD, Lindholm A, Hyllegerg B, Round P. Improved glycemic control with insulin aspart: a multicenter randomized double-blind crossover trial in type 1 diabetic patients. UK Insulin Aspart Study Group. Diabetes Care. 1998;21:1904-1909.

11 Lindholm A, McEwen J, Riis AP. Improved postprandial glycemic control with insulin aspart. A randomized double-blind trial cross-over trial in type 1 diabetes. Diabetes Care. 1999;22:801-805.

12 Mudaliar SR, Lindberg FA, Joyce M, et al. Insulin aspart (B28 asp-insulin): a fast-acting analogue of human insulin. Diabetes Care. 1999;22:1501-1506.

13 Bode BW, Strange P. Efficacy, safety, and pump compatibility of insulin aspart used in continuous subcutaneous insulin infusion therapy in patients with type 1 diabetes. Diabetes Care. 2001;24:69-72.

14 Rosskamp RH, Park G. Long-acting insulin analogues. Diabetes Care. 1999;22(suppl 2):B109-B113.

15 Lepore M, Pampanelli S, Fanelli C, et al. Pharmacokinetics and pharmacodynamics of subcutaneous injection of long-acting human insulin analog glargine, NPH insulin, and ultralente human insulin and continuous subcutaneous infusion of insulin lispro. Diabetes. 2000;49:2142-2148.

16 Raskin P, Klaff L, Bergenstal R, Halle J-P, Donley D, Mecca T. A 16-week comparison of the novel insulin analogue insulin glargine (HOE 901) and NPH human insulin used with insulin lispro in patients with type 1 diabetes. Diabetes Care. 2000;23:1666-1671.

17 Rosenstock J, Schwartz SL, Clark CM, Park GD, Donley DW, Edwards MB. Basal insulin therapy in type 2 diabetes. 28-week comparison of insulin glargine (HOE 901) and NPH insulin. Diabetes Care. 2001;24:631-636.

18 Lantus Package Insert. Kansas City: Aventis; 2000.

19 Vague P, Selam J-L, Skeje S, et al. Insulin detemir is associated with more predictable glycemic control and reduced risk of hypoglycemia than NPH insulin in patients with type 1 diabetes on a basal-bolus regimen with premeal insulin aspart. Diabetes Care. 2003;26:590-596.

20 American Diabetes Association. Insulin administration (position statement). Diabetes Care. 2003(suppl 1):S121-S124.

21 American Diabetes Association. Continuous subcutaneous insulin infusion (position statement). Diabetes Care. 2003(suppl 1):S125.

22 Bolognia JL, Braverman IM. Skin and subcutaneous tissues. In: Lebovitz HE, ed. Therapy for Diabetes Mellitus and Related Disorders. 3rd ed. Alexandria, Va: American Diabetes Association; 1998:290-303.

23 White JR Jr, Hartman J, Campbell RK. Drug interactions in diabetic patients. Postgrad Med. 1993;93:131-139.

24 Skyler JS, ed. Medical Management of Type 1 Diabetes. 3rd ed. Alexandria, Va: American Diabetes Association; 1998.

25 Zimmerman BR, ed. Medical Management of Type 2 Diabetes. 4th ed. Alexandria, Va: American Diabetes Association; 1998.

26 Jovanovic L, ed. Medical Management of Pregnancy Complicated by Diabetes. 3rd ed. Alexandria, Va: American Diabetes Association; 2000.

27 Seigler DE, Olsson GM, Skyler JS. Morning versus bedtime isophane insulin in type 2 (non-insulin dependent) diabetes mellitus. Diabetic Med. 1992;9:826-833.

28 Roach P, Yue L, Arora V, the Humalog Mix25 Study Group. Improved postprandial glycemic control during treatment with Humalog Mix25, a novel protamine-based insulin lispro formulation. Diabetes Care. 1999;22:1258-1261.

29 DeWitt DE, Hirsch IB. Outpatient insulin therapy in type 1 and type 2 diabetes mellitus. JAMA. 2003;289:2254-2264.

30 White JR Jr, Campbell RK. Inhaled insulin: an overview. Clinical Diabetes. 2001;19: 13-16.

31 Cappelleri JC, Cefalu WT, Rosenstock J, Kourides LA, Gerber RA. Treatment satisfaction in type 2 diabetes: a comparison between inhaled insulin regimen and a subcutaneous insulin regimen. Clin Ther. 2002;24:552-564.

32 Skyler JS, Cefalu WT, Kourides IA, et al. Efficacy of inhaled insulin in type 1 diabetes mellitus: a randomized proof-of-concept study. Lancet. 2001;357:324-325.

33 White JR Jr. Combination oral agent/insulin therapy in patients with type II diabetes mellitus. Clinical Diabetes. 1997;15:102-112.

34 Mudaliar S, Henry RR. Combination therapy for type 2 diabetes. Endocr Pract. 1999;5:208-219.

35 DeFronzo RA. Pharmacologic therapy for type 2 diabetes mellitus. Ann Intern Med. 1999;131:281-303.

36 Campbell RK, White JR. Medications for the Treatment of Diabetes. Alexandria, Va: American Diabetes Association; 2000.

37 Lebovitz HE. Insulin secretagogues: sulfonylureas and repaglinide. In: Lebovitz HE, ed. Therapy for Diabetes Mellitus and Related Disorders. 3rd ed. Alexandria, Va: American Diabetes Association; 1998;160-170.

38 Halter JB. Geriatric patients. In: Lebovitz HE, ed. Therapy for Diabetes Mellitus and Related Disorders. 3rd ed. Alexandria, Va: American Diabetes Association; 1998:234-240.

39 White JR Jr. The pharmacologic management of patients with type II diabetes mellitus in the era of new oral agents and insulin analogues. Diabetes Spectrum. 1996;9:227-234.

40 Gerich JE. Oral hypoglycemic agents. N Engl J Med. 1989;321:1231-1245.

41 Stenman S, Melander A, Groop P, Groop LC. What is the benefit of increasing the sulfonylurea dose? Ann of Intern Med. 1993;118:169-172.

42 Damsbo P, Clauson P, Marbury TC, Windfeld K. A double-blind randomized comparison of meal-related glycemic control by repaglinide and glyburide in well-controlled type 2 diabetic patients. Diabetes Care. 1999;22:789-794.

43 Moses RG, Gomis R, Frandsen KB, Schlienger J-L, Dedov I. Flexible meal-related dosing with repaglinide facilitates glycemic control in therapy-naïve type 2 diabetes. Diabetes Care. 2001;24:11-15.

44 Raskin P, Jovanovic L, Berger S, Schwartz S, Woo V, Ratner R. Repaglinide/troglitazone combination therapy. Improved glycemic control in type 2 diabetes. Diabetes Care. 2000;23:979-983.

45 Prandin Package Insert. Princeton, NJ: Novo Nordisk; 1997.

46 Kalbag JB, Walter YH, Nedelman JR, McLeod JF. Mealtime glucose regulation with nateglinide in healthy volunteers. Diabetes Care. 2001;24:73-77.

47 Keilson L, Mather S, Walter YH, Subramanian S, McLeod JF. Synergistic effects of nateglinide and meal administration on insulin secretion in patients with type 2 diabetes mellitus. J Clin Endocrinol Metab. 2000;85:1081-1086.

48 Horton ES, Clinkingbeard C, Gatlin M, Foley J, Mallows S, Shen S. Nateglinide alone and in combination with metformin improves glycemic control by reducing mealtime glucose levels in type 2 diabetes. Diabetes Care. 2000;23:1660-1665.

49 Dunn CJ, Faulds D. Nateglinide. Drugs. 2000;60:607-615.

50 Starlix Package Insert. East Hanover, NJ: Novartis Pharmaceuticals Corporation; 2000.

51 Bailey CJ. Metformin: an update. Gen Pharmacol. 1993;24:1299-1309.

52 DeFronzo RA, Goodman AM. Multicenter Metformin Study Group. Efficacy of metformin in patients with non-insulin-dependent diabetes mellitus. N Eng J Med. 1995;333:541-549.

53 Wu MS, Johnston P, Sheu WHH, et al. Effects of metformin on carbohydrate and lipoprotein metabolism in NIDDM patients. Diabetes Care. 1990;13:1-8.

54 Stumvoll M, Nurijhan N, Perriello G, et al. Metabolic effects of metformin on non-insulin-dependent diabetes mellitus. N Engl J Med. 1995;333:550-554.

55 DeFronzo RA, Barzilai N, Simonson DC. Mechanism of metformin action in obese and lean non-insulin dependent diabetic subjects. J Clin Endocrinol Metab. 1991;73:1294-1301.

56 Hundal RS, Krssak M, Dufour S, et al. Mechanism by which metformin reduces glucose production in type 2 diabetes. Diabetes. 2000;49:2063-2069.

57 Glucophage, Glucophage XR Package Insert. Princeton, NJ: Bristol-Meyers Squibb Company; 2000.

58 Glucovance Package Insert. Princeton, NJ: Bristol-Meyers Squibb Company; 2000.

59 Dandona P, Fonseca V, Mier A, et al. Diarrhea and metformin in a diabetic clinic. Diabetes Care. 1983;6:472-474.

60 Stang M, Wysowski DK, Butler Jones D. Incidence of lactic acidosis in metformin users. Diabetes Care. 1999;22:925-957.

61 Aviles-Santa L, Sinding J, Raskin P. Effects of metformin in patients with poorly controlled, insulin-treated type 2 diabetes mellitus. Ann Intern Med. 1999;131:182-188.

62 Saltiel AR, Olefsky JM. Thiazolidinediones in the treatment of insulin resistance and type II diabetes. Diabetes. 1996;45:1661-1664.

63 Glitazones. In: White J, Campbell RK. Medications for the Treatment of Diabetes, Alexandria, Va: American Diabetes Association; 2000;71-86.

64 Actos Package Insert. Indianapolis: Eli Lilly; 1999.

65 Avandia Package Insert. Philadelphia: SmithKline Beecham; 1999.

66 Aronoff S, Rosenblatt S, Braithwaite S, Egan JW, Mathisen AL, Schneider RL, The Pioglitazone 001 Study Group. Pioglitazone hydrochloride monotherapy improves glycemic control in the treatment of patients with type 2 diabetes: 6 month randomized placebo-controlled dose response study. Diabetes Care. 2000;23:1605-1611.

67 Phillips LS, Grunberger G, Miller E, Patwadhan R, Rappaport EB, Salzman A, for the Rosiglitazone Clinical Trials Study Group. Once- and twice-daily dosing with rosiglitazone improves glycemic control in patients with type 2 diabetes. Diabetes Care. 2001;24:308-315.

68 Santeusanio F, Compagnucci P. A risk-benefit appraisal of acarbose in the management of non-insulin-dependent diabetes mellitus. Drug Safety. 1994;11:432-444.

69 Alpha-glucosidase inhibitors. In: White J, Campbell RK. Medications for the Treatment of Diabetes. Alexandria, Va: American Diabetes Association; 2000:57-70.

70 Chiasson JL, Josse RG, Hunt JA, et al. The efficacy of acarbose in the treatment of patients with non-insulin-dependent diabetes mellitus. Ann Intern Med. 1994;121:928-935.

71 Lebovitz H. Alpha-glucosidase inhibitors in treatment of hyperglycemia. Lebovitz HE, ed. In: Therapy for Diabetes Mellitus and Related Disorders. 3rd ed. Alexandria, Va: American Diabetes Association; 1998: 176-180.

72 Shmitz O, Nyholm B, Orskov L, et al. Effects of amylin and the amylin agonist pramlintide on glucose metabolism. Diabet Med. 1997;14(suppl 2):S19-S23.

73 Thompson RG, Peterson J, Gottlieb A, et al. Effects of pramlintide, an analogue of human amylin, on the plasma glucose profiles in patients with IDDM: results of a multicenter trial. Diabetes. 1997;46:632-636.

74 Thompson RG, Pearson L, Schoenfeld SL, et al. The pramlintide in type 2 diabetes group: pramlintide, a synthetic analogue of human amylin, improves the metabolic profile of patients with type 2 diabetes using insulin. Diabetes Care. 1998;21:987-993.

Suggested Readings

American Diabetes Association Vital Statistics. Alexandria, Va: American Diabetes Association; 2000.

Bell DH, Mayo MS. Outcome of metformin-facilitated reinitiating of oral diabetic therapy in insulin-treated patients with non-insulin-dependent diabetes mellitus. Endocr Pract. 1997;3:73-76.

Bohannon NJ. Benefits of lispro insulin. Postgrad Med. 1997;101:73-80.

DeWitt D, Dugdale DC. Using new insulin strategies in the outpatient treatment of diabetes: clinical applications. JAMA. 2003;289:2265-2269.

Fleming DR, Jacober SJ, Vandenberg MA, Fitzgerald JT, Grunberger G. The safety of injecting insulin through clothing. Diabetes Care. 1997;20:245-248.

Garber AJ, Duncan TG, Goodman AM, et al. Efficacy of metformin in type II diabetes: results of a double-blind, placebo-controlled, dose-response trial. Am J Med. 1997;103:491-497.

Inzucchi SE. Oral antihyperglycemic therapy for type 2 diabetes. A scientific review. JAMA. 2002;287:360-372.

White J, Campbell RK. Medications for the Treatment of Diabetes. Alexandria, Va: American Diabetes Association; 2000.

White JR Jr, Campbell RK, Hirsch I. Insulin analogues. Postgrad Med. 1997;101:58-70.

Young DS. Effects of Drugs on Clinical Laboratory Tests. 4th ed. Washington, DC: American Association for Clinical Chemistry Press; 1995:274-281.

Learning Assessment: Post-Test Questions

Pharmacologic Therapies for Glucose Management   3

1   Insulin exerts all of the following effects on the body tissues except:
   A   Stimulate entry of glucose into muscle cells for utilization as an energy source
   B   Enhance fat storage
   C   Promote breakdown of liver glycogen to maintain blood glucose levels
   D   Stimulate entry of amino acids into cells enhancing protein biosynthesis

2   When the pancreas is stimulated by an elevated blood glucose level, insulin enters the blood stream:
   A   In equimolar quantities with proinsulin
   B   In equimolar quantities with C-peptide
   C   In equimolar quantities with glucagon
   D   With a small amount of C-peptide

3   Lispro and aspart insulin analogs are a:
   A   Rapid-acting insulin which has an onset of action in 15 to 30 minutes, reaches a peak in 1 to 2 hours, and has a therapeutic duration of 3 to 4 hours
   B   Long-acting insulin which has an onset of action in 4 to 6 hours, reaches a peak in 18 hours, and has a therapeutic duration of 24 to 36 hours
   C   Intermediate-acting insulin which has an onset of 1 to 4 hours, reaches a peak in 8 hours, and has a therapeutic duration of 10 to 16 hours
   D   Rapid-acting insulin which has an onset of 30 minutes to 1 hour, reaches a peak in 2 to 4 hours, and has a therapeutic duration of 6 to 8 hours

4   MJ is planning a trip to Europe for 21 days. She asks how her insulin should be stored while traveling. Which of the following is the best advice for MJ?
   A   "Carry ice packs to keep your insulin at 36°F to 46°F."
   B   "Store your open insulin at room temperature for 7 days, after which time it must be discarded."
   C   "Insulin may be stored at 59°F to 86° F for the entire trip provided it is used within 1 month."
   D   "People with diabetes in all foreign countries use U-100 insulin, so there should be no difficulty obtaining insulin when traveling in Europe."

5   A patient asks you if she can reuse her syringes and needles. Which of the following is the best answer?
   A   "Needles and syringes should never be reused because of increased risk of infection."
   B   "Needles and syringes may be used indefinitely since the new needles are thin and never become dull."
   C   "Needles and syringes may be reused provided they are kept refrigerated."
   D   "Syringes and needles can be reused. The needle should be safely recapped and the syringe should be stored at room temperature."

6   A primary action of thiazolidinediones is to:
   A   Decrease gluconeogenesis
   B   Stimulate the beta cells of the islets of Langerhans to produce more insulin
   C   Inhibit alpha-glucosidase
   D   Enhance insulin-stimulated glucose transport into muscle cells

7   The most acutely dangerous complication of sulfonylurea therapy is:
   A   Weight gain
   B   Skin rashes
   C   Gastrointestinal disturbance
   D   Hypoglycemia

8 GW, a 70-year-old patient with type 2 diabetes, has a blood creatinine level of 3.0 mg/dL. Which of the following drugs is contraindicated for GW?
A Pioglitazone
B Glipizide
C Glyburide
D Metformin

9 Thiazolidinediones should be used with caution in patients with:
A Hepatic dysfunction
B Renal dysfunction
C Hypoglycemia
D Dyslipidemia

10 An oral agent for diabetes that may be especially useful in patients who have type 2 disease with elevated triglycerides and LDL cholesterol is:
A Glyburide
B Glimepiride
C Metformin
D Acarbose

11 The role of exogenous glucagon is to:
A Stimulate hepatic glucose release
B Counteract hyperglycemia
C Delay gastric emptying
D Increase the postprandial glucose levels

12 When should combination therapy for persons with type 2 diabetes be considered?
A Two years following diagnosis
B Only after a person develops 2 or more complications
C When sulfonylurea dose approaches half of the maximum dose
D When sulfonylurea dose is at the maximum dose

See next page for answer key.

Post-Test Answer Key

Pharmacologic Therapies for Glucose Management 3

1	C	7	D
2	B	8	D
3	A	9	A
4	C	10	C
5	D	11	A
6	D	12	D

A Core Curriculum for Diabetes Education
Diabetes Management Therapies

Pharmacologic Therapies for Hypertension and Dyslipidemia

4

John V. St. Peter, PharmD, BCPS
Hennepin Center for Diabetes and Endocrinology
College of Pharmacy, University of Minnesota
Minneapolis, Minnesota

Tommy Johnson, PharmD, CDE
University of Georgia College of Pharmacy
Athens, Georgia

Introduction

1 Atherosclerotic cardiovascular disease is the most common cause of morbidity and mortality in persons with diabetes.[1,2] Diabetes is now recognized as a coronary heart disease (CHD) risk equivalent.[3] A gender disparity also may exist among those with type 2 diabetes such that women exhibit higher risk for CHD than men.

    A Dyslipidemia, hypertension, obesity, and smoking are known to increase the risk of CHD in persons with either type 1 or type 2 diabetes.[4,5] The risk of CHD in persons with type 2 diabetes is 2 to 3 times greater than in those without diabetes.[6,7]

    B Metabolic syndrome is a comorbid condition in most persons with type 2 diabetes and a major contributor to significant CHD.[8]

2 Hypertriglyceridemia and hypertension are common comorbid conditions in both type 1 and type 2 diabetes. However, consistent with differences in pathophysiology, persons with type 2 diabetes more commonly present with a greater degree and number of the components of the metabolic syndrome (low HDL cholesterol; small, dense LDL cholesterol; increased apolipoprotein B; insulin resistance; central obesity; and a family history of CHD). Hypertension is commonly part of the metabolic syndrome in those with type 2 diabetes, whereas blood pressure elevations in patients with type 1 diabetes may be related to the presence or development of other comorbidities such as nephropathy.

3 Aggressive risk factor management and treatment, in addition to intensive glycemic management, is necessary to reduce macrovascular disease risk in persons with diabetes.[9] Pharmacotherapies should be implemented in addition to or in conjunction with adequate trials of recommended lifestyle modifications (eg, medical nutrition therapy, weight loss, smoking cessation, physical activity, and moderation of alcohol intake).

4 Successful management of multiple risk factors in persons with diabetes routinely requires the application of multiple pharmacologic therapies. Many professional organizations and national committees have made recommendations for the treatment of hypertension, dyslipidemia, and metabolic syndrome. Recommendations may vary slightly among these organizations and committees.

5 Diabetes educators can assist and support persons with diabetes with the implementation of multiple risk factor interventions by being familiar with some of the general aspects of commonly employed pharmacotherapies for hypertension and dyslipidemia.

Objectives

Upon completion of the chapter, the learner will be able to

1 List sources of recommendations and practice guidelines for the treatment of hypertension and dyslipidemia.

2 Determine the stage of hypertension based on the person's systolic and diastolic blood pressure.

3 State the categories of pharmacotherapies used to treat hypertension and dyslipidemia.

4 State the preferred pharmacotherapy for hypertension based on the American Diabetes Association recommendations.

5 State the preferred pharmacotherapy for dyslipidemia based on the American Diabetes Association recommendations.

6 Identify treatment set points and goals for drug therapy related to hypertension and dyslipidemia in persons with diabetes.

7 Describe common laboratory tests and/or physiologic measurements that are routinely performed prior to and after implementing selected pharmacotherapies for hypertension and dyslipidemia.

8 List critical side effects and/or conditions that can occur secondary to selected pharmacotherapies for hypertension and dyslipidemia.

Practice Guidelines and Position Statements for the Treatment and Management of Associated Comorbid Conditions in Diabetes

1 Recommendations are available for the implementation and application of therapies for hypertension, dyslipidemia, metabolic syndrome, and related comorbid conditions.

A The American Diabetes Association annually publishes a position statement, "Standards of Medical Care for Patients With Diabetes Mellitus," which includes recommendations for glycemic control and the prevention and management of diabetes complications.[10]

B The American Association of Clinical Endocrinologists (AACE) and the American College of Endocrinology developed 2 documents, "Medical Guidelines for the Management of Diabetes: The AACE System of Intensive Diabetes Self-Management"[11] and "Medical Guidelines for the Clinical Practice for the Diagnosis and Treatment of Dyslipidemia and Prevention of Atherogenesis."[12] These guidelines include recommendations for glycemic control and intensive treatment of comorbid complications.

C The National Cholesterol Education Program Expert Panel published a report, "Third Report on Detection, Evaluation, and Treatment of High Blood Cholesterol in Adults,"[3] which includes recommendations for managing lipids, diabetes, and the metabolic syndrome.

D The 7th report of the Joint National Committee on Prevention, Detection, Evaluation, and Treatment of High Blood Pressure focuses on recommendations for managing hypertension.[13]

E The National Kidney Foundation published "Clinical Practice Guidelines for Chronic Kidney Disease: Evaluation, Classification, and Stratification."[14]

Pharmacologic Treatment of Hypertension in Persons With Diabetes: Classification and Treatment Goals

1 Aggressive treatment of hypertension is recommended for persons with diabetes.[13]

2 Blood pressure is divided into 4 distinct categories: normal, prehypertension, stage 1 hypertension, and stage 2 hypertension (see Table 4.1). For the purpose of determining the stage or category of hypertension, blood pressure should be

A Measured in the seated position

B Determined as the average of 2 blood pressure readings obtained at 2 separate clinic visits

3 The blood pressure goal for people with diabetes is less than 130 mm Hg systolic and less than 80 mm Hg diastolic. Some authorities recommend lower pressures depending on the presence of comorbid conditions, such as nephropathy, and the tolerance of the person to whom the therapies are being employed.

4 Pharmacotherapy should be initiated when blood pressure remains consistently above a systolic pressure of 130 mm Hg and/or a diastolic pressure of 80 mm Hg. For those with diabetes, pharmacotherapy is initiated at a blood pressure that is within the range of the prehypertension stage. This level is lower than the blood pressure level at which treatment is recommended for persons without diabetes because of the greater risk of cardiovascular disease in persons with diabetes.

5 Initiation of pharmacotherapy is appropriate after inadequate response to or concurrent with lifestyle modifications, such as modest weight reduction; the DASH (dietary approaches to stop hypertension) diet, a meal planning approach that emphasizes whole grains, fruits, vegetables, low-fat dairy products, beans, and seeds; dietary sodium restriction; adequate physical activity; and moderation of alcohol intake.

Table 4.1. Classification of Blood Pressure[1]

Hypertension Stage[2]	Pressure (mm Hg)	
	Systolic	Diastolic
Normal	Less than 120	Less than 80
Prehypertension	120–139	80–89[3]
1	140–159	90–99
2	160 or greater	100 or greater

1 Seated blood pressure, mean of 2 measurements on at least 2 separate office visits.
2 Stage and treatment are based upon the highest of either systolic or diastolic pressure.
3 Pharmacotherapy may be initiated in persons with diabetes when blood pressure consistently exceeds 130/80 mm Hg.

Pharmacologic Agents Used in the Treatment of Hypertension

1 Multiple classes of antihypertensive medications are currently available for the treatment of hypertension. The general pharmacologic categories and examples in each category are shown in Table 4.2. Any class of agent may be used alone or in combination to treat hypertension in persons with diabetes.[15] Persons with diabetes and hypertension routinely require at least 2 medications from different classes to adequately control their blood pressure.[10,13]

2 Several classes of agents are recognized as preferred over others when treating hypertension in persons with diabetes.

   A Angiotensin-converting enzyme (ACE) inhibitors and angiotensin II receptor blockers (ARBs) slow the progression of nephropathy. Based upon current evidence, the initial choice of an ACE inhibitor versus ARBs depends on age, the presence of hypertension, the type of diabetes, the degree of albuminuria, the presence of renal insufficiency, other cardiovascular risk factors, and tolerance to the drug.[15] If the person is intolerant to the initial choice of an ACE inhibitor or ARB, then an alternate ACE inhibitor or ARB should be considered. Special laboratory monitoring of serum potassium and renal function may be needed before and during therapy.

B ß-receptor blockers (ß-blockers) without intrinsic sympathomimetic activity (eg, metoprolol or atenolol) are indicated to reduce mortality in persons with recent myocardial infarction, regardless of diabetes status.

C Diuretics effectively reduce cardiovascular events and can be used by persons with diabetes. Special laboratory monitoring of serum potassium and renal function may be needed before and during therapy.

D Nondihydropyridine calcium channel blockers (CCBs) (eg, verapamil or diltiazem) or ß-blockers should be considered for persons with diabetes and albuminuria when ACE inhibitors or ARBs are not tolerated.

3 Many over-the-counter cough and cold preparations, weight-loss products, and herbal therapies contain substances that can reduce the effectiveness of antihypertensive therapies. Examples include ephedrine or ephedra-based substances and caffeine.

A Ma huang is a natural substance that is metabolized to ephedrine.

B Many natural products and foods contain or are metabolized to caffeine, including many types of chocolate, guarana, and various tea extracts.

Diuretics

1 Diuretics are generally classified based on the site and/or mechanism of action. There are 4 major groups of diuretics: thiazide-type, loop, potassium-sparing, and carbonic anhydrase inhibitors (see Table 4.2). Thiazide-type (eg, hydrochlorothiazide or chlorthalidone) and loop diuretics (eg, furosemide or bumetanide) are commonly employed in the treatment of high blood pressure. Carbonic anhydrase inhibitors are not typically used in the treatment of hypertension.

2 The degree of renal function is an important factor in determining the most appropriate diuretic to treat high blood pressure. Thiazide-type agents are weaker diuretics than the loop agents but are more potent for lowering blood pressure when the glomerular filtration rate (GFR) exceeds 30 mL/minute. Thiazide-type diuretics are relatively ineffective when GFR falls below 30 mL/minute due to excess accumulation of sodium and water. Loop agents are preferred when GFR falls below 30 mL/minute.

3 Diuretics are formulated for oral use as single entities or in fixed-dose combinations with other antihypertensive agents.

A Hydrochlorothiazide and chlorthalidone are the 2 most frequently prescribed diuretics for treating high blood pressure.

B Hydrochlorothiazide (but not chlorthalidone) is commonly combined in fixed-dose combination with ACE inhibitors, ARBs, ß-blockers, centrally acting agents, and other diuretics (commonly potassium-sparing diuretics).

C When diuretics are used in combination with other therapies, the greatest antihypertensive efficacy and fewest side effects are seen with low doses of hydrochlorothiazide ranging from 6.25 to 25 mg/day.[16-18]

Table 4.2. Major Classes of Agents Used to Treat High Blood Pressure

Angiotensin-converting enzyme (ACE) inhibitors
Benazepril, captopril, enalapril, fosinopril, lisinopril, moexipril, perindopril, quinapril, ramipril, trandolapril

Angiotensin II receptor blockers (ARBs)
Candesartan, eprosartan, irbesartan, losartan, olmesartan, telmisartan, valsartan

Calcium channel blockers (CCBs)
Nondihydropyridine: Diltiazem, verapamil
Dihydropyridine: Amlodipine, felodipine, isradipine, nicardinipine, nifedipine, nisoldipine

ß-receptor blockers (ß-blockers)
Relatively nonselective ß-receptor blockers: Nadolol, propranolol, timolol
Relatively cardioselective ß-receptor blockers: Acebutolol, atenolol, bisoprolol, metoprolol
ß-receptor blockers with intrinsic sympathomimetic activity (ISA): Acebutolol, pindolol

Combined α- and ß-receptor blockers
Carvedilol, labetalol

α₁.- receptor blockers
Doxazosin, prazosin, terazosin

Centrally acting agents
Clonidine, methyldopa

Direct vasodilators
Hydralazine, minoxidil

Diuretics
Thiazide-type diuretics: Chlorthalidone, hydrochlorathiazide, metolazone
Loop diuretics: Bumetanide, furosemide, torsemide
Potassium-sparing diuretics: Amiloride, spironolactone, triamterene

4 The major mechanisms of blood-pressure-lowering action with diuretics are different for acute and chronic use and are thought to include the following

  A Acutely, diuretics act by decreasing plasma volume. Blood pressure is lowered as a result of decreased stroke volume and cardiac output that results from declining plasma volume.

  B With chronic use, diuretics lower blood pressure by decreasing peripheral vascular resistance. Thiazide diuretics are thought to lower vascular resistance by mobilizing sodium and water from arteriolar walls and effectively increasing luminal diameter.

5 There are differences in the pharmacokinetics and pharmacodynamics of the thiazide diuretics. However, these differences seem to be of little clinical consequence because they appear to have a similar capacity to lower blood pressure. The blood-pressure-lowering effects are generally detectable after 3 to 4 days of therapy. Hypotensive effects may persist for up to 1 week after discontinuing thiazide diuretics. Food decreases the serum concentrations of thiazide diuretics but, in general, has minimal clinically significant effects on blood pressure lowering.

6 Routine clinical monitoring is recommended with diuretic use.

    A Blood pressure and serum electrolytes should be measured before and periodically during therapy. Hypokalemia and hypomagnesemia can result in muscle cramps and fatigue. Serious cardiac arrhythmias can occur in susceptible patients.

    B Serum uric acid should be measured before and periodically during therapy. In persons with preexisting gout or uric acid stone disease, hyperuricemia related to diuretic use can exacerbate gouty arthritis and uric acid stones. Problems with hyperuricemia related to diuretic use are uncommon in persons with no previous history of gout or uric acid stone disease.

    C Persons with diabetes may require increased monitoring of plasma glucose and lipid concentrations when initiating diuretic therapy.

    D Seated and orthostatic blood pressure should be measured.

7 Cautions and contraindications related to diuretics include the fact that thiazide-like drugs are contraindicated in persons with known hypersensitivity to sulfonamides. The absolute risk of cross-sensitivity between sulfa-containing compounds is not well defined and may, in fact, be quite low. However, extreme caution is advised in the presence of a documented history of allergic reaction.[19]

8 Adverse effects associated with diuretics include serum chemistry and electrolyte disturbances (eg, hyperglycemia, hyperuricemia, hypokalemia, hypomagnesemia, and hypercalcemia). Both thiazide and loop diuretics can cause disorders of serum chemistry and electrolytes; however, loop diuretics appear to have less effect on glucose and lipid concentrations. Thiazide-diuretic-induced changes in chemistries and electrolytes are more common at higher doses (eg, 100 mg/day) and occur less frequently than the currently recommended antihypertensive doses of 6.25 to 25 mg/day.

9 Clinically significant drug or dietary interactions with diuretics can occur.

    A Concurrent use of nonsteroidal antiinflammatory agents (eg, ibuprofen-like drugs) can decrease the antihypertensive effect of diuretics.

    B Sodium intake can significantly affect the blood-pressure-lowering effects of diuretics; high sodium intake can reverse the blood-pressure-lowering effects and low sodium intake can enhance the blood-pressure-lowering effects.

    C Hypotension can result when diuretics are used in combination with other blood pressure-lowering agents.

10 Most persons with diabetes require multiple agents to control their blood pressure, and diuretics are acceptable agents to use in this patient group.

    A The thiazide-type diuretics are a commonly employed diuretic for the treatment of hypertension. Thiazide diuretics are typically used in combination with an ACE inhibitor, ARBs, or ß-blockers.

    B Thiazide diuretics have the potential to adversely affect both glucose and lipid levels in persons with diabetes. However, these effects occur infrequently at the low doses of 6.25 to 25 mg/day that are recommended for the treatment of hypertension.

C Persons with diabetes may require additional biochemical monitoring when diuretics are used to treat hypertension.

Angiotensin-Converting Enzyme (ACE) Inhibitors

1 There are more than 10 angiotensin-converting enzyme (ACE) inhibitors currently marketed in the United States either as single entities or in combination with other antihypertensive agents. With ACE inhibitor/diuretic combination drug formulations, the hydrochlorothiazide doses can range from 6.25 to 25 mg. With ACE inhibitor/calcium channel blocker (CCB) combination drug formulations, either a nondihydropyridine (verapamil) or dihydropyridine CCB (felodipine or amlodipine) is used.

2 There are several major pharmacologic effects of ACE inhibitors.

   A In normotensive and hypertensive individuals, blood pressure reduction is thought to be related to decreasing concentrations of the potent vasoconstrictor angiotensin II. ACE inhibitors block angiotensin II production via the renin-angiotensin system, which is one of the 2 major pathways of angiotensin production. Blood pressure is also reduced by direct inhibition of arterial wall or kidney tissues by the renin-angiotensin systems.

   B Renal function (glomerular filtration rate) can increase or decrease with the initiation of ACE inhibitor therapy; therefore, persons with diabetes require increased vigilance when initially exposed to these agents. Decreasing renal function is more common in those with preexisting renal impairment. Serum potassium and urinary sodium excretion may increase due to changes in aldosterone secretion.

3 The pharmacokinetics and pharmacodynamics of ACE inhibitors are relatively consistent throughout the drug class. Many of the ACE inhibitors are formulated as highly absorbed prodrugs that are rapidly metabolized to active forms after absorption. Food does not appear to extensively alter ACE inhibitor absorption.

   A Blood pressure lowering is usually evident within 1 hour of dosing, and maximum effects are seen at 6 to 8 hours. Most ACE inhibitors are administered once or twice daily given that the blood pressure effects generally persist for 12 to 24 hours after dosing.

   B Both systolic and diastolic blood pressures usually decrease. However, using ACE inhibitors as a single agent to treat hypertension may be less effective in African Americans than in Caucasian populations.[20]

   C Orthostatic hypotension and reflex tachycardia are generally uncommon but can occur in hypovolemic patients.

4 Routine clinical monitoring is recommended with ACE inhibitors.

   A Blood pressure and serum electrolytes should be measured before and periodically during therapy. Hyperkalemia can occur soon after initiation of therapy. Potassium levels should be monitored 2 to 4 weeks after initiating therapy.

   B Renal function should be assessed before and periodically during therapy. Because impaired renal function can occur soon after initiation of therapy, persons taking ACE inhibitors should be monitored closely during initiation and dose titration.

5 There are certain cautions, contraindications, and precautions related to therapy with ACE inhibitors.

   A ACE inhibitor use is contraindicated during pregnancy because it has resulted in serious neonatal complications and death.

   B In persons with bilateral renal artery stenosis or unilateral stenosis of a single, functioning kidney, ACE inhibitor use can cause dilation of the efferent arteriolar circulation, which can result in acute renal failure.

6 Certain adverse effects are associated with ACE inhibitors.

   A Hyperkalemia can occur with ACE inhibitors. Multiple etiologies for the increases in serum potassium are possible, especially in persons with diabetes and preexisting renal dysfunction. Elevated serum potassium concentrations do not always necessitate discontinuance of ACE inhibitors, but critical assessment by primary care providers is required. Significant increases in serum potassium can occur with concurrent use of nonsteroidal antiinflammatory agents, potassium-sparing diuretics, and potassium supplements.

   B Acute hypotension is an adverse effect that occurs commonly during initiation of therapy in persons who are extremely volume- or sodium-depleted.

   C About 10% to 20% of persons who take ACE inhibitors develop a persistent cough that sometimes resolves by switching to another ACE inhibitor or to an ARB.

   D Extreme decreases in renal function may require discontinuation of ACE inhibitor therapy. However, decrements in renal function do not always necessitate discontinuance of ACE inhibitors; they do, however, require critical assessment by primary care providers.

   E Angioedema is an infrequent but severe complication that appears to occur more commonly in African Americans than in Caucasians. This adverse effect commonly involves the facial area and resolves with discontinuation of the drug. Laryngeal edema requires emergency management. Cross-reactivity between ACE inhibitors and ARBs is known to occur.[21]

   F Hematologic side effects include neutropenia and agranulocytosis.

   G Persons with preexisting connective tissue or renal disease appear to have skin rashes and taste disturbances (dysgeusia) with ACE inhibitors. This is an infrequent occurrence overall and may be more common with captopril, which contains a sulfhydryl group that is not present in other ACE inhibitors.

7 ACE inhibitors have an important role in the treatment of hypertension in persons with diabetes.

   A ACE inhibitors are preferred agents for treating hypertension, not only for their effects on blood pressure but additionally for their direct renoprotective effects.

   B For those with type 1 diabetes with or without hypertension and any degree of albuminuria, ACE inhibitors slow the progression of nephropathy.

   C For those with type 2 diabetes and hypertension, ACE inhibitors slow progression of microalbuminuria to macroalbuminuria.

   D When ACE inhibitors are not tolerated, ARBs should be considered.

Angiotensin II Receptor Blockers (ARBs) "sartan"

1 Multiple members of the angiotensin II receptor blockers (ARB) class are currently marketed in the United States either as single entities or in combination with other antihypertensive agents. With ARB/diuretic combination drug formulations, the hydrochlorothiazide doses can range from 12.5 to 25 mg.

2 A major pharmacologic effect of ARBs is to lower blood pressure by blocking the AT_1 receptor. Angiotensin II stimulation of the AT_1 receptor causes vasoconstriction, release of antidiuretic hormone and aldosterone, and activation of the sympathetic nervous system.

3 The pharmacokinetics and pharmacodynamics of ARBs are similar to those of the ACE inhibitors; however, distinct differences exist. As a group, the ARBs appear to have similar antihypertensive effects. Relatively small changes in blood pressure are seen when ARB doses are increased from low to moderate because of the relatively flat dose-response curve of these agents. Greater decrements in blood pressure are seen when ARBs are used in combination with low doses of thiazide-type diuretics. Food appears to have minimal effects on the absorption of ARBs.

4 Routine clinical monitoring with ARBs is similar to that required with ACE inhibitors and includes measuring blood pressure and serum electrolytes before and periodically during therapy. Hyperkalemia can occur soon after initiation of therapy. Renal function should be assessed before and periodically during therapy because impaired renal function can occur soon after initiation of therapy.

5 Certain contraindications and precautions are associated with ARBs.
   A As with ACE inhibitors, ARBs are contraindicated during pregnancy.
   B ARBs are contraindicated in persons with bilateral renal artery stenosis or unilateral stenosis of a single, functioning kidney.
   C ARBs must be used cautiously in the presence of impaired blood flow to the kidney.

6 Adverse effects associated with ARBs include hyperkalemia, renal insufficiency, and cough. The frequency of cough with ARBs is significantly less than that seen with ACE inhibitors. Angioedema also appears to occur even less frequently than with ACE inhibitors; however, reports of cross-reactivity exist.

7 ARBs have an important role in the treatment of hypertension in persons with diabetes.
   A ARBs are preferred agents for treating hypertension, not only for their effects on blood pressure but additionally for their direct renoprotective effects.
   B ARBs are an alternative agent for those who fail to tolerate an ACE inhibitor.
   C ARBs should be considered for persons with type 2 diabetes, hypertension, and nephropathy (with or without macroalbuminuria).

ß-Receptor Blockers

1 ß-receptor blockers are available as single entities or in fixed-dose combination with thiazide-type diuretics. Thiazide-type diuretic doses range from 5 to 25 mg. Several different subclasses of ß-receptor blockers are available and are outlined in Table 4.2.

2 The ß-receptor blockers are effective antihypertensive agents. Several mechanisms by which ß-blockers lower blood pressure have been proposed, including reducing cardiac output, decreasing peripheral resistance, and through various effects on plasma or tissue renin activity. ß-receptor blockers with intrinsic sympathomimetic activity (ISA) may provide less protection against cardiovascular events and may be less desirable for the treatment of hypertension than other ß-receptor blockers.

  A ß-receptor blockers are routinely employed after acute myocardial infarction because they have been shown to reduce the incidence of reinfarction and death when given after acute myocardial infarction.

  B ß-blockers are now commonly given to persons with heart failure. They were originally contraindicated in heart failure conditions, but have been shown to reduce mortality in some patient populations with heart failure.

3 There are differences in the pharmacokinetics and pharmacodynamics of the various ß-blockers, although their ability to lower blood pressure is similar. Both $ß_1$ and $ß_2$ adrenergic receptors are found throughout the body; some tissues and/or organs have higher concentrations of either $ß_1$ or $ß_2$-receptors. The heart and kidney have relatively higher $ß_1$ activity, whereas $ß_2$ activity is more predominant in the pancreas, lungs, liver, and smooth muscle.

  A Some ß-blockers are considered to be cardioselective when they preferentially block $ß_1$ receptors and have little or no effect on $ß_2$ adrenergic receptors.

  B Cardioselectivity refers to the specificity of binding to $ß_1$ adrenergic receptors. Cardioselectivity is seen at low-to-moderate doses only and not at high doses. Table 4.2 outlines agents that are relatively cardioselective.

  C Declines in both systolic and diastolic blood pressure usually occur with ß-blockers.

4 Routine clinical monitoring with ß-receptor blocker use includes measuring heart rate and blood pressure, obtaining a serum lipid profile before beginning therapy and when indicated thereafter, and measuring glycemic control.

5 There are certain cautions, contraindications, and precautions related to therapy with ß-receptor blockers.

  A High doses of ß-blockers should be used cautiously in persons with diabetes because these agents can block symptoms of hypoglycemia, impair insulin secretion, and slow glycogenolysis.

  B Abrupt cessation of ß-receptor blockers is not recommended. A washout period of at least 14 days is recommended to avoid an acute withdrawal syndrome, which sometimes exacerbates existing cardiovascular disease.

6 The following adverse effects are associated with ß-receptor blockers:

  A Bradycardia and other rhythm disorders

   B Congestive heart failure, which occurs most commonly when high doses are used in persons with preexisting left ventricular dysfunction

   C Bronchospasm, which occurs most commonly in persons with preexisting asthma or chronic obstructive pulmonary disease

   D Disorders of glucose metabolism or regulatory feedback; exacerbation of hypoglycemic unawareness can occur because ß-blockers impair several of the symptoms of hypoglycemia that rely on the sympathetic nervous system (both hyperglycemia and prolonged recovery from hypoglycemia can result from ß-blocker inhibition of insulin secretion and glycogenolysis)

   E Elevations in serum lipids and glucose

7 ß-receptor blockers have a role in the treatment of hypertension in persons with diabetes.

   A These agents are effective antihypertensive agents alone or in combination with other agents. Cardioselective agents in relatively lower doses may offer some advantages with respect to hypoglycemia awareness and glucose metabolism.

   B ß-receptor blockers are also indicated to reduce mortality after myocardial infarction.

good for Heart in low dose

Calcium Channel Blockers

1 There are 2 major types of calcium channel blockers (CCBs), nondihydropyridine and dihydropyridine (Table 4.2). CCBs are available as single agents or in fixed-dose combinations with ACE inhibitors.

   A The calcium channel blockers slow the influx of calcium across cell membranes and more specifically block 1 of the 2 major types of calcium channels. CCBs block the L-type calcium channel, which results in vasodilation of both coronary and peripheral vessels.

   B The nondihydropyridine agents have more depressive effects on cardiac conduction.

2 The CCBs demonstrate a wide range of pharmacokinetic effects. Both the nondihydropyridine and dihydropyridine classes have long- and short-acting agents. Sustained-release dosage forms are used in both classes of CCBs. For the treatment of hypertension, a sustained-release dosage form is used for all members of the nondihydropyridine group (diltiazem and verapamil).

3 Routine clinical monitoring with CCBs includes measuring heart rate and blood pressure and monitoring for peripheral edema.

4 Adverse effects associated with CCBs include cardiac conduction abnormalities, which occur infrequently with the nondihydropyridine agents and usually in persons with preexisting conduction problems; dizziness and flushing, which occur more commonly with the dihydropyridine agents; peripheral edema, which occurs with all classes of CCBs; acute hypotension; and constipation, which occurs most commonly with verapamil.

5 CCBs have a limited role in the treatment of hypertension in persons with diabetes.

   A CCBs can be used for the treatment of hypertension but are considered a secondary choice to other agents. Many diabetes experts recommend use of a nondihydropyridine CCB only when patients do not tolerate ACE inhibitors or ARBs.[15]

   B Dihydropyridine CCBs may have less impact on cardiovascular disease progression compared with other agents (ACE inhibitors, ARBs, diuretics, and ß-receptor blockers).

Pharmacologic Treatment of Dyslipidemia in Persons With Diabetes: Priorities and Goals

1 Aggressive treatment of dyslipidemia is recommended in persons with diabetes.[22] Recommendations are based on study results from a small numbers of persons with diabetes who have participated in several major lipid treatment trials. Lipid treatment studies specifically targeting persons with diabetes have yet to be completed.

   A The most common pattern of dyslipidemia in persons with type 2 diabetes is decreased HDL cholesterol and elevated triglycerides. LDL cholesterol, while not excessively elevated, may be more atherogenic due to smaller, dense particle size.

   B Although aggressive glycemic control alone has a significant impact on the development and progression of microvascular disease, it does not appear to similarly decrease macrovascular disease risk. Reduction of cardiovascular disease risk in persons with type 2 diabetes requires managing comorbid conditions such as dyslipidemia.

   C Persons with type 1 diabetes tend to have normal lipid profiles when they have good glycemic control. Aggressive lipid-lowering therapy should be considered in persons with type 1 diabetes when indicated according to treatment guidelines.

2 A priority order of treatment is suggested for managing diabetic dyslipidemia (see Table 4.3). The major goals include lowering LDL cholesterol, increasing HDL cholesterol, and lowering elevated triglycerides. The presence or absence of comorbid vascular disease determines the suggested set points for initiating drug therapy for dyslipidemia in persons with diabetes.

   A Without comorbid coronary heart disease (CHD), cerebrovascular disease (CVD), or peripheral vascular disease (PVD), lipid-lowering drug therapy is recommended when LDL cholesterol is greater than or equal to 130 mg/dL (3.2 mmol/L). Medical nutrition therapy should be implemented prior to or concurrent with drug therapy.

   B With concurrent CHD, CVD, or PVD, lipid-lowering drug therapy is recommended when LDL cholesterol is greater than or equal to 100 mg/dL (2.6 mmol/L). The primary treatment goal is to lower LDL cholesterol to less than 100 mg/dL (2.6 mmol/L). Medical nutrition therapy should be implemented prior to or concurrent with drug therapy.

Table 4.3. Recommended Priorities and Suggested Drug Therapies for the Treatment of Dyslipidemia in Persons With Diabetes

Priority	Dyslipidemia	Desired Action	Preferred Order of Therapy*
1	Elevated LDL-C	Lower LDL-C	1 Statins 2 Fenofibrate or bile acid binding resin
2	Low HDL-C	Raise HDL-C	1 Lifestyle modification 2 Fibrates or niacin
3	Elevated triglycerides	Lower triglycerides	1 Glycemic control 2 Fibrates or statins
4	Combined hyperlipidemia	Combination therapy	1 Glycemic control plus statin 2 Glycemic control plus statin and fibrate 3 Glycemic control plus bile acid binding resin and fibrate 4 Glycemic control plus statin and niacin

LDL-C = LDL cholesterol, HDL-C = HDL cholesterol.
*Drug therapy may not be a preferred choice or option.

C Pharmacotherapy can be considered when HDL cholesterol is less than 40 mg/dL (1.1 mmol/L). The HDL cholesterol goal in men is greater than 40 mg/dL (1.1 mmol/L) and in women is greater than 50 mg/dL (1.4 mmol/L).

D Triglyceride-lowering drug therapy may be considered when serum triglycerides are consistently greater than 200 mg/dL. The triglyceride goal is less than 150 mg/dL (1.7 mmol/L).
  • A non-HDL cholesterol level (total cholesterol minus HDL cholesterol) of less than 130 mg/dL (3.2 mmol/L) is a secondary treatment goal when triglycerides are elevated (>200 mg/dL [2.2 mmol/L]).[3]
  • Various behavioral and lifestyle modification therapies should be maximized prior to initiating triglyceride-lowering drug therapy, including modest weight loss and adequate physical activity.

3 Preference in the selection of lipid-lowering drugs is based on the type of dyslipidemia and currently available outcome data from major lipid-lowering trials that included subpopulations with diabetes.
  A Statins are considered the first-choice agents for lowering LDL cholesterol, and fibric acids are the primary choice for lowering triglycerides.

B Bile acid binding resins are secondary choices for lowering LDL cholesterol, and nicotinic acid is an alternative agent for lowering both LDL cholesterol and triglycerides.

C Combination drug therapy may be required to manage dyslipidemia.[23] Various combinations of statins, fibric acids, and/or niacin can increase risk of serious side effects (eg, myositis and liver dysfunction), and their safe use requires increased clinical monitoring and vigilance. Concurrent renal insufficiency further increases the risk of myositis with combined use of statins and fibric acids. A new class of agents that block cholesterol absorption, ezetimibe, are well tolerated and can be used alone or in combination with statins.

HMG-CoA Reductase Inhibitors (Statins)

1 At least 5 different HMG-CoA reductase inhibitors (statins) are currently available (see Table 4.4). Lowering LDL cholesterol with statins is achieved by changing endogenous cholesterol cycling. Statin effects on other lipid moieties are described in Table 4.4.

A Statins are competitive inhibitors of HMG-CoA reductase. HMG-CoA reductase (3-hydroxy-3-methylglutaryl coenzyme A reductase) is the rate-limiting enzyme involved in cholesterol biosynthesis.

B Statins enhance the catabolism of LDL cholesterol by increasing LDL receptor activity.

Table 4.4. Lipid-Lowering Therapies and Effects on Lipid Profile

Class/Agent	Total Chol	LDL	HDL	Trig
HMG-CoA reductase inhibitors (statins) • Atorvastatin • Fluvastatin • Lovastatin • Pravastatin • Simvastatin	↓↓↓	↓↓↓	↔↑	↔↓
Fibric acids • Clofibrate • Fenofibrate • Gemfibrozil	↓ ↔↑	↓ to ↓↓	↑	↓↓↓
Niacin	↓	↓	↑↑	↓↓↓
Bile acid resins • Cholestyramine • Colesevelam • Colestipol		↓ to ↓↓	↔	↓ or ↑
Cholesterol absorption inhibitors • Ezetimibe	↓ to ↓↓	↓ to ↓↓	↑	↓

The number of arrows indicates the strength of the effect. An arrow pointing sideways indicates a neutral effect.

2 Within the statin drug class are agents that have long and short half-lives and that exhibit variable potency. Agents of this class exhibit different degrees of protein binding. Some have active metabolites while others do not.

A The liver is the major organ of elimination for several of the statins, with 1 exception. Statins with hepatic metabolism via the cytochrome P450 3A4 enzyme system include lovastatin, simvastatin, and atorvastatin. Fluvastatin is more specifically cleared via the cytochrome P450 2C9 enzyme system. Pravastatin does not undergo appreciable hepatic elimination.

B Potency as determined by relative ability to lower LDL cholesterol has been characterized in clinical trials.[24]

C Statins are generally administered once daily.

D Bedtime or nighttime dosing yields maximal lowering of LDL cholesterol at any given dose with several of the lower potency statins (lovastatin, simvastatin, pravastatin, and fluvastatin). This effect is not seen with atorvastatin, which is currently the most potent statin.

3 Routine clinical monitoring with statins is required.

A Serum lipid concentrations should be measured at baseline and as indicated (6-8 weeks after initiation, 3-6 months after attaining the lipid-lowering goal, then annually thereafter) to assess the effect of the statin therapy.

B Liver enzymes should be assessed before beginning statin therapy and periodically thereafter.

- Recommendations for postexposure assessment of serum aminotransferase concentrations [AST (SGOT), ALT (SGPT)] range from 6 to 12 weeks after starting statin therapy or from any dose increase to semiannually for the first year of therapy.
- Some clinicians repeat enzymes at the time that lipid levels are reassessed (eg, 6-8 weeks after initiation, 3-6 months after attaining the lipid-lowering goal, then annually thereafter).

C Complaints of persistent or increasingly severe musculoskeletal symptoms may indicate the need for further laboratory assessment.

4 There are certain cautions, contraindications, and precautions related to lipid-lowering therapy with statins.

A Statin use is contraindicated in pregnancy.

B Statins should be used with caution in patients with impaired renal and/or hepatic function.

C Statins should be used with caution in patients with a history of or who currently have significant alcohol intake.

5 Adverse effects associated with statins are sometimes more common at higher doses or serum concentrations.

A Significant elevations of liver enzymes can occur. Statins should be discontinued when enzyme elevations are greater than 3 times the upper limit of normal.

B Musculoskeletal symptoms such as nonspecific muscle and joint pain are common with statin use. Persistent muscle and joint pain can indicate significant myopathy that must be investigated with further laboratory testing of serum creatinine kinase to rule out risk for rhabdomyolysis.

6 Clinically significant drug or food interactions can occur with statins.

A Statins that undergo hepatic metabolism via the cytochrome P450 3A4 enzyme system can interact with several classes of agents, resulting in excess serum statin concentrations and increased risk of toxicity. The risk of myopathy and/or rhabdomyolysis increases with concurrent use of cyclosporin, fibric acid derivatives, erythromycin, niacin, and some antifungal agents. Statin serum concentrations can increase significantly with concurrent use of nondihydropyridine CCBs.

B Grapefruit juice taken concurrently with some statins (eg, atorvastatin, lovastatin, and simvastatin) can increase statin bioavailability and increase serum concentrations. Consuming a large amount of grapefruit juice (greater than 240 mL) with statin doses should be avoided.

7 Statins have a significant role in the treatment of diabetic dyslipidemia (see Table 4.3).

A Statins are the first-choice drugs for lowering LDL cholesterol. The choice of the statin and the dose depend on the degree of LDL cholesterol lowering needed to attain the lipid goal.[24] Statins can be used in combination with other lipid-lowering therapy.

B Higher statin doses may have some triglyceride-lowering effects.

Fibric Acid Derivatives (Fibrates)

1 Three fibric acid derivatives, or fibrates, are available, of which either gemfibrozil or fenofibrate are commonly used when managing diabetic dyslipidemia (see Table 4.4).

2 Fibrates lower triglycerides and raise HDL cholesterol serum concentrations. LDL cholesterol may increase at the start of therapy depending on the type and extent of dyslipidemia. The exact mechanisms by which fibrates normalize the serum lipid profile are unknown. The following mechanisms have been suggested:

A Increased clearance of triglycerides and very-low-density lipoproteins (VLDL)

B Inhibition of cholesterol biosynthesis

C Decreased free fatty acid release and decreased hepatic secretion of VLDL

3 Routine clinical monitoring is required with the use of fibrates.

A Serum lipid concentrations should be measured at baseline and as indicated to assess the effect of the therapy.

B Liver enzymes should be assessed before the start of therapy and periodically thereafter.

C Musculoskeletal symptoms should be assessed routinely, and complaints of persistent or increasingly severe joint and muscle pain may indicate the need for further laboratory assessment.

D A complete blood count should be performed annually.

4 Fibrates are contraindicated in persons with severe hepatic impairment, severe renal dysfunction, and preexisting gallbladder disease.

5 Certain adverse effects are associated with the use of fibrates.

A Musculoskeletal effects, including myositis, myopathy, and rhabdomyolysis, occur more frequently when fibrates are used in combination with statins or in the presence of renal insufficiency.

B Cholelithiasis occurs infrequently. The use of fibrates can predispose persons to developing gallstones secondary to increased cholesterol excretion in bile.

C Hematologic abnormalities are rare but have occurred, including decreased hemoglobin and hematocrit, thrombocytopenia, and neutropenia.

6 Clinically significant drug interactions may occur with fibrates and oral anticoagulants, resulting in an increased incidence of bleeding. Combined use of statins and fibrates can increase the risk of musculoskeletal effects, including rhabdomyolysis. Use of cyclosporin with fibrates can increase the risk of cyclosporine-related impairment of renal function.

7 Fibrates have a specific role in the treatment of diabetic dyslipidemia (see Table 4.3).

A Fibrates are the primary drug therapy for lowering triglycerides but should only be used after good glycemic control is achieved.

B They are effective for raising HDL cholesterol.

C Fibrates are useful agents in combination with other lipid-lowering therapy. However, concurrent use with statins and niacin requires intensive monitoring.

Niacin

1 Niacin is available in 3 different oral formulations and in a fixed-dose combination with a statin (lovastatin). Formulations include immediate, sustained, and extended release.

2 Niacin favorably alters the lipid profile by reducing hepatic VLDL, which leads to a reduction in LDL cholesterol. Several mechanisms by which niacin alters lipid metabolism have been proposed, including inhibition of lipolysis, decreasing plasma free fatty acids, and direct effects on hepatic production of apolipoprotein B. Niacin also increases HDL cholesterol by reducing the catabolism of HDL cholesterol.

3 The pharmacokinetics and dosing of niacin depend on the type of formulation. Different formulations should not be used interchangeably. Currently, the preferable formulation for persons with diabetes is unclear, with some groups recommending immediate-release preparations (maximum 3 g/day) and others noting favorable effects with sustained-release forms (maximum 2 g/day).

4 Routine clinical monitoring is required with niacin therapy.

A Serum cholesterol and triglyceride concentrations should be measured at baseline and every 3 to 6 months during therapy.

B Liver enzymes should be assessed before starting therapy and periodically thereafter. Recommendations for postexposure assessment of serum aminotransferase concentrations [AST (SGOT), ALT (SGPT)] range from 6 to 12 weeks during the first year of therapy, then semiannually thereafter. Liver enzyme elevations are less frequent with niacin doses under 3 g daily.

C Glycemic control should be assessed routinely. Worsening glucose tolerance has been reported with relatively higher doses of niacin. Some persons with diabetes experience minimal changes in glucose tolerance when exposed to slow titration with sustained-release preparations.[25,26]

D Musculoskeletal symptoms should be assessed periodically. However, these symptoms are much more common when niacin is used in combination with statins or fibrates.

5 Cautions, contraindications, and precautions related to niacin include active liver disease; preexisting gout, which may be exacerbated by niacin use; and worsening of glucose control in persons with diabetes.

6 Certain adverse effects are associated with the use of niacin.
  A Flushing can occur, usually within 20 minutes of dosing with immediate-release preparations and within 2 to 4 hours with extended-release preparations. Symptoms may persist from ½ to 1½ hours. Symptoms usually improve with continued use. Flushing symptoms are thought to be prostaglandin-mediated and may be lessened with use of a nonsteroidal antiinflammatory agent (325 mg aspirin or 200 mg ibuprofen) prior to niacin administration or by taking niacin doses with meals.[27] Slow upward titration of the dose may decrease the flushing frequency and duration.
  B A significant number of individuals experience gastrointestinal effects such as dyspepsia, abdominal pain, and flatulence.
  C Dry eyes have been reported with niacin therapy.
  D Other clinical laboratory abnormalities are elevated plasma uric acid and elevated plasma glucose.

7 Niacin has a specific role in the treatment of diabetic dyslipidemia (see Table 4.3).
  A Niacin is a secondary agent for lowering LDL cholesterol and triglycerides or raising HDL cholesterol.
  B More frequent use of niacin in persons with diabetes may be acceptable.[25,26] Slow titration, lower doses, and the use of some sustained-release preparations may limit the negative effects of niacin on glycemia.
  C Niacin can be used in combination with other lipid-lowering therapies. However, more frequent side effects should be expected with combination therapy and monitoring should be appropriately intense.

Bile Acid Resins (BARs)

1 The available bile acid resins (BARs) are shown in Table 4.4. BARs are administered in 2 different dosage forms. Cholestyramine and colestipol are powders and are ingested as suspensions after dilution. Colesevelam is marketed in tablet form.

2 BARs have mixed effects on the lipid profile.
  A BARs decrease LDL cholesterol by binding bile acids in the gut, decreasing the available bile acids for the production of cholesterol and interrupting enterohepatic circulation of bile acids. This process results in the up-regulation of cholesterol synthesis and coincidentally increases the available LDL receptors and effectively lowers LDL cholesterol.
  B BARs increase triglycerides because VLDL production increases in parallel with the increase in cholesterol synthesis. Consequently, persons with high triglyceride concentrations prior to beginning BARs may experience further elevations after beginning BAR therapy.

3 Certain adverse effects are associated with the use of BARs.
   A Gastrointestinal effects can occur. Constipation is more common with higher BAR doses and in persons with preexisting constipation. Abdominal pain, bloating, and flatulence also occur.
   B Electrolyte disorders have been reported. Persons with renal insufficiency can develop hyperchloremic acidosis.

4 Clinically significant drug interactions can occur with the use of BARs.
   A When coadministered, BARs nonspecifically bind with an extensive number of pharmacologic agents. Therefore, BARs should not be coadministered with other pharmacologic agents. Persons taking BARs should be counseled to take other medications 1 hour before or 4 hours after taking their dose of bile acid resins.
   B Chronic therapy with BARs can result in various vitamin deficiencies, such as reduced absorption of fat-soluble vitamins and folic acid.

5 BARs have a limited role in the treatment of diabetic dyslipidemia (see Table 4.3).
   A BARs are considered secondary agents for lowering LDL cholesterol in persons with diabetes.
   B Although BARs can be used in combination with other lipid-lowering therapies, the timing of ingestion of the agents must be carefully considered to minimize drug binding interactions.

Self-Review Questions

1 What are the 4 stages of hypertension?
2 What is the treatment goal for hypertension?
3 What 4 classes of hypertensive agents are generally prescribed for persons with diabetes?
4 How are diuretics used for antihypertensive therapy in persons with diabetes?
5 Why are ACE inhibitors and ARBs preferred agents for treating hypertension in persons with diabetes?
6 When are ß-receptor blockers and CCBs prescribed for treatment of hypertension in persons with diabetes?
7 What are the treatment priorities and goals for lipid-lowering therapy in diabetic dyslipidemia?
8 Why are statins the first-choice drugs for lowering LDL cholesterol?
9 What is the primary drug therapy for lowering triglycerides?
10 When are niacin and BARs used in the treatment of diabetic dyslipidemia?

Key Educational Considerations

1 As with blood glucose-lowering agents, medications are not a substitute for medical nutrition therapy and physical activity in persons with hypertension and dyslipidemia.

2 Therapy should be individualized for treating hypertension and dyslipidemia based on the person's other comorbidities, laboratory findings, and ability to comply with therapy.

3 The action and interaction of herbal remedies and over-the-counter products on blood glucose, blood pressure, and cholesterol should not be dismissed and must be taken into consideration when determining the effectiveness of prescribed therapy for these conditions.

4 Medications such as hydrochlorothiazide and niacin, which have been considered contraindicated or as causing adverse effects on blood glucose, blood pressure, and cholesterol, may be used, in some cases, without adverse effects when administered in lower doses.

5 When persons are taking certain medications to treat blood glucose, blood pressure, and cholesterol, laboratory monitoring of electrolytes and hepatic and renal function is as important as monitoring of blood glucose, blood pressure, and cholesterol levels.

6 Monotherapy to treat elevations in blood glucose, blood pressure, and cholesterol is usually ineffective. To reach clinical goals, combination therapy using agents with different mechanisms of action is usually required.

Learning Assessment: Case Study 1

FB is a 55-year-old white male with type 2 diabetes that was diagnosed a week ago during his annual employee physical exam. His fasting blood glucose level was 179 mg/dL (9.9 mmol/L)when initially tested and 184 mg/dL (10.2 mmol/L) when rechecked 4 days later. His blood pressure was 165/87 mm Hg during the initial exam and 162/89 mm Hg at the follow-up appointment. The following information summarizes FB's medical history and current health status.

Past medical history
Seasonal allergies
Obesity

Family history
(+) Diabetes
(+) Stroke
(+) Hypertension
(+) Dyslipidemia
(+) Heart failure

Social history
(+) cigarette smoker for 30 years (2 packs per day)
Alcohol, occasionally

Current medications
Fexofenadine D bid (seasonally)
Ephedra/guarana-containing weight-loss/energy capsules

Physical exam
Weight 235 lb (107 kg), decreased by 5 lb over the past 2 months
Height 5 ft 10 in

Waist circumference 43 in
BMI 34 kg/m^2
Pulse 83 bpm
Total cholesterol 215 mg/dL
LDL cholesterol 117 mg/dL
HDL cholesterol 28 mg/dL
Triglycerides 350 mg/dL

Questions for Discussion

1 Is FB currently taking anything that may be adversely affecting his blood pressure?

2 What about his lifestyle would you like to learn more about?

3 Does FB have hypertension based on the information given, and if so, what stage of hypertension does he have (based on the classification guidelines established by the Joint National Committee on the Prevention, Detection and Treatment of High Blood Pressure)?

4 If FB has hypertension, should drug therapy be initiated, and if so, which agent would be the best initial therapy?

5 What other lab test should be performed?

Discussion

1 FB's elevated blood pressure may be due to several factors.

A The decongestant in fexofenadine D contains 120 mg of pseudoephedrine. Oral nasal decongestants may increase blood pressure and should be avoided or used in smaller milligram dosages for a shorter time. An oral antihistamine would be a better option for treating his seasonal allergies. If FB has nasal congestion along with the allergies, a nasal saline spray may be used.

B The ephedra in the weight-loss and energy capsule has been shown to increase blood pressure as well as increase the incidence of stroke. Since 1994, there have been over 100 deaths reported due to the use of these products, and many more cases have probably not been reported. Between 1993 and 2001, the FDA reported that 59% of deaths and 63% of reports of hypertension from dietary supplements were due to products that contain ephedra. Guarana, which is related to caffeine, contains methylxanthine, a stimulant that can increase blood pressure and contains large amounts of theophylline, theobromine, and tannic acids.

2 It would be helpful to learn the following information about FB's lifestyle:

A Physical activity history. If FB has not been exercising recently, he should undergo an exercise stress test and get clearance from his physician to begin exercising. An exercise program can be as simple as walking for 5 minutes at a time and increasing the frequency and distance to achieve a goal of 150 minutes per week, or 10 000 steps per day. By increasing his physical activity, FB may decrease his systolic blood pressure by 4 to 9 mm Hg.

B Whether FB has been following a diet and what type. An individualized meal assessment can be performed and a meal plan can be developed incorporating the DASH (Dietary Approaches to Stop Hypertension) diet principles. A decrease in systolic blood pressure of 8 to 14 mm Hg can be obtained with the DASH diet. FB's carbohydrate consumption should be assessed and recommendations should be made for the appropriate amount of carbohydrates in his diet.

C What stage FB is in with regard to his cigarette smoking. If he is in the ready phase, enrollment in a smoking cessation program with nicotine replacement therapy may be beneficial.

D Whether FB would want to try to achieve weight loss through lifestyle modification rather than through herbal supplements. Maintaining a body mass index of 18.5 to 24.9 kg/m^2 or achieving a 10-kg weight loss can lower his systolic blood pressure by approximately 5 to 20 mm Hg.

E Whether FB takes other over-the-counter products such as nonsteroidal anti-inflammatory drugs on a chronic basis, consumes large amounts of licorice, or takes any other herbal or natural products.

3 Based on FB's blood pressure readings, he would be classified as having stage 2 hypertension. A new stage called prehypertension has been added for when blood pressure is 120 to 139 mm Hg systolic and 80 to 89 mm Hg diastolic. The blood pressure goal for people with diabetes is less than 130/80 mm Hg.

4 It may be necessary for FB to take more than 1 blood-pressure-lowering agent to reach the goal of 130/80 mm Hg. When the systolic blood pressure is 20 mm Hg above target and the diastolic blood pressure is 10 mm Hg above target, initial therapy with 2 agents should be considered.

A If discontinuing the oral nasal decongestant and weight-loss capsules does not immediately lower his blood pressure to within target ranges, and if other lifestyle modifications are unsuccessful, several options for initial antihypertensive agents may be started.

- Thiazide diuretics in low doses, such as hydrochlorothiazide 12.5 to 25 mg or chlorthalidone 12.5 to 25 mg daily, can be used without affecting glucose tolerance or adversely affecting lipid or uric acid levels.
- Thiazide diuretics, along with beta blockers, calcium channel blockers, angiotensin-converting enzyme (ACE) inhibitors, and angiotensin receptor blockers (ARBs), are beneficial for decreasing the incidence of stroke and cardiovascular disease.
- There are several studies that show that the use of some ACE inhibitors and some ARBs can decrease blood pressure, slow the progression of nephropathy, and reduce albuminuria.

B It would be helpful to have information about FB's health insurance to determine if the ability to afford his medications is or will become a compliance issue. If he does not have insurance, or if the copayments are too high, use of generic medications should be considered.

5 Other lab tests that may be considered include urinalysis; hematocrit; serum potassium, calcium, sodium, and creatinine; and thyroid function tests.

Learning Assessment: Case Study 2

TO is a 43-year-old Hispanic male who has had type 2 diabetes for 4 years and has never had a fasting lipid panel performed. He just returned from his first diabetes education training session and is anxious to find out what his cholesterol readings are after learning about lipids in the class. When TO asks his healthcare provider for the results, he learns that his readings are as follows:

Weight 265 lb (120 kg), increased by 5 lb over the past 4 months
Height 5 ft 4 in
Waist circumference 56 in
BMI 46 kg/m²
Blood pressure 127/79 mm Hg
Pulse 89 bpm
Total cholesterol 300 mg/dL
LDL cholesterol 222 mg/dL
HDL cholesterol 28 mg/dL
Triglycerides 250 mg/dL

Questions for Discussion

1 What other information would you want to gather from TO to assist in determining his therapy?

2 What would be the most appropriate initial therapy to treat TO's dyslipidemia?

3 Would a bile acid sequestrant be a proper choice of a lipid-lowering agent for TO?

Discussion

1 TO's living arrangements should be assessed to determine whether he prepares his meals. A meal recall would also be helpful for determining if his meal plan is adversely contributing to his increased weight and elevated lipid levels.

2 Assess TO's level of physical activity to see if he is getting an adequate amount of exercise. If it has been a while since TO exercised on a regular basis, advise him to obtain medical clearance to do so.

3 Review his financial resources and insurance status to determine if either of these areas is a potential barrier to treatment.

4 Assess his use of alcohol and tobacco products.

5 Perform other lab tests such as liver function tests, thyroid function tests, and repeat fasting lipid profiles.

6 TO's dyslipidemia therapy should be initiated with a statin to lower his LDL cholesterol levels. Statin therapy may further improve TO's lipid profile by raising HDL cholesterol and possibly lowering triglycerides.

7 Niacin can be used in persons with diabetes, although some reports of therapeutic doses of 2 to 3 g/day have indicated aggravation of insulin resistance. Other reports indicate that these adverse effects are transient and, with proper dose titration and time, the use of niacin should not be a concern. Additional blood glucose monitoring may be needed to assess the individual impact on blood glucose levels. Flushing of the face and trunk is a common side effect that can be decreased by taking a 325-mg aspirin 30 minutes before taking the dose of niacin.

8 Fibric acid derivatives such as gemfibrozil and fenofibrate are used mainly to decrease triglyceride levels, which are commonly elevated in persons with type 2 diabetes. It has been recently found that persons taking gemfibrozil and repaglinide may be at risk for hypoglycemia due to the potential of gemfibrozil to prolong the duration of action of repaglinide.

9 Bile acid resins should not be used in persons with diabetes when their triglycerides are elevated because these agents can increase triglyceride levels. The common lipid profile for persons with type 2 diabetes includes low HDL cholesterol and high triglycerides. Another common problem is the ability of bile acid resins to bind to other drugs, making it necessary to take other medications 1 hour before or 4 hours after the bile acid resins. Gastrointestinal side effects are common.[28]

References

1 West KM, Ahuja MM, Bennett PH, et al. The role of circulating glucose and triglyceride concentrations and their interactions with other "risk factors" as determinants of arterial disease in nine diabetic population samples from the WHO Multinational Study. Diabetes Care. 1983;6:361-369.

2 Krolewski AS, Kosinski EJ, Warram JH, et al. Magnitude and determinants of coronary artery disease in juvenile-onset, insulin-dependent diabetes mellitus. Am J Cardiol. 1987;59:750-755.

3 National Cholesterol Education Program (NCEP) Expert Panel on Detection, Evaluation, and Treatment of High Blood Cholesterol in Adults (Adult Treatment Panel III). Executive summary of the 3rd report of the National Cholesterol Education Program (NCEP) Expert Panel on Detection, Evaluation, and Treatment of High Blood Cholesterol in Adults (Adult Treatment Panel III) final report. Circulation. 2002; 106:3143-3421.

4 Kannel WB, McGee DL. Diabetes and glucose tolerance as risk factors for cardiovascular disease: the Framingham Study. Diabetes Care. 1979;2:120-126.

5 Wingard DL, Barrett-Connor E. Heart disease and diabetes. In: Harris MI, ed. Diabetes in America. Bethesda, Md: National Institutes of Health, National Institute of Diabetes and Digestive and Kidney Diseases;1995:429-448.

6 Kannel WB, McGee DL. Diabetes and cardiovascular disease. The Framingham Study. JAMA. 1979; 241:2035-2038.

7 Laakso M, Lehto S. Epidemiology of macrovascular disease in diabetes. Diabetes Rev. 1979;5:294-315.

8 Alexander CM, Landsman PB, Teutsch SM, Haffner SM. NCEP-defined metabolic syndrome, diabetes, and prevalence of coronary heart disease among NHANES III participants age 50 years and older. Diabetes. 2003;52:1210-1214.

9 Gaede P, Vedel P, Larsen N, Jensen GV, Parving HH, Pedersen O. Multifactorial intervention and cardiovascular disease in patients with type 2 diabetes [comment]. N Engl J Med. 2003;348:383-393.

10 American Diabetes Association. Standards of medical care for patients with diabetes mellitus (position statement). Diabetes Care. 2003;26(suppl 1):S33-S50.

11 American Association of Clinical Endocrinologists and American College of Endocrinology. The American Association of Clinical Endocrinologists medical guidelines for the management of diabetes: the AACE system of intensive diabetes self-management—2002 update. Endocr Pract. 2002;8(suppl 1):41-82.

12 Jellinger PS, Dickey RA, Ganda OP, et al. The American Association of Clinical Endocrinologists medical guidelines for clinical practice for the diagnosis and treatment of dyslipidemia and prevention of atherogenesis 2002 amended version. Endocr Pract. 2000;6:3-52.

13 Chobanian AV, Bakris GL, Black HR, et al; National Heart, Lung, and Blood Institute Joint National Committee on Prevention, Detection, Evaluation and Treatment of High Blood Pressure. The 7th report of the Joint National Committee on Prevention, Detection, Evaluation, and Treatment of High Blood Pressure: the JNC 7 report. JAMA. 2003;289:2560-2572.

14 National Kidney Foundation. K/DOQI clinical practice guidelines for managing dyslipidemia in chronic kidney disease. Am J Kidney Dis. 2002;39(suppl 2):S1-S246.

15 American Diabetes Association. Treatment of hypertension in adults with diabetes (position statement). Diabetes Care. 2003; 26(suppl 1):S80-S82.

16 Savage PJ, Pressel SL, Curb JD, et al. Influence of long-term, low-dose, diuretic-based, antihypertensive therapy on glucose, lipid, uric acid, and potassium levels in older men and women with isolated systolic hypertension: The Systolic Hypertension in the Elderly Program. SHEP Cooperative Research Group. Arch Intern Med. 1998;158:741-751.

17 Lakshman MR, Reda DJ, Materson BJ, Cushman WC, Freis ED. Diuretics and beta-blockers do not have adverse effects at 1 year on plasma lipid and lipoprotein profiles in men with hypertension. Department of Veterans Affairs Cooperative Study Group on Antihypertensive Agents. Arch Intern Med. 1999;159:551-558.

18 Grimm RH Jr, Flack JM, Grandits GA, et al. Long-term effects on plasma lipids of diet and drugs to treat hypertension. Treatment of Mild Hypertension Study (TOMHS) Research Group [comment]. JAMA. 1996;275:1549-1556.

19 Sullivan TJ. Cross-reactions among furosemide, hydrochlorothiazide, and sulfonamides. JAMA. 1991;265:120-121.

20 Douglas JG, Bakris GL, Epstein M, et al. Management of high blood pressure in African Americans: consensus statement of the Hypertension in African Americans Working Group of the International Society on Hypertension in Blacks. Arch Intern Med. 2003;163:525-541.

21 Rivera JO. Losartan-induced angioedema. Ann Pharmacother. 1999;33:933-935.

22 American Diabetes Association. Management of dyslipidemia in adults with diabetes (position statement). Diabetes Care. 2003;26(suppl 1):S83-S86.

23 Worz CR, Bottorff M. Treating dyslipidemic patients with lipid-modifying and combination therapies. Pharmacotherapy. 2003;23:625-637.

24 Jones P, Kafonek S, Laurora I, Hunninghake D. Comparative dose efficacy study of atorvastatin versus simvastatin, pravastatin, lovastatin, and fluvastatin in patients with hypercholesterolemia (the CURVES Study)[erratum appears in Am J Cardiol. 1998;82:128]. Am J Cardiol. 1998;81:582-587.

25 Elam MB, Hunninghake DB, Davis KB, et al. Effect of niacin on lipid and lipoprotein levels and glycemic control in patients with diabetes and peripheral arterial disease: the ADMIT Study: A randomized trial. Arterial Disease Multiple Intervention Trial. JAMA. 2000;284:1263-1270.

26 Grundy SM, Vega GL, McGovern ME, et al. Efficacy, safety, and tolerability of once-daily niacin for the treatment of dyslipidemia associated with type 2 diabetes: results of the Assessment of Diabetes Control and Evaluation of the Efficacy of Niaspan Trial. Arch Intern Med. 2002;162:1568-1576.

27 Whelan AM, Price SO, Fowler SF, Hainer BL. The effect of aspirin on niacin-induced cutaneous reactions. J Fam Pract. 1992;34:165-168.

28 Niemi M, Backman JT, Neuvonen M, Neuvonen PJ. Effects of gemfibrozil, itraconazole, and their combination on the pharmacokinetics and pharmacodynamics of repaglinide: Potentially hazardous interaction between gemfibrozil and repaglinide. Diabetologia. 2003;46(6):347-51.

Suggested Readings

Carter BL, Saseen JL. Hypertension. In: Dipiro JT, Talbert RL, Yee GC, Matzke GR, Wells BG, Posey LM, eds. Pharmacotherapy: A Pathophysiologic Approach. 5th ed. New York: McGraw-Hill; 2002:157-183.

Talbert RL. Hyperlipidemia. In: Dipiro JT, Talbert RL, Yee GC, Matzke GR, Wells BG, Posey LM, eds. Pharmacotherapy: A Pathophysiologic Approach. 5th ed. New York: McGraw-Hill; 2002:395-417.

American Hospital Formulary Service Drug Information 2002. Bethesda, Md: American Society of Health-System Pharmacists; 2002 (see also www.ashp.org and www.ahfs-druginformation.com)

Internet Resources

American Association of Clinical Endocrinologists
http://www.aace.com/clin/guidelines/diabetes_2002.pdf

American Diabetes Association
http://www.diabetes.org/

Learning Assessment: Post-Test Questions

Pharmacologic Therapies for Hypertension and Dyslipidemia

4

1 LB is a 53-year-old African-American male who has a family history of hypertension. At his latest visit to his physician his blood pressure was 143/87 mm Hg. According to national blood pressure guidelines, how would LB's blood pressure be classified?
A Normal
B Prehypertension
C Stage 1 hypertension
D Stage 2 hypertension

2 The blood pressure goal for people with diabetes is
A <120/80 mm Hg
B <130/80 mm Hg
C >140/90 mm Hg
D 160/100 mm Hg

3 Which of the following statements about the treatment of hypertension in persons with diabetes is not true?
A ACE inhibitors are the drug of choice for treating hypertension in persons with diabetes and are the only blood-pressure-lowering agents that should be used in this population
B Combination therapy is often needed for persons to reach their blood pressure goal and may include agents such as ß-receptor blockers, thiazide diuretics, and calcium channel blockers
C Thiazide diuretics in doses of 6.25 to 25 mg daily can be safely used in people with diabetes
D Laboratory testing, including electrolytes, is often needed in persons who are being medically treated for hypertension

4 The major pharmacologic effects of ACE inhibitors are thought to include
A Decreasing concentrations of the potent vasoconstrictor angiotensin II through blockade of angiotensin II production via the renin-angiotensin system
B Direct inhibition of arterial wall and kidney tissue by the renin-angiotensin systems
C Blood pressure lowering within 1 hour of dosing, and maximal effects at 6 to 8 hours
D All of the above are true about ACE inhibitors

5 JB is a 47-year-old white female who has just returned from her healthcare provider's office. She had a fasting lipid profile done as part of a physical that is required for her new job. She has diabetes and is prescribed erythromycin for an infection (due to her penicillin allergy) and ketoconazole for a fungal infection. Her lipid panel results are as follows:

Total cholesterol	212 mg/dL
LDL cholesterol	124 mg/dL
HDL cholesterol	34 mg/dL
Triglycerides	270 mg/dL

What would be the best next step in JB's treatment?
A Use therapeutic lifestyle changes for 6 months, then consider medications
B Since her LDL cholesterol is already over 100 mg/dL, start her on a fibric acid derivative as first-line therapy
C Since her LDL cholesterol is already over 100 mg/dL, start her on simvastatin
D Due to the potential drug interactions between certain HMG-CoA (statins) therapies, JB should be started on pravastatin and have liver function tests performed if they have not been done already

6 The most common laboratory profile of diabetic dyslipidemia in persons with type 2 diabetes is
  A High HDL cholesterol and LDL cholesterol
  B High LDL cholesterol and low triglycerides
  C Low LDL cholesterol and low HDL cholesterol
  D Low HDL cholesterol and high triglycerides

7 Contraindications and potential side effects of treatment with angiotensin converting enzyme (ACE) inhibitors include all of the following except
  A A dry, hacking cough
  B Use during pregnancy
  C Bilateral renal artery stenosis or unilateral stenosis of a single, functioning kidney
  D Weight gain with worsening glycemic control

8 Fibric acid derivatives such as fenofibrate and gemfibrozil primarily lower
  A LDL cholesterol
  B HDL cholesterol
  C Triglycerides
  D Small, dense LDL cholesterol particles

9 Which of the following statements about the use of nicotinic acid (niacin) is not true?
  A Niacin is contraindicated in persons with diabetes because of worsening insulin resistance
  B Niacin may be used in persons with diabetes; dosages should be slowly titrated to 2 g daily and blood glucose levels should be monitored closely
  C Niacin effectively lowers LDL cholesterol and triglyceride levels and raises HDL cholesterol levels
  D Niacin-related flushing may be decreased by taking doses with meals or taking a 325-mg aspirin 30 minutes before the niacin dose

10 Which of the following is a true statement about HMG-CoA inhibitors (statins)?
  A Statins are the preferred agent for lowering LDL cholesterol in persons with diabetes
  B Testing liver function at baseline, when dosage increases are made, and periodically is not necessary
  C All statins should be given at bedtime since more cholesterol synthesis occurs during the night
  D Statins can be used safely by children and by women who become pregnant

11 When using drug therapy for dyslipidemia, the treatment goal for triglyceride concentrations
  A Should be <150 mg/dL for persons with diabetes
  B Is the same for people with and without diabetes
  C Is not important, only the lowering of LDL cholesterol is important
  D Should be >40 mg/dL for men and women

12 When using ß-blockers in persons with diabetes,
  A Worsening of hypoglycemic unawareness can occur as ß-blockers mask symptoms of hypoglycemia that are mediated by the sympathetic nervous system
  B Neither hyperglycemia or prolonged recovery from hypoglycemia can result from ß-blocker inhibition of insulin secretion and glycogenolysis
  C Elevations in serum lipids and glucose are usually not a concern
  D Cardioselective ß-blockers (eg, bisoprolol or atenolol), in relatively lower doses, do not offer any advantages with respect to hypoglycemia awareness and glucose metabolism

13 Which group of blood-pressure-lowering agents has been shown to decrease blood pressure, slow the progression of nephropathy, and reduce albuminuria in people with diabetes?
  A Thiazide diuretics
  B Loop diuretics
  C Angiotensin II receptor blockers
  D Calcium channel blockers

See next page for answer key.

Post-Test Answer Key

Pharmacologic Therapies for Hypertension and Dyslipidemia

4

1	C	**8**	C
2	B	**9**	A
3	A	**10**	A
4	D	**11**	A
5	D	**12**	A
6	D	**13**	C
7	D		

A Core Curriculum for Diabetes Education
Diabetes Management Therapies

Monitoring 5

Virginia Peragallo-Dittko, APRN, BC-ADM, MA, CDE
Diabetes Education Center
Winthrop-University Hospital
Mineola, New York

Introduction

1 Regular monitoring is an essential component of any diabetes management program.

2 Monitoring by the individual with diabetes includes self-monitoring of blood glucose (SMBG), serum ketones, and urine ketones (and urine glucose, if recommended).

3 Monitoring of metabolic control by the healthcare team involves assessing glycosylated hemoglobin and fructosamine; reviewing blood glucose patterns; assessing growth and patterns of weight change; and monitoring the development and progression of long-term complications, including urinary protein measurements, blood pressure measurements, and lipid levels. This area of diabetes care clearly combines the diabetes educator's skills of management and education.

Objectives

Upon completion of this chapter, the learner will be able to

1 List recommended preprandial and postprandial blood glucose ranges.

2 List factors that affect the accuracy of self-monitoring of blood glucose (SMBG) results.

3 Describe the most common user error related to SMBG.

4 Identify 3 critical uses of SMBG data by persons with diabetes.

5 Describe 2 ways that SMBG results are used to teach an abstract principle of diabetes management.

6 Identify 2 psychosocial adaptations related to SMBG.

7 Identify the SMBG needs of special populations.

8 Explain the measurement methods and target ranges for glycosylated hemoglobin, fructosamine, and urinary protein.

9 List the treatment targets for blood pressure and blood lipids.

10 List the indications for tests of ketonemia, ketonuria, and glycosuria.

11 Identify how to use documentation of weight patterns as a monitoring tool.

Self-Monitoring of Blood Glucose

1 Self-monitoring of blood glucose is an important component of the treatment plan for persons with diabetes mellitus because it provides immediate feedback and data for the following:

A Achieving and maintaining specific glycemic goals.

B Preventing and detecting hypoglycemia and avoiding severe hypoglycemia.

C Adjusting care in response to changes in lifestyle of individuals and the need to add or adjust pharmacologic therapy.

D Determining the need for insulin therapy in gestational diabetes mellitus.[1]

E Evaluating the glycemic response to types and amounts of food and physical activity.

2 It is essential to ensure the accuracy of the blood glucose monitoring values because these values are used to make treatment decisions concerning medication dosage adjustment, food intake or timing, and exercise timing.

A Blood glucose meters designed for home use are not completely accurate. The American Diabetes Association (ADA) recommends that the performance goal for blood glucose meters should be a total error of less than 10% at blood glucose levels of 30 mg/dL to 400 mg/dL (1.7 mmol/L to 22.2 mmol/L), 100% of the time.[1] Many products do not meet this performance goal.

B Accuracy is defined as the "degree of conformity of a measure to a standard or true value." For blood glucose meters, the laboratory is the standard against which they are judged.

- The laboratory measures venous blood glucose and the meter measures capillary blood glucose. By the time blood reaches the veins, some of the glucose in the blood has been transferred to other tissues, so the blood flowing through the veins has less glucose than the blood flowing through the capillaries. After a fast of 8 or more hours, the difference between the level of glucose in capillary blood and in venous blood is very small. After a meal, the difference can be quite large, as blood glucose levels rise and the rate of glucose transfer into the tissue accelerates.

- Another consideration concerning the accuracy of blood glucose meters concerns the difference between whole blood glucose and plasma blood glucose. Whole blood is composed of plasma (serum) and 3 formed elements: red blood cells (erythrocytes), white blood cells (leukocytes), and platelets. The glucose content of red blood cells is about 20% less than the glucose content of plasma, due to the density of the red blood cells. Since whole blood consists of approximately equal portions of plasma and red blood cells, a mixture of the 2 would yield a glucose value about 11% to 15% lower than plasma alone as measured in the laboratory.

- While all meters use a drop of whole blood on the test strip, the majority of the meters read the plasma glucose level or have been programmed to calculate the plasma glucose level. A meter that provides plasma glucose levels will have results that are closer to the laboratory's results.

- Because a meter that reports whole blood values and a meter that reports plasma values will have different results for the same blood sample, there are different preprandial blood glucose treatment goals for whole blood or plasma. The American College of Endocrinology (ACE) recommends a preprandial plasma glucose target value of <110 mg/dL (6.1 mmol/L).[2] The American Diabetes Association recommends a preprandial plasma glucose target between 90 mg/dL and 130 mg/dL (5.0 mmol/L and 7.2 mmol/L).[3] Previously they also included recommendations for whole blood glucose target goals before a meal of between 80 mg/dL and 120 mg/dL (4.4 mmol/L and 6.7 mmol/L).

C Other factors that may influence the results of SMBG systems include variations in the hematocrit (some systems are accurate with hematocrit ranges of 0% to 60%), altitude, environmental temperature and humidity, hypotension, hypoxia, and triglyceride concentrations.[1]

D User error is the most common reason for inaccurate results. Potential sources of user error include strips that are improperly stored, expired, or defective; an uncalibrated meter; a soiled meter; or an inadequate blood sample.

- The strips must be stored according to the manufacturer's guidelines to yield accurate results. These guidelines also refer to avoiding exposure to heat, cold, and humidity during shipping.

- Teach patients to check the expiration date of the strips, especially when a mail-order shipment could include strips that expire within a few months and need to be used immediately. Because strips are costly, patients are commonly tempted to use expired strips. This may lead to inaccurate readings.

- Control solution is a product that is provided by manufacturers to verify that the meter and strips are working properly. This underused method of verifying accuracy operates the same way that the patient monitors a drop of blood. Every manufacturer provides at least 1 control solution and some have low-, normal- and high-level control solutions to test the meter at extremes.

- Calibrating the meter is another way to ensure the most accurate results. Some meters automatically calibrate the strips with the meter, whereas other meters require setting a code or inserting a chip or strip to calibrate the meter.

- With some meters, the blood sample intended for the strip may come in contact with the meter and soil the optic window. This will yield inaccurate results. The manufacturers provide instructions for cleaning the meter.

- An inadequate blood sample is the most frequent cause of inaccurate results and errors in subsequent treatment decisions. Some meters will reject an inadequate sample whereas other meters have a feature that signals the user when the blood sample is not large enough to provide an accurate reading. Unfortunately, this feature creates a false sense of security because users assume that if they do not get the signal, they have given an adequate sample. The meter will only signal the user about a blood sample it cannot process; any other sample—even an inadequate one—will register a reading, but the reading will be inaccurate. Patients should be asked at every opportunity to demonstrate their technique for using their meters. This demonstration gives the educator an opportunity to verify technique, provide advice, or clean a soiled unit.

- Some individuals have difficulty securing a drop of blood and may require guidance in choosing a lancing device or meter. Providing individualized guidance for each person's needs minimizes waste of strips and eases the person's frustration with blood glucose monitoring.

- Guidelines for determining the accuracy of a blood glucose meter are summarized in Table 5.1.[4]

E Persons with diabetes should be taught specific directions for securing an adequate blood sample.[5] For example, when using the fingertips as a puncture site, the person should be aware of the following procedures:

- Vigorously wash hands with warm water to increase circulation to fingertips.

- Try hanging the hand at your side for 30 seconds so the blood can pool in your hand.

- Shake the hand to be pricked as though you were shaking down a thermometer. *pricked*

- Use a lancing device or endcap that will allow a deeper puncture or a larger gauge lancet.

- After your finger is punctured, gently milk the blood from the bottom to the tip of your finger until the blood drop is the correct size. Milking the finger works better than just squeezing the fingertips.

F Meters and strips have been designed to use alternative sites such as the forearm, upper arm, or thigh for puncture.

Table 5.1. Guidelines for Determining Accuracy of a Blood Glucose Meter[4]

1 Blood glucose meter results should be compared against the laboratory values, not against another meter.

2 Compare fasting blood glucose levels only. After-meal levels will differ between capillary blood (as measured on the meter) and venous blood (as measured in the laboratory).

3 To compare meter and laboratory results, the 2 tests must be done at the same time. Patients who measure their blood glucose at home either before or after the venipuncture allow too much time between the readings for a valid comparison.

4 The venous blood must be spun by a centrifuge machine to separate the plasma from the erythrocytes within 30 minutes after the time the blood sample was taken. If it is not spun, the glucose in the blood will begin to break down and the results will not accurately reflect the blood glucose levels at the time the sample was collected.

5 Comparing meter to laboratory involves a fingertip or alternative site puncture and a venipuncture. Applying a drop of blood from the venipuncture needle is not acceptable. Some strips are designed for capillary blood only and will give false readings if venous blood is used.

6 A meter that reports whole blood glucose levels will have a reading 11% to 15% lower than the laboratory.

- There is wide discordance between fingertip and alternative site samples when blood glucose levels are changing rapidly due to circulatory physiology. Blood circulation in the skin of the fingers and palm of the hand is distinctly different from that in the arms and legs. The blood flow through the arteriovenous shunts in the fingertips proceeds at a higher velocity than the flow through other capillaries of the skin. Therefore, the transient difference between alternative site and fingertip during rapid blood glucose changes is a result of this decreased velocity of blood flow to sites such as the forearm.[6]
- When blood glucose concentration is falling rapidly, this lag between alternative site and fingertip could cause a delay in detection of hypoglycemia if an alternative site is being used for measuring glucose levels. In preprandial monitoring, glucose levels are in a steady state, so the difference between alternative site and fingertip samples is small and not clinically significant, but for up to 2 hours postprandially the blood glucose is in flux.[6]
- Alternative site blood glucose monitoring carries a level of risk that requires patients to decide when to use alternative sites safely. Alternative sites may be used before a meal and 2 hours after a meal. Alternative sites should not be used when patients are hypoglycemic, prone to hypoglycemia (during peak activity of an injected basal insulin or up to 2 hours after injecting rapid-acting insulin), after exercise, during illness, when blood glucose levels are rapidly increasing or decreasing (such as any time less than 2 hours after a meal), and before driving.
- Patients with a history of hypoglycemic unawareness should not use alternative sites.

- Because between-site differences of up to 100 mg/dL (5.6 mmol/L) have been reported,[7] documentation by the patient should include not only the result, time, medication, and relevant comments, but also the sampling site used.
- Samples taken from alternative sites less than 2 hours after a meal may reflect the wide discordance between fingertip and alternative site samples. Teach pregnant women who check blood glucose levels 1 hour after a meal this difference between fingertip and alternative site samples.

3 Many patients are trained in the mechanics of using a meter but not how to use the data. This inadequacy may be related to patient education. Harris and associates[8] found that the frequency of monitoring was related to having attended a diabetes patient education class. Diabetes patient education was associated with an almost threefold greater probability that subjects monitored their blood glucose at least once per day.
  A The critical uses of SMBG data by persons with diabetes are shown in Table 5.2.

Table 5.2. Uses of SMBG Data by Persons with Diabetes

- Identifying and treating hypoglycemia
- Making decisions concerning food intake or medication adjustment when exercising
- Determining the effect of food choices or portions on blood glucose levels
- Pattern management
- Managing intercurrent illness
- Managing hypoglycemia unawareness

  B Self-monitoring of blood glucose provides reliable data for problem-solving and decision-making.
  - While some decisions (eg, treating hypoglycemia or determining the need for a snack) require instantaneous feedback for decision-making, most decisions require reviewing numerous readings to identify a pattern (eg, adjusting medication dosages, changing the meal plan, or recognizing the impact of exercise).
  - The memory feature of many meters is not intended to replace the logbook, but rather provide the option of recording readings at a later date.
  - Although a written record and graph of blood glucose readings yields important information, jotting down comments or explanations can be more helpful for teaching the impact of certain decisions related to medication, exercise, or food.
  C Educators and clinicians rely on SMBG to teach problem-solving skills, which are the essence of diabetes self-management, and complex management skills such as blood glucose pattern awareness and insulin dose adjustment (see Chapter 6, Pattern Management of Blood Glucose, in Diabetes Management Therapies, for examples).
  D Diabetes educators use SMBG as the tool that links abstract principles of management with daily decision making.
  - Educators can use blood glucose results to teach the concept of postexercise, late-onset hypoglycemia and the behaviors necessary to prevent this condition.

- Behavior change concerning food choices or portions is facilitated by relating the food or portion to the postprandial blood glucose result.[9,10]
- For persons with type 2 diabetes who are asymptomatic for hyperglycemia, the need for behavior change becomes personally relevant when they monitor and record blood glucose levels.

E Self-monitoring of blood glucose is used by educators to identify and influence psychosocial adaptations.

- Self-monitoring of blood glucose can influence self-efficacy.[11] For example, patients report increased confidence in their problem-solving abilities as a result of using SMBG.
- The act of monitoring can also hold emotional consequences when patients are confronted with an unacceptable number. This phenomenon, called "monitor talk," can help identify psychosocial needs and direct future learning.[12] Educators can discourage value judgment and replace the notion of good and bad readings with the terms "in range" or "out of range." Reference to blood glucose tests can be replaced with the terms "checks" or "measurements."
- Identified barriers to monitoring include the discomfort of lancing the skin, elevated or labile readings, reminder of the diagnosis of diabetes, cost of strips, emotional response to blood letting or skin piercing, and the inconvenience of record keeping. By identifying barriers, the educator can provide direction and support the patient's choice in using this valuable tool.
- Self-monitoring of blood glucose can be used to allay anxiety about hypoglycemia, especially parental anxiety, and is a critical tool for treating fear of hypoglycemia.[13]
- Although the influence of stress and stress management techniques on glycemic control is controversial, individuals may benefit from identifying a physical marker for their psychological distress.

F The frequency and timing of SMBG are determined by how the data will be used.

- More frequent monitoring is beneficial during insulin dose adjustment or when an oral medication is prescribed that has a primary effect on postprandial glucose levels. Periodic postprandial checks may benefit someone who is learning about the glycemic effect of food portions.
- Postprandial monitoring is an essential part of diabetes self-management. Research has demonstrated that any therapy targeted at lowering postprandial blood glucose will also lower A1C level.[14]
- In individuals with type 1 and type 2 diabetes, abnormalities in insulin and glucagon secretion, hepatic glucose uptake, suppression of hepatic glucose production, and peripheral glucose uptake contribute to higher and more prolonged postprandial blood glucose excursions than in nondiabetic individuals.[15]

- In general, a measurement of plasma glucose 2 hours after the start of the meal provides a reasonable assessment of postprandial hyperglycemia. Specific clinical conditions such as gestational diabetes or pregnancy complicated by diabetes may benefit from measuring blood glucose 1 hour after a meal.[15]
- Postprandial plasma glucose targets have been defined. The American College of Endocrinology recommends a treatment-targeted 2-hour postprandial plasma blood glucose level of <140 mg/dL (7.8 mmol/L).[2] The American Diabetes Association recommends treatment aimed at reducing average peak postprandial plasma glucose values <180 mg/dL (10.0 mmol/L) measured 1 to 2 hours after the start of the meal.[3]

- One of the most common barriers to postprandial monitoring is that patients frequently forget to check after a meal because there is no trigger to remind them.
- Monitoring schedules are based on the patient's needs, desires, and use of the data. Although some clinicians have not yet been convinced of the merit of SMBG for patients not treated with insulin, the value of SMBG cannot be overemphasized as a teaching tool, motivator, and reinforcer and as an aid in prescribing appropriate dosages of the various combinations of oral glucose-lowering medications.

G Guidelines for teaching individuals how to use a blood glucose meter are listed in Table 5.3.

Table 5.3. Guidelines for Teaching Individuals How to Use a Blood Glucose Meter

- Use universal precautions: change lancets, endcaps, and gloves for each patient.[16]
- Encourage the patient to lance the finger or alternative site at the beginning of the session to minimize anxiety about the discomfort involved.
- Demonstrate how to check blood glucose using control solution first and then using the individual's blood.
- After demonstrating this technique, ask the individual to provide a return demonstration before teaching about control solution, calibration, cleaning, and using the logbook.
- Explain how to dispose of lancets in an appropriate sharps container.
- Evaluate the individual's technique at every opportunity.

---

4 Educators are frequently asked to provide consultation regarding the choice of a meter for a hospital or other facility. Although the scientific literature contains numerous reports of the statistical accuracy of systems for SMBG, most determine accuracy in ways that may not be clinically useful for these settings. The Error Grid Analysis[17] provides a useful methodological contribution for evaluating accuracy of glucose meters and clinical relevancy of statistical data related to SMBG.

5 Noninvasive monitoring involves measuring the concentration of glucose in the blood without puncturing the skin to obtain a drop of blood.[18] The system detects trends and tracks patterns in blood glucose levels. It is not intended to replace the immediate feedback provided by fingertip or alternative site blood glucose monitoring.

6 Data management systems allow for downloading the memory stored in the meter to a computer (either directly or by modem) for record keeping or plotting the results on a graph. These systems can be accessed via personal computer or the Internet.

A Data summarization alone, however, does not identify the relationship that leads to the observed outcomes (eg, the 4 carbohydrate servings at breakfast that led to postprandial hyperglycemia).

B Data management systems can store hundreds of results and other information entered by the patient such as insulin or medication type and dose, meals, and exercise.

C Blood glucose monitoring manufacturers provide information about compatible computer software on their respective web sites.

◻ Personal Digital Assistants (PDA) are also used as electronic logbooks. Combining the meter with the PDA allows automatic storage of the blood glucose result, and the user can log other helpful data.

7 The Joint Commission for the Accreditation of Health Care Organizations (JCAHO) and the Centers for Medicare and Medicaid Services (CMS) require hospitals and other facilities to have quality assurance programs for bedside blood glucose monitoring.[19] Proficiency testing, use of control solutions, staff training, and correlation studies comparing bedside results with hospital laboratory values are essential elements of the quality assurance process.

▲ The Clinical Laboratory Improvement Amendments of 1988 (CLIA '88)[20] requires all laboratories that examine materials derived from the human body to be certified. This includes physician offices. Glucose tests performed on a meter approved by the Food and Drug Administration (FDA) for home use are waived under CLIA and can be done at any site by any person. Blood glucose meters must have verified accuracy, and the provider's office must enroll in the CLIA program, follow the manufacturers' test recommendations and submit fees for a waived test.

8 Certain populations of people with diabetes have unique needs relating to SMBG.

▲ Elderly people with diabetes remain an underserved population despite the prevalence of diabetes in the elderly and the validity of SMBG as a management tool.

- Age should not be the sole criterion for decisions concerning SMBG. The elderly are a heterogeneous population requiring personalized therapy and monitoring schedules.
- Educators need to consider the unique needs of some of the elderly patients that may influence the choice of products, such as potential limitations in manual dexterity, slowed reaction time or fluctuating vision[21] (for more information, see Chapter 6, Diabetes in Older Adults, Diabetes in the Life Cycle and Research).

■ Children also have unique needs that influence product choice.

- Children especially benefit from strips that require a small sample size of blood and lancing devices that hide the lancet and minimize discomfort.
- Parents benefit from meters that quickly yield results and store at least the last reading in the memory. This latter feature is particularly important because after a skin puncture, parents are focused on comforting their child and the meter may turn off before the parent can write down the result (for more information, see Chapter 2, Type 1 Diabetes in Youth, in Diabetes in the Life Cycle and Research).

◼ Visually impaired persons with diabetes, including those with fluctuating vision to nonfunctional vision, need products that are fully accessible to the visually impaired person; current products fall short of this need. Equipment features that would be of benefit include tactile markings on the strip; clear speech output on a small, portable meter; and a method of consistent placement of the blood sample[22] (for more information, see Chapter 7, Eye Disease and Adaptive Diabetes Education for Visually Impaired Persons, in Diabetes and Complications).

Continuous Glucose Monitoring

1 The continuous glucose monitoring system monitors glucose from interstitial fluid that is converted to an electronic signal. A sensor-type device transmits the signal to a monitor that acquires the data continuously. The typical measurement period is up to 72 hours.

A The continuous glucose monitoring system is intended for diagnostic and prescriptive use and can be helpful to identify glycemic effects of food, exercise, and insulin; previously unrecognized hypoglycemia; proper insulin doses to match food absorption in gastroparesis; and effects of dialysis on glucose levels.

Long-Term Monitoring of Metabolic Control

1 Hemoglobin A1c (A1C), the most abundant minor hemoglobin component in the red blood cell, increases in proportion to the blood glucose level over the preceding 3 to 4 months. Because the red blood cell has a life span of 120 days, this test reflects the blood glucose concentration over that period of time. The A1C test is an accurate, objective measure of chronic glycemia in persons with diabetes. The term HbA1c is now simplified to A1C.

A Glycosylation occurs as glucose in the plasma attaches itself to the hemoglobin component of the red blood cell; this process is irreversible.

- The more glycosylation, the higher the values.
- The glycosylated hemoglobin does not reflect the simple mean but reflects the weighted mean over a long period of time.[23] The traditional idea that glycosylated hemoglobin reflects the simple mean and is referred to as the average of the blood glucose is inaccurate. For example, in an A1C measured on May 1, 50% of the A1C level is determined by the plasma glucose level during the preceding 1-month period (April), 25% of its level is determined by the plasma glucose level during the 1-month period before that (March), and the remaining 25% is determined by the plasma glucose level during the 2-month period before the past 2 months (February and January).

B Glycosylated hemoglobin can be measured by many different methods. Accurate interpretation requires knowledge of the method used to determine the glycosylated hemoglobin level, the component measured, and the normal range for the particular assay.

- Affinity chromatography and colorimetric assay methods measure total glycosylated hemoglobin (GHb), including all fractions of the hemoglobin molecule: HbA1a, HbA1b, and HbA1c.[19] Upper normal values of GHb may be in the range of 8% to 9%.
- Ion-exchange chromatography, high-performance liquid chromatography (HPLC), and immunoassay methods are used to measure A1C. The normal value is usually in the range of 4% to 6%.
- Some laboratories measure total glycosylated hemoglobin, but they report the ADA treatment goal of <7% in the reference range column of the report instead of listing the actual reference range of up to 9%. This may have clinical relevance if healthcare providers compare values from different laboratories. A result of 7.8% would be considered out of range if the reference range is 4.0% to 6.0% and within range if the reference range was 5.0% to 8.0%.
- The National Glycohemoglobin Standardization Program is an effort designed to encourage laboratories to standardized and report all glycosylated hemoglobin assays in values equivalent to the A1C as measured in the Diabetes Control and Complications Trial (DCCT).[24,25]
- Interfering factors (sickle-cell hemoglobin and other hemoglobinopathies) may affect measurement of A1C level depending upon the method.[26]

- A1C measurement is not currently recommended for diagnosis of diabetes.

C Regular measurements of A1C permit timely detection of departures from the target range. In the absence of well-controlled studies that suggest a definite testing protocol, both the ADA[3] and ACE[2] suggest glycosylated hemoglobin testing at least 1 or 2 times a year in patients with a history of stable glycemic control, and at least quarterly assessments in patients whose therapy has changed or who are in poor control.

D Glycemic targets should be individualized for each individual.

- The DCCT[24] conclusively demonstrated, however, that the risk of retinopathy, nephropathy, and neuropathy in individuals with type 1 diabetes is reduced by intensive treatment regimens compared with conventional treatment regimens. These benefits were observed with an average A1C of 7.2% (normal range = 4.0% to 6.0%) in the intensively treated group. The reduction in risk of these complications correlated continuously with the reduction in A1C produced by intensive therapy.[3]
- In the epidemiologic analysis of the UKPDS data, the risk for occurrence of microvascular and macrovascular complications was shown to increase at A1C values of 6.5% or more.[27]
- According to ACE, the recommended target for attainment of glycemic control should be A1C values of 6.5% (reference range 4.0 to 6.0%).[2]
- The ADA recommended target for A1C values is <7.0% (reference range 4.0 to 6.0%).[3]
- A glycosylated hemoglobin result within the nondiabetic reference range may reflect frequent hypoglycemia and requires further evaluation.
- The glycosylated hemoglobin is a strong indicator of blood glucose control when compared with SMBG results.

E Glycosylated hemoglobin is a teaching tool as well as a marker of metabolic control. If a patient monitors only fasting blood glucose levels and finds values in the normal range but has an A1C result of 9.8% (normal range = 4.0% to 6.0%), the educator can encourage the patient to monitor at other times of the day (especially postprandial readings) to uncover periods of elevated blood glucose and identify the factors that may be associated with the elevated results.

- Table 5.4 lists the correlation between A1C levels and mean plasma blood glucose levels based on data from the DCCT. Although this information may be helpful to clinicians in defining the relationship between plasma glucose and A1C, it would not be included in diabetes self-management training (DSMT). For DSMT, the educator would focus on helping a patient develop an action plan designed to bring the A1C closer to goal.
- At-home A1C testing is available. Most products are certified by the National Glycohemoglobin Standardization Program. Insurance reimbursement varies with the insurance plan and the type of product.

2 Glycosylated serum albumin (fructosamine), a glycated serum protein test, measures glycemic control over 2 to 3 weeks.[28] Normal ranges vary among the different methods of measurements. Fructosamine values are used in short-term follow-up of interventions that have been recently implemented to lower blood glucose[1] or when there is a discrepancy between the A1C level and the patient's reported blood glucose readings.

Table 5.4. Correlation Between A1C Level and Mean Plasma Glucose Levels[3]

	Mean Plasma Glucose	
A1C (%)	mg/dL	mmol/L
6	135	7.5
7	170	9.5
8	205	11.5
9	240	13.5
10	275	15.5
11	310	17.5
12	345	19.5

Monitoring for the Prevention and Management of Complications

1 Cardiovascular disease (CVD) is the major cause of mortality for persons with diabetes. Studies have shown the efficacy of reducing cardiovascular risk factors in preventing or slowing CVD. Monitoring blood pressure and blood lipids for the prevention and management of cardiovascular risk is considered part of the management of diabetes.

  A Hypertension is likely to be present in type 2 diabetes as part of the metabolic syndrome that is accompanied by high rates of CVD. In type 1 diabetes, hypertension is often the result of underlying nephropathy.
  • The American Diabetes Association recommends a target blood pressure of 130/80 mm/Hg.[3]

  B Patients with type 2 diabetes have an increased prevalence of lipid abnormalities that contributes to higher rates of CVD. Lipid management aimed at lowering LDL cholesterol, raising HDL cholesterol, and lowering triglycerides has been shown to reduce macrovascular disease and mortality in patients with type 2 diabetes, especially those who have had prior cardiovascular events.
  • Target lipid goals include LDL cholesterol <100 mg/dL (<2.6 mmol/L); HDL cholesterol >40 mg/dL (>1.1 mmol/L) for men and >50 mg/dL (>1.3 mmol/L) for women; and triglycerides <150 mg/dL (<1.7 mmol/L).[3]
  • Following the recommendations of the National Cholesterol Education Program's Report of the Expert Panel of Blood Cholesterol Levels in Children and Adolescents, LDL cholesterol should be lowered to <110 mg/dL (<2.8 mmol/L) in children with cardiovascular risk factors in addition to diabetes.[29]

2 Patients taking thiazolidinediones and HMG-CoA reductase inhibitors require periodic monitoring of liver function.

Ketone Tests

1 Monitoring for the presence of ketones remains an essential component of diabetes care. Individuals with type 1 diabetes are ketosis-prone, whereas those with type 2 diabetes are generally ketosis-resistant.

A Either blood or urinary ketones can be measured. Blood ketones can be measured using a special meter designed for home use, and urinary ketones can be measured using a dipstick and matching the results to a color chart.

B Ketones should be tested routinely during illness by all individuals with diabetes. Individuals with type 2 diabetes can become ketotic during severe stress precipitated by infections or trauma.[30]

- Individuals with type 1 diabetes should test ketones when their blood glucose is consistently elevated (>300 mg/dL [>16.7 mmol/L]). For those using an insulin pump, ketonuria or ketonemia in the presence of hyperglycemia may indicate failure of the insulin delivery system.

- Pregnant women with diabetes (including gestational diabetes) are often advised to monitor urinary ketones every morning. These measurements are useful for detecting inadequate food intake (starvation ketosis) and providing warning of impending metabolic decompensation[31] (for more information, see Chapter 4, Pregnancy With Preexisting Diabetes, in Diabetes in the Life Cycle and Research).

- Urinary ketones also may be measured on a regular schedule in individuals with diabetes who are actively trying to lose weight by calorie restriction. Because ketones are a waste product of fat metabolism, ketonuria in the presence of euglycemia can indicate weight loss, not metabolic decompensation.

- Individuals with type 1 diabetes who are restricting calories to lose weight require decreased dosages of insulin to prevent hypoglycemia. Too much of a reduction of insulin will result in hyperglycemia, ketonuria, and, if not corrected, metabolic decompensation to ketoacidosis.

C Three ketone bodies are formed from the conversion of free fatty acids in the liver: acetoacetate, 3-ß-hydroxybutyrate, and acetone.

- Urinary ketones are detected by the nitroprusside reaction in the treatment of acute diabetic ketoacidosis. The nitroprusside reagent predominantly reacts with acetoacetate and does not react with ß-hydroxybutyrate.

- Following the institution of insulin therapy, the concentration of acetoacetate increases and ß-hydroxybutyrate decreases. This shift accounts for the clinical observation that urine ketone test results may become more positive during the early phase of therapy and indicate clinical improvement rather than deterioration.

D Rapid enzymatic methods have been developed for the quantification of 3-ß-hydroxybutyrate levels in small-volume blood samples. These systems are designed for use at home and can measure 3-ß-hydroxybutyrate levels on finger-stick blood samples.[32]

Urine Tests

1 The ability to detect low levels of albumin in the urine (microalbuminuria) represents an important advancement in the diagnosis and treatment of diabetic nephropathy. The presence of microalbuminuria represents an early phase of nephropathy and is a well-established marker of cardiovascular risk.[33]

A Annual urine microalbumin screening in individuals with type 1 diabetes should begin after 5 years' duration of diabetes. Because of the difficulty in precise dating of type 2 diabetes, urinary microalbumin screening should begin at the time of diagnosis.[3]

B Screening for microalbuminuria can be performed by 3 methods: measurement of the albumin-to-creatinine ratio in a random spot collection; 24-hour collection with creatinine, allowing the simultaneous measurement of creatinine clearance; and timed (eg, 4-hour or overnight) collection (see Table 5.5).

Table 5.5. Definitions of Abnormalities of Albumin Excretion

	Albumin to creatinine ratio random spot collection, μg/mg creatinine	24-h collection, mg/24 h	Timed collection, μg/min
Normal	<30	<30	<20
Microalbuminuria	30 to 299	30 to 299	20 to 199
Clinical albuminuria	≥300	≥300	≥200

Because of variability in urinary albumin excretion, 2 of 3 specimens collected within a 3- to 6-month period should be abnormal before considering a patient to have crossed one of these diagnostic thresholds. Exercise within 24 hours, infection, fever, congestive heart failure, marked hyperglycemia, and marked hypertension may elevate urinary albumin excretion over baseline values.
Source: Reprinted with permission from American Diabetes Association.[3]

C The albustix reagent does not screen for microalbuminuria because it does not become positive until the albumin excretion rate (AER) exceeds 300 mg/24 h (200 μg/min).

D In healthy individuals, small amounts of albumin can be found in the urine with a mean albumin excretion rate of 10 ± 3 mg/day (7 ± 2 μg/min).[34]

E Screening for microalbuminuria should be avoided if the patient has a urinary tract infection, hematuria, fever, congestive heart failure, marked hyperglycemia, or marked hypertension or is menstruating or has exercised within 24 hours.[35]

2 Urine glucose testing was the original method of monitoring glycemic control, but blood glucose monitoring is the preferred method. Urine glucose testing provides retrospective information and does not reflect current blood glucose.

A The results of urine glucose testing should be reported in percent values, not plus (+) values, for continuity of results from 1 method to another.

B The advantages of urine testing for glucose are that it is less expensive than blood glucose monitoring and is noninvasive.

C Urine testing for glucose offers several distinct disadvantages.

- Elevated renal thresholds (blood glucose >180 mg/dL [>10 mmol/L]) that occur with age will give false negative results.
- Renal thresholds may be low in pregnancy.
- Since urine testing gives a delayed picture of what is happening in the blood, it is not indicated in flexible insulin therapy.

- False results (negative or positive) may occur with ingestion of certain medications (cephalosporins, large amounts of ascorbic acid).
- Urine testing can be awkward to do especially when away from home.
- Urine testing is limited to testing for elevated glucose levels.

Assessment of Growth and Weight

1 Monitoring also involves assessment of growth in children and weight and body mass index (BMI) in all patients with diabetes. Waist circumference measurement taken after inspiration and expiration at the midpoint between the lowest rib and iliac crest is helpful in identifying individuals with the metabolic syndrome. A waist circumference of greater than 40 inches (102 cm) in men and 35 inches (88 cm) in women has been identified as a risk factor for the metabolic syndrome.[36]

2 Documentation of weight is considered another indicator for diabetes management.
  A Weight gain may reflect improvement in glycemic control, increased caloric consumption, frequent episodes of hypoglycemia, fluid retention, and eating disorders, among other conditions.
  B Similarly, weight loss may reflect elevated blood glucose levels, decreased caloric consumption, or eating disorders.
  C Fluctuations in weight can occur depending upon the scale used and time of day.

Summary

1 Since self-monitoring of blood glucose is one of the essential tools of self-management, diabetes educators have the unique opportunity and responsibility to provide instruction concerning not only monitoring techniques but use of the data.

2 Diabetes educators can also teach individuals to approach monitoring as feedback (ie, helpful information) rather than evaluation (ie, punishment).

3 Teach individuals that the meaning of the results from the methods used to monitor metabolic control provides more than feedback; it reinforces their active role in self-management and their position as the center of the healthcare team.

Teaching Patients About Monitoring: Basic Education Components

1 Table 5.3 lists guidelines for teaching how to use a blood glucose meter.

2 Focus the teaching session on the meaning of the blood glucose results. Help the patient to the identify target ranges and review the dynamic nature of blood glucose so that the patient will expect fluctuations. Help the patient choose a reasonable monitoring schedule that will provide meaningful data.

3 Guide the patient in choosing a system for documentation of the readings either using a written logbook, electronic logbook, or computer program. Documentation includes more than just the blood glucose reading; it also includes notes concerning food, activity, stress, and medication.

4 Choice of meter will depend on insurance reimbursement and an assessment of manual dexterity and visual acuity plus the individual's unique needs or desires.

5 Create the expectation that the person with diabetes will benefit from knowing the A1C results. Include the current A1C result, normal range, target range, and date for the next A1C test. Together, outline a plan for reaching that person's target range.

6 Ketone testing is part of the basic education for patients with type 1 diabetes, gestational diabetes, and pregnancy with preexising diabetes.

7 Advanced education components include benefits of monitoring urine for protein, ketone monitoring for persons with type 2 diabetes as part of sick-day rules, and use of the data provided by SMBG.

Key Educational Considerations

1 A variety of meters is available for monitoring blood glucose, and each one is unique.
  A It is important to carefully assess the patient's visual acuity and dexterity skills before recommending a specific meter. Let the patient practice using the meter. Demonstration meters and supplies are available from the manufacturer's representative.
  B Diabetes educators are pivotal in guiding patients to select the meter that is most appropriate for them and one for which they easily can obtain supplies. Some insurers only reimburse for certain meters and reagents.

2 Ask patients to bring their meters and all supplies to each visit. The meter can be cleaned, the strips and control solution can be tested, codes can be verified, and an actual blood glucose measurement can be performed.

3 Provide patients with the toll-free customer service number for the manufacturer of their meter. Experts are available at this number 24 hours per day to answer questions and provide assistance.

4 Careful and safe disposal of used lancets is critical. Teach patients to dispose of used lancets in an appropriate sharps container (regulations vary from state to state). When monitoring blood glucose away from home, patients can place their used lancets in an empty pill container or 35-mm film canister.

5 Consider the cost of supplies when patients decide the frequency of monitoring. Be familiar with local suppliers who charge reasonable prices. Refer patients to a social worker or community agency when appropriate.

6 Some individuals benefit from having a second meter that is compact, quick, and simple to use for easily checking their blood glucose level away from home or before driving. Blood glucose monitoring results will be most consistent if the same model of a meter is used all the time. If an individual chooses to use a different model to check the blood glucose before driving, for example, then those readings should either be omitted from the logbook or noted as resulting from a different meter.

7 Postprandial monitoring is effective for teaching the impact of food portions on blood glucose levels. For example, the individual may choose a large portion of frozen yogurt and have an elevated blood glucose reading 2 hours later, whereas after a medium portion of frozen yogurt, the postprandial reading may be in the goal range.

8 Use patient records or logbooks that list glucose levels for a certain time of day in a linear and vertical fashion. This format allows simple visual interpretation of the results.

9 Recording blood glucose levels on a graph, as well as having a numerical listing, provides a useful visual aid for teaching the concept of blood glucose patterns. Computer software marketed by meter manufacturers can be very helpful in providing graphs and other visual representations of the data.

10 If the patient has stopped monitoring, investigate common causes such as emotional reactions to elevated or fluctuating readings, consistent readings within range, discomfort related to lancing the skin, emotional response to blood letting or skin piercing, cost, inconvenience, or collection of meaningless data. As part of the assessment simply ask, "Is it helpful?"

11 Actual blood glucose records of common patterns should be used when teaching self-management.

12 Provide patients with the opportunity to practice testing for urinary or serum ketones during their teaching appointment.

13 A supply sheet, signed by the healthcare provider, can be an effective organizational aid for the person with diabetes and the pharmacist and may serve as a prescription.

14 Teaching the concept of glycosylated hemoglobin can be challenging. This test can be referred to as the blood test with a memory that represents blood glucose levels over the last 3 months. A1C can be thought of as a long-term monitoring method as opposed to the day-to-day self-monitoring measurements that are performed with a home meter.

15 Avoid referring to A1C as an average of blood glucose levels. Besides being technically inaccurate, this language can lead persons to confuse A1C with the average in their meter memory.

16 The educator can use a picture of a pyramid or a thermometer to outline the various A1C levels and then demonstrate the goal range and the individual's most recent result. Ask patients what they think about the results and what they would like to do about them, rather than offering judgments.

Self-Review Questions

1 What factors affect the accuracy of SMBG results?
2 What is the most common user error related to SMBG?
3 List tips that can be followed to secure an adequate blood sample.
4 What are the critical uses of SMBG data by persons with diabetes?
5 Describe ways educators can use SMBG to link the principles of diabetes management with daily decision-making.
6 List the ACE and ADA pre- and postprandial blood glucose target ranges.
7 In what situations should alternative site monitoring be avoided?
8 Describe common psychosocial adaptations related to SMBG.
9 Describe how monitoring schedules are determined.
10 What is a reliable method for evaluating the accuracy of blood glucose meters?
11 List the elements of quality assurance regarding blood glucose meters.
12 Describe the unique SMBG needs of the elderly, children, and visually impaired persons with diabetes.
13 Define glycosylated hemoglobin and the target ranges.
14 Define fructosamine and when this assessment is used.
15 List the lipid and blood pressure goals for persons with diabetes.
16 List the advantages and disadvantages of urine glucose testing.
17 What groups of patients should monitor for ketones?
18 What are 3 methods of screening for microalbuminuria and the target ranges?
19 When should screening for microalbuminuria be avoided?
20 Describe the role of documenting weight changes in the management of diabetes.

Learning Assessment: Case Study 1

AD sees the diabetes educator regularly following a visit with his physician. At each visit with the educator, he brings both of his meters (from 2 different manufacturers) and presents different scenarios concerning the discrepancies between the 2 meters or between the lab and each meter. He keeps no records and barely checks his blood glucose because "he is not confident of the results." The diabetes educator dutifully verifies the accuracy of the meters and spends the entire visit defending the meters. When reviewing the documentation of these visits, the diabetes educator realizes that there has been no diabetes education and looks to colleagues for advice.

Questions for Discussion

1 What are the dynamics of these visits?
2 What are possible explanations for this person's behavior?
3 How can the educator alter the pattern of the visits?
4 What content is generally included when teaching about blood glucose monitoring?

Discussion

1 AD may be using the meters as an effective smoke screen.
   A If AD organizes the visits around the meters, then nothing else is discussed. He may have lost confidence in the meters, but verifying accuracy and defending the meters is not helping him regain his confidence.

■ When interactions with patients become frustrating, reflecting on the experience and seeking the advice of colleagues often helps to bring a different perspective to the situation. As a result of her thoughts and discussions, the educator recognizes her role in perpetuating this pattern. While she knows she cannot change AD's behavior, she can change her own.

2 To alter the pattern of visits, the educator decides to develop a specific plan of action. When making the plan, she realizes that she needs to be sure that it is designed to meet AD's needs and includes strategies that keep him in control of the visit, such as asking questions and seeking his opinions rather than just offering advice. The important thing is to create a different, more functional partnership with him.

A Because this might represent avoidance behavior, the educator needs to assess what AD is trying to avoid in order to more effectively meet his needs. This task will no doubt be challenging, but one technique for inviting discussion is to say, "It seems like we spend all of our time on this topic and I am concerned that you are not getting what you need from me. Could we start with your other concerns?"

B If he is unable to identify concerns, you could share the barriers to self-care that others have identified and ask if he has had similar experiences or if there are other things about his diabetes care that are hard for him.

C Another option would be to ask AD if the physician made any treatment changes during the last visit, offer to review these changes with AD, and use them as a springboard for teaching new content. The issues surrounding monitoring still need to be discussed, but focusing on another area of AD's concerns may decrease frustration for him and the educator. Generally, once the patient's technique in using the meter has been assessed (strip storage, expiration date, and so on), teach how to record blood glucose readings, target ranges, and, most importantly, how to use the data.

Learning Assessment: Case Study 2

JD is a 26-year-old male who was diagnosed with type 1 diabetes 6 months ago. He vacationed in another state and presented in the emergency department with a hypoglycemic seizure. His blood glucose log revealed readings that were either elevated or within range. This person's goal was euglycemia and he would adjust his insulin dosages based on his premeal blood glucose readings. The evening before the seizure, he participated in a family meal that included large portions of food and alcohol. In anticipation of an elevated bedtime blood glucose, he injected extra units of rapid-acting insulin immediately before the meal and again before going to bed. His wife was so frightened by the seizure that she cannot sleep and encourages him to eat more at night to prevent hypoglycemia.

He returned for his follow-up visit with the diabetes educator a week after seeing his endocrinologist. In February, his A1C level was 6.2% (reference range 4.0% to 6.0%) and in May the A1C level was 4.7% with the same reference range. The result was confirmed 1 week later. His endocrinologist congratulated him on the tight control. At the visit with the educator, his prelunch blood glucose was 102 mg/dL (5.7 mmol/L) using the educator's supplies, and he demonstrated accurate technique.

Questions for Discussion

1 What clues are provided by his story and the recent A1C result?

2 What does the educator still need to assess?

3 How can the educator help JD's wife?

Discussion

1 A low A1C result is often achieved at the expense of frequent hypoglycemia. A low result should signal the educator to assess for the frequency and severity of hypoglycemia keeping in mind that many patients underreport the frequency of hypoglycemia if they successfully managed the episode. It would be helpful to assess JD's understanding of the impact of alcohol on the blood glucose, especially the hypoglycemic effects of alcohol. It would also be prudent to review JD's guidelines for deciding on a premeal dose of rapid-acting insulin.

2 Part of the assessment of the patient's technique involves checking the meter to see if it is soiled (when applicable) and inquiring about strip storage. JD found the vial of strips that accompany his meter to be bulky so he decided to store them out of the vial. This practice yielded inaccurate results. Unfortunately, JD was adjusting his insulin based on inaccurate results.

3 JD's wife might be comforted when she learns that incorrect storage of the strips contributed to JD's hypoglycemic seizure. Since she did not attend the visit, the educator could arrange to meet with JD's wife or telephone her to listen to her concerns. If applicable, the educator could reinforce the safety guidelines for insulin adjustment and nighttime snacking as prevention of nocturnal hypoglycemia. The educator could also reinforce how excessive nighttime snacking would not serve JD's needs and may create conflict.

References

1 American Diabetes Association. Self-monitoring of blood glucose (consensus statement). Diabetes Care. 1994;17:81-86.

2 American College of Endocrinology. Guidelines for glycemic control (consensus statement). Endocrine Practice. 2002;8(suppl 1):6-11.

3 American Diabetes Association. Standards of medical care for patients with diabetes mellitus (position statement). Diabetes Care. 2003;26(suppl 1):S33-S50.

4 Peragallo-Dittko V. How accurate is your meter? Diabetes Self-Manage. 2000;17(5):78-85.

5 Peragallo-Dittko V. The lowdown on lancets and lancing devices. Diabetes Self-Manage. 1999;16(3):64-71.

6 McGarraugh G, Price D, Schwartz S, et al. Physiological influences on off-finger glucose testing. Diabetes Technol Ther. 2001;3:367-376.

7 Jungheim K, Koschinsky T. Risky delay of hypoglycemia detection by glucose monitoring at the arm [letter]. Diabetes Care. 2001;24:1303-1306.

8 Harris MI, Crowe CC, Howie LJ. Self-monitoring of blood glucose by adults with diabetes in the United States population. Diabetes Care. 1993;16:1116-1123.

9 Babione L. SMBG: the underused nutrition counseling tool in diabetes management. Diabetes Spectrum. 1994;7:196-197.

10 Ahern JA, Gatcomb PM, Held NA, Petit WA Jr, Tamborlane WV. Exaggerated hyperglycemia after a pizza meal in well-controlled diabetes. Diabetes Care. 1993;16:578-580.

11 Rubin RR, Peyrot M, Saudek CD. The effect of a diabetes education program incorporating coping skills training on emotional well-being and diabetes self-efficacy. Diabetes Educ. 1993;19:210-214.

12 Price MJ. Qualitative analysis of the patient-provider interactions: the patient's perspective. Diabetes Educ. 1989;15:144-148.

13 Cox DJ, Irvine A, Gonder-Frederick L, Nowacek G, Butterfield J. Fear of hypoglycemia: quantification, validation and utilization. Diabetes Care. 1987;10:617-621.

14 Bastyr EJ III, Stuart CA, Broddows RG, Schwartz S, Graf CJ, Zagar A, Robertson KE. Therapy focused on lowering postprandial glucose, not fasting glucose, may be superior for lowering HbA1c. Diabetes Care. 2000;23:1236-1241.

15 American Diabetes Association. Postprandial blood glucose (consensus statement). Diabetes Care. 2001;24:775-778.

16 American Association of Diabetes Educators. Educating providers and persons with diabetes to prevent the transmission of bloodborne infections and avoid injuries from sharps [position statement]. Diabetes Educ. 1997;23:401-403.

17 Clarke WL, Cox D, Gonder-Frederick LA, Carter W, Pohl SL. Evaluating clinical accuracy of systems for self-monitoring of blood glucose. Diabetes Care. 1987;10:622-628.

18 Klonoff DC. Noninvasive blood glucose monitoring. Diabetes Care. 1997;20:433-437.

19 Walker EA. Quality assurance for blood glucose monitoring. Nurs Clin North Am. 1993;28:61-70.

20 American Diabetes Association. CLIA guidelines implemented. Diabetes Rev. 1993; 1:130.

21 Peragallo-Dittko V. Clinical and educational usefulness of SMBG with the elderly. Diabetes Spectrum. 1995;8:17-19.

22 Bernbaum M, Albert SG, Brusca S, et al. Effectiveness of glucose monitoring systems modified for the visually impaired. Diabetes Care. 1993;16:1363-1366.

23 Tahara Y, Shima K. Kinetics of HbA1c, glycated albumin, and fructosamine and analysis of their weight functions against preceding plasma glucose level. Diabetes Care. 1995;18;440-447.

24 The Diabetes Control and Complications Trial Research Group. The effect of intensive treatment of diabetes on the development and progression of long-term complications of insulin-dependent diabetes. N Engl J Med. 1993;329:77-86.

25 American Diabetes Association. Tests of glycemia in diabetes (position statement). Diabetes Care. 2003;26(suppl 1):S106-S108.

26 Goldstein DE, Little RR. More than you ever wanted to know (but need to know) about glycohemoglobin testing. Diabetes Care. 1994;17:938-939.

27 Stratton IM, Adler AI, Neil HA, et al. Association of glycaemia with macrovascular and microvascular complications of type 2 diabetes (UKPDS 35): prospective observational study. BMJ. 2000;321:405-412.

28 Negoro H, Morley JE, Rosenthal MJ. Utility of serum fructosamine as a measure of glycemia in young and old diabetic and non-diabetic subjects. Am J Med. 1988;85:360-364.

29 The Expert Panel of Blood Cholesterol Levels in Children and Adolescents. Treatment recommendations of the National Cholesterol Education Program Report of the Expert Panel on Blood Cholesterol Levels in Children and Adolescents. Pediatrics. 1992;89(suppl):525-584.

30 Fajans SS. Classification and diagnosis of diabetes. In: Porte D Jr, Sherwin RS, eds. Ellenberg and Rifkin's Diabetes Mellitus: Theory and Practice. 5th ed. Stamford, Ct: Appleton and Lang; 1997:357-372.

31 Metzger BE, Phelps RL, Dooley SL. The mother in pregnancies complicated by diabetes mellitus. In: Porte D Jr, Sherwin RS, eds. Ellenberg and Rifkin's Diabetes Mellitus: Theory and Practice. 5th ed. Stamford, Ct: Appleton and Lange; 1997: 887-915.

32 Laffel L. Ketone bodies: a review of physiology, pathophysiology and application of monitoring to diabetes. Diabetes Metab Res Rev. 1999;15:412-426.

33 Gall MA, Hougaard P, Borch-Johnsen K, et al. Risk factors for development of incipient and overt diabetic nephropathy in patients with non-insulin dependent diabetes mellitus: prospective, observational study. BMJ. 1997;314:783-788.

34 DeFronzo RA. Diabetic nephropathy. In: Porte D, Jr, Sherwin RS, eds. Ellenberg and Rifkin's Diabetes Mellitus: Theory and Practice. 5th ed. Stamford, Ct: Appleton and Lange; 1997:971-1008.

35 Morgensen CE, Vestbo E, Poulsen PL, et al. Microalbuminuria and potential confounders. Diabetes Care. 1995;18:572-581.

36 National Institutes of Health, National Heart, Lung, and Blood Institute. Clinical guidelines on the identification, evaluation, and treatment of overweight and obesity in adults—the evidence report. Obes Res. 1998;6:51S-209S.

Suggested Readings

Atkin SH, Dasmahapatra A, Jaker MA, Chorost MI, Reddy S. Finger-stick glucose determination in shock. Ann Intern Med. 1991;114:1020-1024.

Bina DM, Anderson RL, Johnson ML, Bergenstal RM, Kendall DM. Clinical impact of prandial state, exercise, and site preparation on the equivalence of alternative-site blood glucose testing. Diabetes Care. 2003;26:981-985.

Wedman B, Michael SR. Tool chest: glycosylated hemoglobin models. Diabetes Educ. 1988;14:280-282.

For a listing of currently available meters, refer to Diabetes Forecast: Resource Guide (Annual Issue) and Diabetes Self-Management.

Learning Assessment: Post-Test Questions

Monitoring   5

1 The most important benefit to patients of SMBG is:

   A It facilitates problem-solving and decision-making skills

   B It decreases the number of medical visits they make

   C It enables them to make medication adjustments based on a single reading

   D It may reveal psychosocial issues

2 What is a decision concerning diabetes control that can be made from a single blood glucose reading?

   A Adjustment of a patient's split insulin regimen

   B Treatment of a blood glucose reading less than 70 mg/dL

   C Understanding the impact of a daily walking program

   D Adjustment of meal plan

3 The most common SMBG user error is:

   A Using an insufficient blood sample

   B Improper storage of meter and equipment

   C Failure to calibrate the meter

   D Inadequate reporting of high and low BG values

4 Which of the following is not a factor that can affect the accuracy of SMBG systems?

   A Altitude

   B Temperature and humidity

   C Microalbuminuria

   D Hypoxia and hypotension

5 A1C:

   A Represents an average blood glucose concentration within a defined period of time

   B Is a weighted mean over a relative period of time

   C Should be measured at the onset of symptoms and during each routine medical checkup

   D Is easily measured by a single method with a known range using a defined component

6 JG brings in her blood glucose monitor to a diabetes education session. She states that it has not worked properly since she purchased it through a mail-order discount device company. What would be the educator's first assessment step to determine the problem?

   A Demonstrate proper technique of the meter and give the patient a videotape of instructions

   B Use the glucose control solution to determine the meter's accuracy

   C Ask the patient to demonstrate SMBG using her meter

   D Get a venipuncture to determine the patient's random blood glucose level

7 The expiration date on JG's reagent strip container indicates that her strips are current. Could they still be a source of error in SMBG determinations?

   A No, strips are extremely durable and rarely are a source of SMBG error

   B No, even expired strips are commonly used by patients with diabetes

   C Yes, the manufacturer could print the date wrong

   D Yes, environmental changes in temperature and atmosphere during shipping could degrade strips

8 An effective approach for teaching patients how to use a blood glucose meter is:

   A Show how to calibrate the meter before demonstrating its use

   B Change your gloves every hour

   C Evaluate the patient's technique whenever hyperglycemia occurs

   D Teach the patient how to check the blood glucose before teaching meter cleaning and record keeping

9 Urine testing of ketones using the nitro-prusside reaction primarily measures which of the following ketone bodies?
A Acetone
B Acetoacetate
C ß-hydroxybutyrate
D Ketone

10 Blood glucose results measured by a meter designed for home use can be influenced by all of the following except:
A Measurement of whole blood versus plasma
B Measurement of capillary versus venous blood after a meal
C Measurement using different finger-tips for puncture
D Measurement using strips stored outside of the vial or foil wrapper

See next page for answer key.

Post-Test Answer Key

Monitoring

5

1	A		6	C
2	B		7	D
3	A		8	D
4	C		9	B
5	B		10	C

A Core Curriculum for Diabetes Education
Diabetes Management Therapies

Pattern Management of Blood Glucose　　　　6

Deborah A. Hinnen, MN, ARNP, BC-ADM, CDE
Via Christi Regional Medical Center
Wichita, Kansas

Diana W. Guthrie, PhD, ARNP, FAAN, BC-ADM, CDE
Professor Emeritus, University of Kansas School of Medicine
Wichita, Kansas

Belinda P. Childs, MN, ARNP, CDE
Mid-America Diabetes Associates
Wichita, Kansas

Judy Friesen, RD, LD, FADA, CDE
Via Christi Regional Medical Center
Wichita, Kansas

Diana Speelman Rhiley, EdS, LCMFT, CDE
Via Christi Regional Medical Center
Wichita, Kansas

Richard A. Guthrie, MD, CDE, FAACE
Mid-America Diabetes Associates
Via Christi Regional Medical Center
University of Kansas School of Medicine
Wichita, Kansas

Introduction

1 Pattern management is the application of a systematic analysis of data by both persons with diabetes and healthcare providers in the daily, weekly, and long-term management of blood glucose levels.

2 It is often used with intensive management therapies to achieve euglycemia with the ultimate goal of preventing the chronic complications of diabetes.[1-3] It can also be used with more basic therapies, especially in persons with type 2 diabetes.

3 This chapter addresses pattern management as a way to analyze the data collected through self-monitoring of blood glucose (SMBG) in a logical and methodical manner, thus allowing carefully planned changes to the treatment program.

4 An expected benefit is more consistency in analysis of the variables of diabetes self-management This may lead to increased awareness of causes of glycemic fluctuations.

Objectives

Upon completion of this chapter, the learner will be able to

1 List concepts of pattern management.

2 Identify strategies utilized in pattern management.

3 Describe algorithms for making insulin adjustments.

4 Describe changes in insulin regimens to accommodate special situations (eg, travel, shift work).

5 Describe how pattern management may be utilized in persons with type 2 diabetes whether on oral agents or insulin.

Concepts of Pattern Management

1 Pattern management is a comprehensive approach to blood glucose management that includes all aspects of current diabetes therapy.[4] While this approach is typically identified with intensive or flexible insulin therapy, pattern management can also include changes in nonpharmacologic therapies (ie, nutrition therapy and physical activity) and utilization of many pharmacologic combinations to improve glycemic control.

2 Combinations of multiple oral glucose-lowering agents can be used to address the specific pathophysiologic problems of insulin resistance, insulin secretory defect, and excessive hepatic glucose production. This further enhances the opportunity to personalize and intensify diabetes management for persons with type 2 diabetes.

3 Improvements in monitoring tools increase the potential for gathering the information necessary to appropriately apply nutrition therapy, physical activity, and medications in order to attain blood glucose goals established by the individual with diabetes and the diabetes care team (see Chapter 5, Monitoring, in Diabetes Management Therapies, for recommended glucose goals for adults and Chapter 2, Type 1 Diabetes in Youth, in Diabetes in the Life Cycle and Research, for glucose goal ranges for children and adolescents).

4 Elements of pattern management include

  A Self-identified desire of the person with diabetes to be an active participant in care.

  B Identification of individualized blood glucose goals by the person with diabetes and diabetes care team.

  C Frequent self-monitoring of blood glucose (SMBG) written in a record book to provide data for making adjustments.

  D A food/meal plan to follow and consistency in carbohydrate intake are basic skills for pattern management. Determining insulin-to-carbohydrate ratios is an advanced skill to adjust insulin based on carbohydrate intake. Insulin-to-carbohydrate ratios are developed by determining the amount of insulin needed to cover usual carbohydrate intake.[5]

  E Multiple injections of insulin, insulin pump therapy, combinations of oral glucose-lowering medications, or oral glucose-lowering medications and insulin.

  F Self-adjustments, based on blood glucose monitoring data, of food intake, physical activity, and medication(s) to achieve glycemic goals.

  G Frequent interaction between individuals with diabetes and the diabetes care team. Telephone, fax, and e-mail can be used to discuss glucose values between visits.

  H Self-management training, including
- Comprehensive and interactive coverage of the content education areas identified by the National Standards for Diabetes Self-Management Education[6]
- The relationship of glucose levels, food, activity, and medications
- The impact of elements of control on personal glucose levels for prevention of hypoglycemia or hyperglycemia or for prediction of medication changes.
- Purpose, strategies, and value of pattern management for intensive therapy to achieve blood glucose goals
- Empowerment of patient through education for decision-making and problem-solving, goal setting, and long-term motivation
- An understanding of personal belief systems related to the value of health and intensive diabetes management
- Personal diabetes and health-related supplies

  I Support systems to provide emotional and management support
- Diabetes care team with on-call clinical support
- Family or care partners
- Support groups (ie, American Diabetes Association, hospital, education center)
- Other community diabetes educational activities

Strategies for Pattern Management

1 Pattern management involves reviewing several days of glucose records and making adjustments in diabetes therapies based on trends, rather than reacting to a single high or low blood glucose reading. Adding supplemental or sliding-scale insulin at the time of the elevated glucose level solves the problem only for that particular point in time but does not prevent the problem from occurring again.

2 The patient must have a food plan that he or she can follow consistently. The number of carbohydrate servings is determined by the person with diabetes. To determine patterns, the person's food intake, physical activity, and insulin or other medications must be as consistent as possible. This helps prevent blood glucose fluctuations that can mask true patterns.

3 Pattern management includes a review of all variables that affect blood glucose levels—food, physical activity, stress, and illness—not just insulin or other medication adjustments.[7]

   A In persons using insulin, if blood glucose levels are out of goal range, consider whether

- The individual prefers to change carbohydrate intake or physical activity, or adjust insulin or other medications. Often it is easier to make insulin or other medication adjustments. However, weight management must be a consideration. Increasing insulin to cover extra food carbohydrates will increase calories and potentially weight.
- The individual is on enough insulin, too much insulin, or on the wrong insulin regimen.

   B In persons with type 2 diabetes, if blood glucose levels are out of goal range, consider whether

- The individual has a food/meal plan that he or she is able to follow.
- The individual requires a change in medication dose or addition of a second or third oral medication, the addition of evening insulin to oral medications, or a change to an insulin regimen.

4 The first step in pattern management is to identify blood glucose goals and for the person to monitor blood glucose levels 4 to 6 times a day. The frequency of monitoring is based on the management regimen. Food records with the number of carbohydrate servings and blood glucose readings are then analyzed once or twice a week. Questions to ask when evaluating blood glucose readings are listed in Table 6.1. When looking for patterns, read down the columns of blood glucose checks to review all the readings at each time. Three high readings at the same time each day is a pattern of highs. Two low readings at the same time is a pattern of lows.[7]

Table 6.1. Questions to Ask When Evaluating Blood Glucose Readings

1 Is there a pattern upon examination of 3 to 5 days of blood glucose readings?

2 Does something happen at the same time every day, such as an insulin reaction or high glucose after breakfast?

3 Are there blood glucose readings representing all "times" of the day?

4 Are there blood glucose readings representing the "peak" times of each medication (insulins and/or oral agents)?

5 Are there readings to represent peak glucose readings after all meals?

6 Are there "other notes" or "changes" such as meal times, carbohydrate or calorie variances, exercise changes, unusual hours of work or school, stress, or illness?

7 Is prevention of weight gain or weight loss important for the patient? If so, consideration must be given to trying to reduce the use of hypoglycemic medications (ie, insulin or insulin secretagogues), especially if low blood glucose levels are occurring routinely.

8 Does the patient have a history of weight gain? Is the weight gain the result of frequent episodes of hypoglycemia with overtreatment?

9 Does the patient have a history of weight loss? Is the weight loss caused by poor glycemic control?

A If blood glucose readings are high for 3 to 5 days at a specific time—ie, a repeated pattern—potential causes for the elevated levels are examined so the problem can be corrected. Causes of high blood glucose levels can be
- Eating too much carbohydrate or more calories than usual
- Doing less physical activity than usual
- Taking too little insulin; missing an insulin dose; or problems with the dose, type, or combination of oral medications
- Using expired or improperly stored insulin, not taking oral agents as prescribed
- Experiencing emotional or physical stress, including illness
- Rebound response from the liver releasing excessive amounts of glucose from glycogen as a result of hypoglycemia
- Overtreatment of hypoglycemia

B If blood glucose levels are low for 2 days at the same time of day, potential causes are examined. Low blood glucose levels are usually corrected before highs. Hypoglycemia can cause a rebound glucose response which causes hyperglycemia to occur later. Causes of low blood glucose levels can be
- Eating too little carbohydrate or less than usual; too few calories
- Doing more physical activity than usual
- Taking too much insulin or oral medications
- Experiencing hot weather or taking a hot bath

C This method of managing diabetes has been used since the 1930s, originally with children and later with adults with type 1 or type 2 diabetes.[8]

5 Patient ownership in this intensive management approach is essential. Commitment to long-term self-care is enhanced by the patient being educated to fully understand the rationale and the goals. This empowers the patient to set personal short- and long-term goals and to discuss with others how obstacles will be dealt with, including the challenge of maintaining long-term motivation.

Glucose Monitoring

1 Self-monitoring of blood glucose (SMBG) is critical for pattern management. The frequency and timing of blood glucose monitoring is variable depending on the pharmacologic therapy and glucose goals. When insulin doses are being adjusted, SMBG may be required 6 to 8 times per day until doses are adequately titrated and glucose goals are attained. SMBG should be done premeal, 2 <u>hours after the</u> start of the meal, at bedtime, and periodically between 2 and 3 AM.

2 SMBG is done fasting, premeals, and at the peak effect of the medication (typically 2 hours postprandially) so that insulin or medications can be adjusted appropriately (see the Problem-Solving Practice section of this chapter for examples).

A Premeal glucose measurements are needed to monitor basal (or background) insulin dose(s) (eg, NPH, glargine, or Ultralente). (See Tables 6.2 and 6.3.) If fasting or predinner readings are out of target range, consider adjusting basal insulin doses. Premeal testing may also be used to determine a supplemental/correction insulin dose to add or subtract from the bolus dose.

B Two-hour postprandial (pp) glucose readings are needed to titrate rapid-acting insulin (eg, lispro insulin or aspart insulin) for mealtime injections. (See Tables 6.4, 6.5, and 6.6.) If the difference in premeal and pp glucose readings is greater than 20 to 40 mg/dL (1.1 to 2.2 mmol/L), consider adjusting the mealtime rapid-acting insulin.

C Two-hour postprandial readings are also used to evaluate the effectiveness of thiazolidinediones (TZDs), glipizide, glyburide, repaglinide, nateglinide, alpha-glucosidase inhibitors, and other glucose-lowering agents.

3 Elevated fasting glucose levels require 3 AM testing and recording for at least once a week to determine the cause. High fasting glucose levels can be caused by

[handwritten margin note: ✳ Somogi]

A Overnight lows that trigger the liver to release glucose (Somogyi or rebound effect)

B Normal hormonal changes that trigger the liver to release excessive glucose in the early morning (dawn phenomenon)

C Insufficient basal or background insulin

D In youth, growth hormone secreted at night during the growth spurt

4 Flexible insulin regimens using basal and bolus insulin injections and insulin pump therapy require SMBG levels 4 to 6 times per day to determine the effectiveness of the basal dose and the amount of each bolus dose.

5 During acute illness, premeal or hourly testing is needed to determine the need for and dose of any supplemental insulin. (See Chapter 9, Illness and Surgery, in Diabetes Management Therapies.)

6 Asymptomatic hypoglycemia requires more frequent and regular testing on a daily basis, particularly at peak insulin times and before driving, as a precaution for recognizing low blood glucose levels. (See Chapter 8, Hypoglycemia, in Diabetes Management Therapies.)

7 Pregnancy requires frequent SMBG (eg, 5 to 6 times per day) in order to make the adjustments needed for tight blood glucose control (see Chapter 3, Pregnancy With Preexisting Diabetes, in Diabetes in the Life Cycle and Research).

8 Unusual schedules present special challenges to glycemic control. The use of pattern management can help to maintain consistent blood glucose levels. SMBG is essential for decision making, and use of basal/bolus regimens can reduce the difficulties of scheduling dilemmas to a great extent.

A Some challenging situations include travel across time zones, working night or swing shifts, farming, business schedules, and college student schedules. Food intake varies and may not always be able to be scheduled. Eating out makes it difficult to estimate portions or carbohydrate content. Physical activity opportunities are also quite variable.

B Each situation requires flexibility and individual planning. Understanding medications and their actions, especially insulin action, is critical. Start with the individual's plan and factor in special situations related to food intake, meal patterns, medication, and physical activity.

C If the individual is unable to eat (especially children) or is hypoglycemic, rapid-acting insulin may be given at the end of the meal.

9 Objective summary assessment of glycemia is needed in addition to SMBG data.
  A Glycosylated hemoglobin (A1C) is measured quarterly until goals are reached and then at least 2 times per year.[9]
  B Glycosylated albumin (fructosamine) may be used for biweekly testing during pregnancy[10] and at other times when a more rapid assessment of overall glycemic control is needed.

Insulin Algorithms

1 Insulin therapy options can include algorithm approaches or individualized pattern management. The algorithm approach to insulin therapy is used to provide variation in the usual insulin dose; supplemental insulin doses are utilized.

2 Algorithm approaches may be compensatory or anticipatory.
  A Compensatory insulin changes are added insulin supplements used to correct unusual hyperglycemia in response to an unanticipated event (eg, acute illness). Medical centers use different methods to determine the compensatory insulin dose.
    • Some centers may develop an individualized table listing mealtime blood glucose levels above (or below) target goal ranges and the number of units of mealtime rapid-acting or short-acting insulin that should be added (or subtracted) from the usual mealtime insulin dose. For example, if the premeal glucose level is 50 mg/dL (2.7 mmol/L) higher than the target blood glucose goal, the individual is instructed to take an additional 1 unit of insulin. If there is a consistent pattern of increasing or decreasing insulin doses, a change should be made in the insulin affecting that time period.
    • Other centers may use other methods. An example of formulas used to compensate for a high blood glucose are the 1500 rule for short-acting insulin (regular) and the 1800 rule for rapid-acting insulin. These formulas are used to determine the insulin sensitivity factor. The insulin sensitivity factor defines how many mg/dL a unit of short-acting insulin or rapid-acting insulin will lower blood glucose levels. Use of this formula provides a starting point for lowering glucose elevations.
    • 1500 rule: 1500 ÷ total daily insulin dose = mg/dL drop in blood glucose from 1 unit of short-acting insulin (sensitivity factor); for example, 1500 ÷ 50 units of total insulin = 30 mg/dL (sensitivity factor) drop in blood glucose from 1 unit of short-acting insulin. To determine the supplemental dose, subtract from the actual blood glucose the goal blood glucose level and divide by the sensitivity factor.
    • 1800 rule: 1800 ÷ total daily insulin dose = mg/dL drop in blood glucose from 1 unit of rapid-acting insulin (sensitivity factor); for example, 1800 ÷ 50 units of total insulin = 36 mg/dL (sensitivity factor) drop in blood glucose from 1 unit of rapid-acting insulin. To determine the supplemental dose, subtract from the actual blood glucose the goal blood glucose and divide by the sensitivity factor.
    • Compensatory insulin changes can also be made if the premeal insulin is low. In this case, the rapid-acting insulin dose may be decreased, given at the time the person eats, or given at the end of the meal.

■ Anticipatory insulin changes are supplements added to the insulin administered before expected increases in carbohydrate intake. Various formulas are available for calculating insulin-to-carbohydrate ratios (see Chapter 1, Medical Nutrition Therapy for Diabetes, and Chapter 7, Insulin Pump Therapy and Carbohydrate Counting for Pump Therapy: Insulin-to-Carbohydrate Ratios, in Diabetes Management Therapies). One unit of rapid-acting or short-acting insulin per 10 to 15 g of carbohydrate is a common starting point (1:10 or 1:15).

  • Insulin-to-carbohydrate ratios may differ for different meals. For example: 1 unit for 10 g of carbohydrate (1:10) for breakfast versus 1 unit to 15 g carbohydrate (1:15) for the lunch and dinner. Preprandial and postprandial glucose testing is essential in determining appropriate insulin-to-carbohydrate ratios.

3 The sliding-scale approach tries to solve the problem only for a particular point in time but does not prevent the problem from occurring again. This method should be discontinued. Sliding scales are not part of pattern management.

  A Sliding-scale doses are given in addition to the usual insulin dose. The supplements are given in relation to a range of preset blood glucose values.

  B A typical sliding-scale program suggests a preset amount of insulin based on glucose readings, regardless of age or weight. The result is often a roller coaster–like shift between hypoglycemia and hyperglycemia, a situation that does nothing to contribute to overall health or feelings of well-being for the patient.

Pattern Management for Insulin Users

1 Blood glucose monitoring data is used in pattern management to make decisions on variables that can be changed to improve glycemic control.

  A Tables 6.2 to 6.6 give guidelines for adjusting insulin (or carbohydrate) based on blood glucose monitoring data for different insulin regimens.

  • Table 6.2 is for pattern management using premeal SMBG and 2 to 3 injections of insulin per day.

  • Table 6.3 is for pattern management using premeal SMBG and 4 injections of insulin per day.

  • Table 6.4 is for pattern management using premeal and 2-hour postmeal SMBG and 2 injections of insulin per day.

  • Table 6.5 is for pattern management using premeal and 2-hour SMBG and 3 injections of insulin per day.

  • Table 6.6 is for pattern management using premeal and 2-hour SMBG and 4 injections of insulin per day.

2 Before using pattern management to make adjustments in insulin, evaluate the following:

  A Consistency in variables that affect blood glucose concentrations. Patterns are only revealed if the person with diabetes is keeping food intake, physical activity, and insulin doses consistent. Consistency helps prevent blood glucose fluctuations that can mask true patterns. Therefore, when making insulin adjustments based on blood glucose patterns, encourage the patient to

  • Eat consistent amounts of carbohydrate at consistent times each day

  • Maintain a consistent schedule of physical activity

  • Take prescribed insulin doses consistently

■ Level of overall glucose control.[7] If the majority of blood glucose checks are over 200 mg/dL (11.1 mmol/L), the regimen may need a significant adjustment.

C Appropriateness of the insulin regimen. In general, 50% of the total insulin dose is needed for basal insulin and 50% for mealtime insulin (divided between 3 meals).

  • Patients may be on a fixed (basic) insulin regimen, but they will have a more physiologic insulin regimen with an intensive (flexible) insulin regimen. An intensive regimen will also give them more flexibilty.

  • If the patient has made frequent adjustments in mealtime insulin doses, the balance between basal (background) and bolus (mealtime) insulin may no longer be appropriate. For example, the mealtime insulin may be 70% of the total insulin dose instead of approximately 50%.

3 The tables are designed to assist in looking for patterns and choosing and making insulin (or carbohydrate) adjustments. If an appropriate food/meal plan has been designed and is being used by the person with diabetes, insulin adjustments are often easier and more appropriate than carbohydrate adjustments. Adjustments in the regimen are meant to gradually move blood glucose checks into the goal ranges. Adjustments should be maintained for 3 days before making additional changes (unless the change has caused frequent hypoglycemia). Follow-up and support of the person with diabetes is essential for successful pattern management.

Table 6.2. Pattern Management—Premeal Monitoring for 2 to 3 Insulin Injections Per Day

Lispro, aspart, or regular insulin mixed with NPH insulin, AM dose
Lispro, aspart, or regular insulin, dinner dose
NPH insulin, bedtime dose
Or
70/30, Novolog Mix 70/30, or Humalog Mix 75/25, AM and dinner doses

Evaluate Blood Glucose (BG) Patterns

1 Adjust insulin based on 2- to 3-day BG patterns.
2 Determine which insulin is responsible for the pattern.
3 Adjust insulin 10% to 20%.
4 2-hour pp blood glucose tests needed for lispro or aspart titration. If using lispro or aspart, 1 injection of NPH insulin may not provide 24-hour basal coverage in insulinopenic patients.

AM	Below Target Blood Glucose	Above Target Blood Glucose
Dose affecting	*Bedtime NPH insulin* 1 Evaluate nocturnal hypoglycemia (check 3 AM BG). 2 Determine if low blood glucose is occurring during or after exercise. 3 Consider decreasing bedtime NPH insulin. 4 Consider increasing carbohydrate content of the evening snack.	*Bedtime NPH insulin* 1 Evaluate nocturnal hypoglycemia or hyperglycemia (check 3 AM BG). 2 Consider increasing bedtime NPH insulin. 3 Consider decreasing carbohydrate content of the evening snack. 4 Check time patient is giving bedtime insulin injection.

Midday Prelunch	Below Target Blood Glucose	Above Target Blood Glucose
Dose affecting	*AM lispro, aspart, or regular insulin* 1 Consider increasing carbohydrate content of breakfast or add midmorning snack or increase carbohydrate content of midmorning snack. 2 Determine if low blood glucose is occurring during or after exercise. 3 Consider decreasing AM lispro, aspart, or regular insulin. 4 Decrease insulin-to-carbohydrate ratio.	*AM lispro, aspart, or regular insulin* 1 Consider decreasing carbohydrate content of breakfast or eliminate midmorning snack. 2 Increase insulin-to-carbohydrate ratio. 3 Consider adjusting exercise times or adding exercise. 4 Consider increasing AM lispro, aspart, or regular insulin. 5 If regular insulin, snack may need to be adjusted.

PM Predinner	Below Target Blood Glucose	Above Target Blood Glucose
Dose affecting	*AM NPH insulin* 1 Consider adding an afternoon snack or increasing carbohydrate content of afternoon snack. 2 Determine if low blood glucose is occurring during or after exercise. 3 Consider decreasing AM NPH insulin.	*AM NPH insulin* 1 Consider eliminating afternoon snack or decreasing carbohydrate content of the midafternoon snack. 2 Consider adjusting exercise times or adding exercise. 3 Consider increasing AM NPH insulin. 4 If pp are out of target, consider increasing insulin-to-carbohydrate ratio at dinner. 5 Check time of lunch and carbohydrate content.

Bedtime	Below Target Blood Glucose	Above Target Blood Glucose
Dose affecting	*PM lispro, aspart, or regular insulin* 1 Consider increasing carbohydrate content at dinner. 2 Determine if low blood glucose is occurring during or after exercise. 3 Consider decreasing predinner lispro, aspart, or regular insulin. 4 Decrease insulin-to-carbohydrate ratio.	*PM lispro, aspart, or regular insulin* 1 Consider decreasing carbohydrate content at dinner. 2 Consider adjusting exercise times or adding exercise. 3 Consider increasing predinner lispro, aspart, or regular insulin. 4 Increase insulin-to-carbohydrate ratio.

Table 6.3. Pattern Management—Premeal Monitoring for 4 Insulin Injections per Day

Lispro, aspart, or regular insulin, AM dose
Lispro, aspart, or regular insulin, lunch dose
Lispro, aspart, or regular insulin, dinner dose
NPH or glargine insulin, bedtime dose or Ultralente, dinner dose

Evaluate Blood Glucose (BG) Patterns

1 Adjust insulin based on 2- to 3-day BG patterns.
2 Determine which insulin is responsible for the pattern.
3 Adjust insulin 10% to 20%.
4 2-hour pp blood glucose testing is needed for lispro or aspart titration.
5 If using lispro or aspart, 1 injection of NPH insulin may not provide 24-hour basal coverage in insulinopenic patients.
6 With glargine, snacks are optional. Clinical experience suggests more than 15 g carbohydrate or more than 100 calories, may require additional rapid-acting insulin.

AM	Below Target Blood Glucose	Above Target Blood Glucose
Dose affecting	*Bedtime NPH or glargine insulin or supper Ultralente* 1 Evaluate nocturnal hypoglycemia (check 3 AM BG). 2 Consider decreasing bedtime NPH, glargine, or Ultralente insulin. 3 Consider adding or increasing carbohydrate content of evening snack.	*Bedtime NPH or glargine insulin or supper Ultralente* 1 Evaluate nocturnal hypoglycemia or hyperglycemia (check 3 AM BG). 2 Consider increasing bedtime NPH, glargine, or Ultralente insulin. 3 Consider decreasing carbohydrate content of evening snack.

Midday Prelunch	Below Target Blood Glucose	Above Target Blood Glucose
Dose affecting	AM *lispro, aspart, or regular insulin* 1 If on regular insulin, consider increasing carbohydrate content of midmorning snack. 2 Determine if low blood glucose is occurring during or after exercise. 3 Consider decreasing AM lispro, aspart, or regular insulin. 4 Decrease insulin-to-carbohydrate ratio.	AM *lispro, aspart, or regular insulin* 1 If on regular insulin, consider decreasing carbohydrate content of midmorning snack. 2 Consider adjusting exercise times or adding exercise. 3 Consider increasing AM lispro, aspart, or regular insulin. 4 Increase insulin-to-carbohydrate ratio.

PM Predinner	Below Target Blood Glucose	Above Target Blood Glucose
Dose affecting	*Lunch lispro, aspart, or regular insulin* 1 If on regular insulin, consider increasing carbohydrate content of the afternoon snack. 2 Determine if low blood glucose is occurring during or after exercise. 3 Consider decreasing AM NPH insulin. 4 Decrease insulin-to-carbohydrate ratio.	*Lunch lispro, aspart, or regular insulin* 1 If on regular insulin, consider decreasing carbohydrate content of the afternoon snack. 2 Consider adjusting exercise times or adding exercise. 3 Consider increasing AM NPH insulin. 4 Increase insulin-to-carbohydrate ratio.

Bedtime	Below Target Blood Glucose	Above Target Blood Glucose
Dose affecting	*Dinner lispro, aspart, or regular insulin* 1 Consider increasing carbohydrate content at dinner. 2 Determine if low blood glucose is occurring during or after exercise. 3 Consider decreasing dinner lispro, aspart, or regular insulin. 4 Decrease insulin-to-carbohydrate ratio.	*Dinner lispro, aspart, or regular insulin* 1 Consider decreasing carbohydrate content at dinner. 2 Consider adjusting exercise times or adding exercise. 3 Consider increasing dinner lispro, aspart, or regular insulin. 4 Increase insulin-to-carbohydrate ratio.

Table 6.4. Pattern Management—Premeal and 2-Hour Postmeal Monitoring for 2 Injections per Day

Lispro, aspart, or regular insulin/NPH, AM dose
Lispro, aspart, or regular insulin/NPH, PM dose

Evaluate Blood Glucose (BG) Patterns

1 Adjust insulin based on 2- to 3-day BG patterns.
2 Determine which insulin is responsible for the pattern.
3 Adjust insulin by 10% to 20% of total daily dose.
4 Premeal and 2-hour pp blood glucose testing needed for lispro or aspart titration.
5 If using lispro or aspart, 1 injection of NPH insulin may not provide 24-hour basal coverage for insulinopenic patients.

2-h pp Breakfast	Below Target Blood Glucose	Above Target Blood Glucose
Dose affecting	AM *lispro, aspart, or regular insulin* **1** Consider decreasing AM lispro, aspart, or regular insulin. **2** Determine if low blood glucose is occurring during or after exercise. **3** Consider increasing carbohydrate content of breakfast. **4** Decrease insulin-to-carbohydrate ratio.	AM *lispro, aspart, or regular insulin* **1** Consider increasing AM lispro, aspart, or regular insulin. **2** Consider adjusting exercise times or adding exercise. **3** Consider giving regular injection 45 minutes before meal. **4** Consider decreasing carbohydrate content at breakfast. **5** Increase insulin-to-carbohydrate ratio.

2-h pp Lunch	Below Target Blood Glucose	Above Target Blood Glucose
Dose affecting	AM *NPH insulin* **1** Consider increasing carbohydrate content at lunch. **2** Determine if low blood glucose is occurring during or after exercise. **3** Consider decreasing AM NPH insulin.	AM *NPH insulin* **1** Consider decreasing carbohydrate content at lunch. **2** Consider adjusting exercise times or adding exercise. **3** Consider increasing AM NPH insulin.

2-h pp Dinner	Below Target Blood Glucose	Above Target Blood Glucose
Dose affecting	*Dinner lispro, aspart, or regular insulin* **1** Consider decreasing dinner lispro, aspart, or regular insulin. **2** Determine if low blood glucose is occurring during or after exercise. **3** Consider increasing carbohydrate content at dinner. **4** Decrease insulin-to-carbohydrate ratio.	*Dinner lispro, aspart, or regular insulin* **1** Consider increasing dinner lispro, aspart, or regular insulin. **2** Consider adjusting exercise times or adding exercise. **3** Consider giving regular injection 45 minutes before meal. **4** Consider decreasing carbohydrate content at dinner. **5** Increase insulin-to-carbohydrate ratio.

Table 6.5. Pattern Management—Premeal and 2-Hour Postmeal Monitoring for 3 Insulin Injections per Day

Lispro, aspart, or regular/NPH insulin, AM dose
Lispro, aspart, or regular insulin, dinner dose
NPH insulin, bedtime dose

Evaluate Blood Glucose (BG) Patterns

1 Adjust insulin based on 2- to 3-day BG patterns.
2 Determine which insulin is responsible for the pattern.
3 Adjust insulin 10% to 20%.
4 Premeal and 2-hour pp blood glucose testing needed for lispro or aspart titration.
5 If using lispro or aspart, 1 injection of NPH insulin may not provide 24-hour basal coverage for insulinopenic patients.

2-h pp Breakfast	Below Target Blood Glucose	Above Target Blood Glucose
Dose affecting	AM *lispro, aspart, or regular insulin* 1 Consider decreasing AM lispro, aspart, or regular insulin. 2 Determine if low blood glucose is occurring during or after exercise. 3 Consider increasing carbohydrate content of breakfast. 4 Decrease insulin-to-carbohydrate ratio.	AM *lispro, aspart, or regular insulin* 1 Consider increasing AM lispro, aspart, or regular insulin. 2 Consider adjusting exercise times or adding exercise. 3 Consider giving regular injection 45 minutes before meal. 4 Consider decreasing carbohydrate content at breakfast. 5 Increase insulin-to-carbohydrate ratio.

2-h pp Lunch	Below Target Blood Glucose	Above Target Blood Glucose
Dose affecting	AM *NPH insulin* 1 Consider increasing carbohydrate content at lunch. 2 Determine if low blood glucose is occurring during or after exercise. 3 Consider decreasing NPH insulin.	AM *NPH insulin* 1 Consider decreasing carbohydrate content at lunch. 2 Consider adjusting exercise times or adding exercise. 3 Consider increasing NPH insulin.

2-h pp Dinner	Below Target Blood Glucose	Above Target Blood Glucose
Dose affecting	*Dinner lispro, aspart, or regular insulin* 1 Consider decreasing lispro, aspart, or regular insulin. 2 Determine if low blood glucose is occurring during or after exercise. 3 Consider increasing carbohydrate content at dinner. 4 Decrease insulin-to-carbohydrate ratio.	*Dinner lispro, aspart, or regular insulin* 1 Consider increasing PM lispro, aspart, or regular insulin. 2 Consider adjusting exercise times or adding exercise. 3 Consider giving regular injection 45 minutes before meal. 4 Consider decreasing carbohydrate content at dinner. 5 Increase insulin-to-carbohydrate ratio.

Table 6.6. Pattern Management—Premeal and 2-Hour Postmeal Monitoring for 4 Injections per Day

Lispro, aspart, or regular insulin, AM dose
Lispro, aspart, or regular insulin, lunch dose
Lispro, aspart, or regular insulin, dinner dose
Glargine insulin or NPH, bedtime dose or Ultralente, dinner dose

Evaluate Blood Glucose (BG) Patterns

1 Adjust insulin based on 2- to 3-day BG patterns.
2 Determine which insulin is responsible for the pattern.
3 Adjust insulin 10% to 20%.
4 Premeal and 2-hour pp blood glucose testing needed for lispro or aspart titration.
5 If using lispro or aspart, 1 injection of NPH insulin may not provide 24-hour basal coverage for insulinopenic patients.

2-h pp Breakfast	Below Target Blood Glucose	Above Target Blood Glucose
Dose affecting	AM *lispro, aspart, or regular insulin* **1** Consider decreasing AM lispro, aspart, or regular insulin. **2** Determine if low blood glucose is occurring during or after exercise. **3** Consider increasing carbohydrate content of breakfast. **4** Decrease insulin-to-carbohydrate ratio.	AM *lispro, aspart, or regular insulin* **1** Consider increasing AM lispro, aspart or regular insulin. **2** Consider adjusting exercise times or adding exercise. **3** Consider giving regular injection 45 minutes before meal. **4** Consider decreasing carbohydrate content at breakfast. **5** Increase insulin-to-carbohydrate ratio.

2-h pp Lunch	Below Target Blood Glucose	Above Target Blood Glucose
Dose affecting	Midday *lispro, aspart, or regular insulin* **1** Consider decreasing midday lispro, aspart, or regular insulin. **2** Determine if low blood glucose is occurring during or after exercise. **3** Consider increasing carbohydrate content at lunch. **4** Decrease insulin-to-carbohydrate ratio.	Midday *lispro, aspart, or regular insulin* **1** Consider increasing midday lispro, aspart, or regular insulin. **2** Consider adjusting exercise times or adding exercise. **3** Consider giving regular injection 45 minutes before meal. **4** Consider decreasing carbohydrate content at lunch. **5** Increase insulin-to-carbohydrate ratio.

2-h pp Dinner	Below Target Blood Glucose	Above Target Blood Glucose
Dose affecting	Dinner *lispro, aspart, or regular insulin* **1** Consider decreasing dinner lispro, aspart, or regular insulin. **2** Determine if low blood glucose is occurring during or after exercise. **3** Consider increasing carbohydrate content at dinner. **4** Decrease insulin-to-carbohydrate ratio.	Dinner *lispro, aspart, or regular insulin* **1** Consider increasing dinner aspart, lispro, or regular insulin. **2** Consider adjusting exercise times or adding exercise. **3** Consider giving regular injection 45 minutes before meal. **4** Consider decreasing carbohydrate content at dinner. **5** Increase insulin-to-carbohydrate ratio.

Problem-Solving Practice: Persons Using Insulin

1 This section is designed to provide practice in pattern management through the evaluation of blood glucose records and determination of problems, possible causes, and options for adjustments. The following guidelines can be used for all of these situations.

2 Goals when well: Blood glucose levels in target range without significant hypoglycemic episodes; no ketones. The following steps are used by the person with diabetes and the healthcare provider:

A Monitor fasting, premeal, and 2-hour postprandial blood glucose levels. Blood glucose monitoring is done 4 to 6 times a day based on the insulin regimen.

B Record food intake, count carbohydrate servings or grams, and record blood glucose data. Analyze records once or twice per week.

C For type 1 diabetes, aim for 75% to 85% in the target range. If the majority of checks are out of goal range, consider whether a change in the insulin regimen is needed.

D Evaluate food intake and carbohydrate consistency. Person with diabetes decides if increasing or decreasing carbohydrate intake is the first change to try or if insulin should be adjusted.

E Evaluate physical activity amount and timing.

F Change insulin dose in amounts of 10%. (This individualizes the dose and accounts for insulin resistance and other sensitivity issues.)

G If fasting blood glucose levels are elevated, consider adding a 3 AM check to determine if it is caused by the Somogyi (rebound) syndrome, dawn phenomenon, or insufficient insulin. If blood glucose levels are erratic due to Somogyi (rebound) syndrome, consider decreasing insulin dose by approximately 10%.

H Evaluate sites and timing of injections. (Hypertrophy occurs more commonly than expected if rotation of sites is not implemented.)

I Evaluate if problems with blood glucose are related to stress and if there is a need for stress management.

Case Studies in Insulin Users

Sean

Type 1 diabetes
- Breakfast—12 units lispro/8 units NPH
- Lunch—10 units lispro
- Dinner—14 units lispro
- Bedtime—11 units NPH
- 2600 calories—3 meals, 1 snack
  2 units lispro = 1 carbohydrate serving (15 g) (2:15)

Time	Mon	Thurs	Sun
Fasting	100 mg/dL	110 mg/dL	103 mg/dL
2 hours after breakfast	322	284	250
Before lunch			
After lunch	280	246	150
Before dinner			
2 hours after dinner	148	131	133
Changes in Schedule/Routine			
Food	+2 milk	pancakes, OJ	+1 toast
Insulin/Medication			
Reactions			
Activity	⬆		
Remarks	7 PM football		

Key:　Food changes/time　　　Activity　　　　　　　Reaction/Illness
　　　+1 = 1 extra CHO (15 g)　⬆ increased activity　　M = mild　　S = severe
　　　−1 = 1 less CHO (15 g)　⬇ decreased activity　　Mo = moderate

Problem

- Pattern of high blood glucose levels after breakfast (and lunch)

Possible Causes

- Too much carbohydrate at breakfast/lunch for the current insulin, or stated another way,
- Not enough insulin before breakfast/lunch
- Insulin-to-carbohydrate ratio is wrong, needs to be recalculated
- Not counting carbohydrate correctly
- Not using insulin-to-carbohydrate ratio

Options

- Consider changing something in routine before the high tests:
  —Increase lispro insulin before breakfast/lunch
  —Increase the insulin-to-carbohydrate ratio at breakfast (for example, 2.5 units lispro
    for 1 carbohydrate serving) (2.5:15); recalculate insulin-to-carbohydrate ratio
  —Decrease total carbohydrate at breakfast/lunch
  —Include exercise after breakfast

Mark (construction worker)

Type 1 diabetes
- Breakfast—34 units 70/30 Novolog Mix
- Dinner—6 units Novolog
- Bedtime—11 units NPH
- 2700 calories—3 meals, 3 snacks

Schedule	Tues	Thurs	Sat
Fasting	106 mg/dL	110 mg/dL	117 mg/dL
2 hours after breakfast	175	341	148
Before lunch			
2 hours after lunch	151	150	229
Before dinner			
2 hours after dinner	135	153	210
Changes in Schedule/Routine			
Food	No change	No change	No change
Insulin/Medication			
Reactions			
Activity	Usual	Usual	Usual
Remarks			

Key: Food changes/time   Activity   Reaction/Illness
      +1 = 1 extra CHO (15 g)   ⬆ increased activity   M = mild   S = severe
      −1 = 1 less CHO (15 g)   ⬇ decreased activity   Mo = moderate

Problem

- Erratic blood glucose levels

Possible Causes

- Injection sites (hypertrophy)
- Stress (need to meet job deadlines)
- Somogyi (rebound, overinsulinization)

Options

- No change in dose, as 75% are in target ranges
- Consider changing insulin regimen to rapid-acting insulin at mealtime for greater food flexibility and a long-acting basal, such as glargine, at bedtime to allow increased flexibility in timing and food/meal intake

Melissa

Type 1 diabetes
- Breakfast—2 units lispro for 4 carbohydrate servings
- Lunch—3 units lispro for 6 carbohydrate servings
- Dinner—3 units lispro for 6 carbohydrate servings
- 10 PM—8 units glargine
- 1800 calories
  ½ unit lispro = 1 carbohydrate (15 g) (0.5:15)

Schedule	Thurs	Sat	Sun
Fasting	110 mg/dL	150 mg/dL	163 mg/dL
2 hours after breakfast	132	191	198
Before lunch			
2 hours after lunch	163	161	185
Before dinner			
2 hours after dinner	128	230	236
Changes in Schedule/Routine			
Food			
Insulin/Medication			
Reactions			
Activity	Usual	Usual	Usual
Remarks			

Key: Food changes/time   Activity   Reaction/Illness
       +1 = 1 extra CHO (15 g)   ⬆ increased activity   M = mild   S = severe
       −1 = 1 less CHO (15 g)   ⬇ decreased activity   Mo = moderate

Problem

- Gradual increase in overall blood glucose levels

Possible Causes

- Type 1 diabetes remission ending (out of "honeymoon" stage)
- Illness or low-grade infection
- Pregnancy, growth spurts. puberty and increased stressors at work, school, or home all cause fluctuations and elevations in blood glucose levels. Insulin losing its potency (temperature too high [>86 degrees]) and weekend grazing are other potential contributors to hyperglycemia. However, they would be reflected in overall elevated glucose levels and A1C and in 3-day patterns.

Options

- For adults: Consider decreasing carbohydrate intake or food intake by 100 to 200 calories and/or increase physical activity. However, most women with type 1 diabetes eat at least 1800 calories.
- For children or adults: Consider increasing insulin 10% overall. Try this dose for 2 to 3 days. Increase again if blood glucose is still high. If 3 dose adjustments do not decrease blood glucose levels, instruct patient to call the diabetes care team.

Pattern Management for Type 2 Diabetes

1 In the 1980s, combination therapy was limited to insulin and sulfonylurea combinations. The recent availability of multiple oral glucose-lowering agents for the treatment of type 2 diabetes has created many new therapeutic options. Knowing the pathology of diabetes is critical. The primary defects of 1) decreased or absent beta cell functioning, 2) increased hepatic glucose release, and 3) peripheral insulin resistance may be determined by observing glucose patterns. This will give clinical support for decisions of which oral glucose-lowering agents to initiate and in which combinations. Multiple defects suggest the need for multiple oral agents.

2 A common clinical practice is initiating monotherapy with either an insulin secretagogue or metformin and adding the other agent when the doses approach half maximum to maximum therapeutic limits. This approach requires specific clinical considerations.

   A Careful patient selection for use of metformin and thiazolidinediones is necessary; liver, renal, cardiac, and respiratory function must be assessed

   B Prevention of possible hypoglycemia with insulin secretagogues (sulfonylureas, repaglinide, nateglinide) and insulin injections

   C Use of postprandial SMBG for dose titration

   D Excess flatulence or diarrhea or edema are side effects that should be evaluated if reported by patients (see Chapter 3, Pharmacologic Therapies for Glucose Management, in Diabetes Management Therapies)

   E Guidelines relating to when oral agents should be taken in relation to meals should be provided. For example: sulfonylureas are generally taken 30 minutes prior to the meal; meglitinides are usually taken 5 to 15 minutes before meals; and metformin is taken with the meal to reduce gastrointestinal disturbances and enhance medication action.[11]

3 The thiazolidinediones (TZDs) primarily improve glycemic control by reducing insulin resistance.[12,13] Pioglitazone HCl (Actos) and rosiglitazone maleate (Avandia) are approved for use in combination with insulin. Recent studies have demonstrated TZDs effectiveness for other indications.

   A Because the time to therapeutic response can be 6 to 8 weeks, other agents may need to be implemented initially to control hyperglycemia.

   B After the glycemic benefit occurs, doses of insulin or other oral agents may be titrated downward.

   C TZDs appear to be more effective when used in combination with other agents (see Chapter 3, Pharmacologic Therapies for Glucose Management, in Diabetes Management Therapies, for additional information).

4 Repaglinide and nateglinide provide additional options for combination therapies with metformin and/or TZDs.

5 Alpha-glucosidase inhibitors may be added as a third agent or used as monotherapy; taking with meals enhances medication action and reduces the frequently significant gastrointestinal side effects.

6 Postprandial glucose monitoring provides the most information for dose titration for all oral agents except metformin. Metformin's primary action is to decrease nocturnal hepatic glucose release (gluconeogenesis and glycogenolysis); thus, its effect is most reflected in the fasting glucose value.

7 Because of the progressive nature of type 2 diabetes, combination therapies using oral agents often progress to combination therapy with insulin. Insulin therapy may begin by the addition of an evening dose of glargine (Lantus) or NPH to the oral agents to control fasting blood glucose concentrations.

    A If fasting blood glucose concentrations are consistently >200 mg/dL (11.1 mmol/L) after combining 2 oral agents, adding a third oral agent is unlikely to achieve the desired glucose control. At this point, insulin should be considered.

    B Eventually attempts to duplicate physiologic insulin action should be made. At this time, most persons with type 2 diabetes will benefit from basal (background) and bolus (mealtime) insulin regimens. Pattern recognition will assist in achieving glucose goals.

    C Higher doses of insulin are generally required in persons with type 2 diabetes compared to persons with type 1 diabetes to achieve control. Average insulin doses of approximately 1.2 units/kg/day may be needed to achieve an A1C value <7%.

    D The basal insulin dose is approximately 50% of the total insulin dose. The other 50% is for bolus or mealtime insulin doses, which is divided between breakfast, lunch, and dinner.

Problem-Solving Practice: Persons With Type 2 Diabetes

1 This section is designed to provide practice in pattern management through the evaluation of blood glucose records and determination of problems, possible causes, and options for adjustments. Use the following as a guide for all of these situations.

2 Goals when well: Blood glucose levels in target range without significant hypoglycemic episodes. The following steps are used by the person with diabetes and the healthcare provider:

    A Monitor fasting, premeal, and 2-hour postprandial blood glucose levels. Blood glucose monitoring is done 3 to 4 times a day based on the treatment regimen.

    B Record food intake, count carbohydrate servings or grams, and record blood glucose data. Analyze records once or twice per week.

    C Evaluate food intake and carbohydrate consistency. Consider if the person with diabetes is able to follow the food/meal plan and count carbohydrate servings.

    D For type 2 diabetes, aim for 95% to 100% in the target range. If the majority of checks are out of goal range, consider whether a change in medications is needed.

    E Evaluate physical activity amount and timing.

    F If fasting blood glucose are elevated, consider adding a 3 AM check to determine if it is caused by the dawn phenomenon or insufficient insulin.

    G Evaluate if problems with blood glucose are related to stress and if there is a need for stress management.

    H Consider the need to add a second (or third) oral agent or insulin to the treatment regimen.

Case Studies in Persons With Type 2 Diabetes

Ethel

Type 2 diabetes
- Glipizide 10 mg bid
- Metformin 1000 mg bid
- 1400 calories

Time	Mon	Wed	Sat
Fasting	72 mg/dL	60 mg/dL	71 mg/dL
After breakfast	100	53	67
Before lunch			
2 hrs after lunch	64	55	90
Before supper			
2 hrs after supper	80	66	91
Changes in Schedule/Routine			
Food	+½ c. OJ	+½ milk	+½ honey
Insulin/Medication			
Reactions	2:30 PM M	9:15 AM M	11:30 AM M
Activity		Usual	Usual
Remarks	Yardwork	Picking beans	

Key: Food changes/time   ↑ Activity   Reaction/Illness
      +1 = 1 extra CHO (15 g)   ↓ increased activity   M = mild   S = severe
      −1 = 1 less CHO (15 g)   decreased activity   Mo = moderate

Problem

- Reactions/hypoglycemia too often throughout the day

Possible Causes

- Too much medication
- Inadequate carbohydrate or total food intake

Options

- Consider decreasing sulfonylurea until blood glucose is >100 mg/dL postprandially (individuals who do not want to gain weight) or
- Increase food 100 to 200 calories (individuals who want to gain weight). Example: 100 calories = 1½ carbohydrate servings or 1½ meat; distribute throughout the day.
- Evaluate food intake and understanding of the food/meal plan; ask if Ethel is skipping meals to try and control blood glucose levels and weight.

Mary

Type 2 diabetes
- Pioglitazone (Actos) 45 mg (for 1 week)
- 1600 calories

Schedule	Tues	Thurs	Sat
Fasting	314 mg/dL	288 mg/dL	301 mg/dL
After breakfast	282	214	285
Before lunch			
2 hours after lunch	296	322	274
Before supper			
2 hours after supper	252	297	244
Changes in Schedule/Routine			
Food	Birthday party	Church lunch	Very careful
	8 PM		
Insulin/Medication	X	X	After breakfast
Reactions			
Activity	Shopping		
Remarks		Tired	

Key: Food changes/time   Activity   Reaction/Illness
      +1 = 1 extra CHO (15 g)   ↑ increased activity   M = mild   S = severe
      −1 = 1 less CHO (15 g)   ↓ decreased activity   Mo = moderate

Problem

- Blood glucose levels are too high

Possible Cause

- TZD not taken long enough to provide full glycemic benefit

Options

- Consider adding another oral glucose-lowering medication
- Consider adding sulfonylurea or insulin for 4 to 6 weeks, then reevaluate

John

Type 2 diabetes
- AM—20 mg glucotrol, 1000 mg metformin
- PM—20 mg glucotrol, 1000 mg metformin
- 1800 calories

Schedule	Mon	Wed	Sat
Fasting	180 mg/dL	192 mg/dL	219 mg/dL
2 hours after breakfast	145	154	138
Before lunch			
2 hours after lunch	162	143	121
Before supper			
2 hours after supper	129	116	95
Changes in Schedule/Routine			
Diet	2000		
Insulin/Medication	X	X	X
Reactions			
Activity	Work at airplane factory	Work	"Honey do" list and football
Remarks			

Key: Food changes/time   Activity   Reaction/Illness
      +1 = 1 extra CHO (15 g)   ↑ increased activity   M = mild   S = severe
      −1 = 1 less CHO (15 g)   ↓ decreased activity   Mo = moderate

Problem

- High fasting blood glucose levels

Possible Cause

- Inadequate medication in evening or at bedtime to prevent dawn phenomenon or excessive hepatic glucose release

Options

- Assure individual the high fasting glucose levels are not because he/she ate too much at dinner or during the evening. Explain that food eaten is used or stored in 4 to 5 hours. Explain how the liver releases excessive glucose in the early morning hours if adequate insulin is not available.
- Consider adding bedtime NPH or glargine insulin dose (initiate bedtime basal dose at 10% of total body weight).
- Consider splitting dinner meds.

Summary of Pattern Management Concepts

1 Diabetes therapy using pattern management is more specific to the physiologic or genetic problems causing hyperglycemia.

2 New insulins and oral agents are emerging that allow treatment of the specific causes of the hyperglycemia from insulin resistance to hepatic glucose output or beta cell secretory defects.

A Insulin analogs allow precise treatment based on lifestyles and variables in eating and exercise routines.

B Insulin pump therapy is changing due to use of insulin analogs. New basal insulins that are more consistent have decreased pump initiation in some instances.

3 The success of this complex therapy depends on the skill and expertise of the educator and care team in presenting and verifying understanding of self-management skills needed by the individual with diabetes.

4 Adjustments in therapy can be made to improve blood glucose control. To accomplish this, persons with diabetes must monitor blood glucose, keep records, eat carbohydrate consistently, analyze data, and make changes in insulin or medication(s) when needed.

5 Healthcare providers will require continuing education, protocols, and support from diabetes experts if these new therapies are to be effective for improving patient outcomes and quality of life.

Key Educational Considerations

1 Pattern management can be used by persons with both type 1 and type 2 diabetes. Careful assessment of the patient's readiness to participate actively in such a program is critical to the success of pattern management.

2 Comprehensive self-management training and education is essential to achieve success in pattern management techniques. Particular emphasis for education includes

A Monitoring and recording blood glucose results.

B Appropriate use of medications.

C Blood glucose testing done at planned times to validate efficacy.

D Nutrition therapy and an understanding of why consistency in carbohydrate is important and/or insulin-to-carbohydrate ratios.

E Physical activity at consistent times and with appropriate adjustments in medication(s), insulin, and/or carbohydrate.

F Appropriate treatment of hypoglycemia.

G Guidelines for short-term sick-day care.

H Understanding of the psychosocial implications of having diabetes.

I Empowerment of the individual with diabetes in self-management.

J Team care provided by healthcare providers.

3 Engage individuals with diabetes in problem-solving situations during instruction to teach pattern recognition and application of appropriate options. Empower patients to make small adjustments.

4 Assure individuals with diabetes that they will be able to access their healthcare team when necessary to establish confidence that self-initiated changes can be made safely.

Self-Review Questions

1 If a patient's fasting blood glucose levels are elevated, what would you do to determine the cause?

2 If you determine that a patient's elevated fasting glucose level is due to low blood glucose levels during the night, what therapy changes could be made?

3 Why is it important to be consistent in carbohydrate intake when making insulin adjustments? How are insulin-to-carbohydrate ratios determined?

4 If a patient has persistently elevated glucose readings at midmorning or prelunch, what adjustment could be made?

5 If a patient's predinner glucose level is elevated, what options are available to improve that blood glucose?

Learning Assessment: Case Study 1

KS, a 14-year-old adolescent with type 1 diabetes, is on the volleyball team. Her games are at 5:30 PM. KS takes her insulin (28 units NPH and 10 units of lispro) at 4:30 PM, eats dinner, and then plays volleyball. However, KS is having low blood glucose levels during every game. Her fasting glucose levels (at 7 AM) are always above 170 mg/dL. She usually takes her morning injection of 28 units NPH and 12 units lispro at 7:30 AM.

Questions for Discussion

1 What are reasons for KS's elevated fasting glucose levels?

2 What could you suggest that would provide increased flexibility and help KS meet her glycemic goals?

Discussion

1 KS has a hectic schedule and would likely benefit from moving the NPH to 10 PM. Her dinnertime insulin and dinner could be after the volleyball game.

2 Giving the NPH at 10 PM would shift its peak to early morning. That single change may correct her elevated fasting level. If not, the bedtime NPH dose could be increased by 1 to 2 units every 2 to 3 days until the fasting blood glucose levels are within range.

3 The rationale behind KS's current use of NPH and lispro insulin must be explored as there may be personal, emotional, or developmental issues in conflict with KS's pursuit of other options that are available for improved glycemic control. For instance, is giving an injection at noon an insurmountable problem?

4 A switch to a lispro insulin at all meals and glargine at 10 PM would allow her greater flexibility in meal times and carbohydrate amounts.

Learning Assessment: Case Study 2

SA is taking 40 mg of glipizide. Her doctor tells her she could stop taking this medication if she could lose 75 lb. At her annual physical last week, the doctor said her laboratory values were good, except for her fasting blood glucose of 248 mg/dL, and her A1C level was 11.3%. He recommends insulin injections, but SA does not want to give herself injections.

Questions for Discussion

1 What do you say to SA about the advice to lose 75 lb?

2 Are there other oral agents that might be effective?

3 What lab work is needed prior to initiating TZD or metformin?

Discussion

1 Explain to SA that improving blood glucose is more important than losing weight. Even if individuals lose 75 lb, most individuals cannot maintain that level of weight loss long-term. However, even a weight loss of 10 lb can be helpful. Explain to SA the progressive nature of type 2 diabetes and the need to change medical therapies and potentially the need for insulin due to beta cell failure.

2 SA might be a candidate for metformin. If her creatinine is <1.4 mg/dL, she might start with 500 mg at dinner, with the next weekly increase of 500 mg at breakfast, then increase by 500 mg per week until she reaches the clinically therapeutic dose of 2000 mg/day or until she reaches her blood glucose goals.

3 SA may also be a candidate for adding a TZD if her liver function studies are within normal limits. However, it may take 6 to 8 weeks at starting doses to obtain full glycemic response.

4 Repaglinide before meals may also be a consideration in lieu of glyburide. While similar to a sulfonylurea, it differs by increasing first-phase insulin release for patients who still have endogenous insulin-producing ability.

References

1 The Diabetes Control and Complications Trial Research Group. The effect of intensive treatment of diabetes on the development and progression of long-term complications in insulin-dependent diabetes mellitus. N Engl J Med. 1993;329:977-986.

2 UK Prospective Diabetes Study (UKPDS) Group. Intensive blood-glucose control with sulfonylureas or insulin compared with conventional treatment and risk of complications in patients with type 2 diabetes (UKPDS 33). Lancet. 1998;352:837-853.

3 Ohkubo Y, Kishikawa H, Araki E, et al. Intensive insulin therapy prevents the progression of diabetic microvascular complications in Japanese patients with non-insulin-dependent diabetes mellitus: a randomized prospective 6-year study. Diabetes Res Clin Pract. 1995;28:103-117.

4 Hirsch I. Implementation of intensive diabetes therapy for IDDM. Diabetes Rev. 1995;3:288-307.

5 American Dietetic Association, American Diabetes Association. Advanced Carbohydrate Counting. Chicago and Alexandria, Va: American Dietetic Association and American Diabetes Association. 2003.

6 American Diabetes Association. National standards for diabetes self-management education programs. Diabetes Care. 2003;26(suppl 1):S149-S156.

7 Davidson J, Reader D, Rickheim P. Blood Glucose Patterns. A Guide to Achieving Targets. Minneapolis: International Diabetes Center, Park Nicollet Institute; 2003.

8 Guthrie DW, Guthrie RA, eds. Nursing Management of Diabetes Mellitus. 4th ed. New York: Springer; 1997.

9 American Diabetes Association. Standards of medical care for patients with diabetes mellitus (position statement). Diabetes Care. 2003;26(suppl 1):S33-S50.

10 American Diabetes Association. Tests of glycemia in diabetes (position statement). Diabetes Care. 2003;26(suppl 1):S106-S108.

11 Childs BP, Guthrie RA, Carr M, McDaniel J, Rhiley D. Incorporating new diabetes oral agents into clinical practice. Diabetes Spectrum. 1996;9:266-268.

12 Aronoff S, Rosenblatt S, Braithwaite S, Egan JW, Mathisen AL, Schneider RL, the Pioglitazone Study Group. Pioglitazone hydrochloride monotherapy improves glycemic control in the treatment of patients with type 2 diabetes. Diabetes Care. 2000;23:1605-1611.

13 Phillips LS, Grunberger G, Miller E, Patwadhan R, Rappaport EB, Salzman A, for the Rosiglitazone Clinical Trial Study Group. Once and twice daily dosing with rosiglitazone improves glycemic control in patients with type 2 diabetes. Diabetes Care. 2001;24:308-315.

Suggested Readings

Advanced Carbohydrate Counting. Alexandria, Va and Chicago: American Diabetes Association and American Dietetic Association; 2003.

Anderson B, Funnell M. The Art of Empowerment: Stories and Strategies for Diabetes Educators. Alexandria, Va: American Diabetes Association; 2000.

Avignon A, Radauceanu A, Monnier L. Nonfasting plasma glucose is a better marker of diabetic control than fasting plasma glucose. Diabetes Care. 1997;20:1822-1826.

Bell D, Ovalle F, Shadmany S. Postprandial rather than preprandial glucose levels should be used for adjustment of rapid-acting insulins. Endocrine Practice. 2000;6:477-478.

Bergenstal R, Fish L, List S. The insulin sliding scale is not dead. Arch Intern Med. 1998;158:298-301.

Bolli G. Clinical strategies for controlling peaks and valleys: type 1 diabetes. International Journal of Clinical Practice. 2002;120(suppl):65-74.

Brewer KW, Chase HP, Owen S, Garg SK. Slicing the pie. Correlating HbA1c values with average blood glucose values in a pie chart form. Diabetes Care. 1998;21:209-212.

Brunelle BL, Llewelyn J, Anderson JH, Gale EA. Meta-analysis of the effect of insulin lispro on severe hypoglycemia in patients with type 1 diabetes. Diabetes Care. 1998;21:1726-1831.

DAFNE Study Group. Training in flexible, intensive insulin management to enable dietary freedom in people with type 1 diabetes: dose adjustment for normal eating (DAFNE) randomized controlled trial. BMJ. 2002;325:746-752.

Davidson J, Reader D, Rickheim P. Blood Glucose Patterns. A Guide to Achieving Targets. Minneapolis: International Diabetes Center, Park Nicollet Institute; 2003.

Farkas-Hirsch R, ed. Intensive Diabetes Management. 2nd ed. Alexandria, Va: American Diabetes Association; 1998.

Guthrie DW, Guthrie RA, eds. Nursing Management of Diabetes Mellitus. 5th ed. New York: Springer; 2002.

Guthrie DW, Guthrie RA. Approach to management. Diabetes Educ. 1990;16:401-406.

Hirsch IB, Farkas-Hirsch R. Sliding scale or sliding scare: it's all sliding nonsense. Diabetes Spectrum. 2001;14:79-81.

Jackson RL, Guthrie RA. Physiologic Management of Diabetes in Children. New York: Medical Examination Publishers. 1986;80-157.

Jackson RL, Kelly HG. Growth of children with diabetes mellitus in relationship to level of control of the disease. J Pediatr. 1946;29:316.

Kalbag JB, Walter YH, Nedelman JR, McLeod JF. Mealtime glucose regulation with nateglinide in healthy volunteers: comparison with repaglinide and placebo. Diabetes Care. 2001;24:73-77.

Klohn M, Castle G, Gerken S. Carbohydrate Counting. Minneapolis: International Diabetes Center, Park Nicollet Foundation; 2002.

Koivisto VA, Tuominen JA, Ebeling P. Lispro Mix25 insulin as premeal therapy in type 2 diabetic patients. Diabetes Care. 1999;22:459-462.

Lalli C, Ciofetta M, Del Sindaco P, et al. Long term intensive treatment of type 1 diabetes with the short-acting insulin analog lispro in variable combination with NPH insulin at mealtime. Diabetes Care. 1999;22;468-477.

Lindholm A, McEwen J, Riis AP. Improved postprandial glycemic control with insulin aspart. A randomized double-blind cross-over trial in type 1 diabetes. Diabetes Care. 1999;22:801-805.

Norris S, Engelgau M, Narayan V. Effectiveness of self-management training in type 2 diabetes: a systematic review of randomized controlled trials. Diabetes Care. 2001; 24: 561-587.

Pearson J, Bergenstal R. Fine-tuning control: pattern management versus supplementation. Diabetes Spectrum. 2001;14:75-78.

Pieber TR, Brunner GA, Schnedl WJ, Schattenberg S, Kaufmann P, Krejs GJ. Evaluation of a structured outpatient group education program for intensive insulin therapy. Diabetes Care. 1995;18:625-630.

Polonsky W. Diabetes Burnout: What to do When You Can't Take it Anymore. Alexandria, Va: American Diabetes Association; 1999.

Queale WS, Seidler AJ, Brancati FL. Glycemic control and sliding scale insulin use in medical inpatients with diabetes mellitus. Arch Intern Med. 1997;157:545-552.

Rabasa-Lhoret R, Garon J, Langlier H, Poisson D, Chiasson J-L. Effects of meal carbohydrate on insulin requirements in type 1 diabetic patients treated intensively with the basal-bolus (Ultralente-regular) insulin regimen. Diabetes Care. 1999;22:667-673.

Sawin CT. Action without benefit: the sliding scale of insulin use. Arch Intern Med. 1997;157:489-491.

Shagan BP. Does anyone here know how to make insulin work backwards? Why sliding-scale insulin coverage doesn't work. Practical Diabetol. 1990;9(3):1-4.

Learning Assessment: Post-Test Questions

Pattern Management of Blood Glucose   6

1 Components of an intensive diabetes management program can include:
  A Generalized glycemic goals that follow a preestablished pattern
  B Interaction with the healthcare team 2 to 3 times a year
  C Self-monitoring of blood glucose levels when symptoms occur
  D Self-management education and reliable support systems

2 The main reason to use an algorithmic approach to insulin therapy is to:
  A Increase insulin dosages by 10% to 20% to avoid hyperglycemia
  B Provide flexibility in usual insulin dosages to maintain euglycemia
  C Decrease insulin dosages by 10% to 20% to avoid hypoglycemia
  D Avoid using a meal plan and offset eating as desired

3 An adult on multiple insulin doses with previously controlled diabetes has been experiencing hyperglycemia with blood glucose values over 225 mg/dL 2 hours after every meal for the past 2 weeks. Which would be the best initial action for the diabetes educator to take?
  A Evaluate food consumption of the person, especially protein intakes
  B Encourage more vigorous aerobic exercise be done by the individual
  C Review meter technique
  D Check the appearance and expiration date of the individual's insulin

4 Effectiveness of lispro insulin is best determined by measuring:
  A Premeal glucoses
  B Fasting glucoses
  C 2-hour postprandial glucoses
  D 3 AM glucoses

5 Pattern management of blood glucose levels involves reviewing:
  A Several days of glucose records and making changes in the diabetes management program when a problem persists
  B Sporadic glucose records and making corrections in the diabetes management program after problems have occurred
  C Glycosolated hemoglobin values and making adjustments in diabetes management before the onset of long-term complications
  D Fasting serum glucose values and making modifications in diabetes management before a problem surfaces

6 One reason sliding-scale insulin administration is less desirable as a pattern management approach is:
  A It is based on patient's current weight
  B It varies according to patient's food intake
  C It may contribute to rapid shifts in glucose levels
  D It may confuse patients trying to remember amount of insulin to administer

7 Pattern management for an adult with type 2 diabetes is likely to be:
  A Testing only fasting and premeal blood glucose levels
  B Analyzing food and blood glucose records once or twice a week
  C Testing urine for ketones
  D Sliding scale plan to cover blood glucose shifts

8 Which of the following statements about combination therapy (oral medications) is most accurate?

A Addition of TZD to existing therapy produces a therapeutic response within a week

B Combination therapy improves glycemic control in persons with type 1 diabetes

C When oral agents are combined, the medications should be taken 1 hour before meals

D Individuals starting combination therapy will need to monitor postprandial blood glucose levels

9 Examples of SMBG data that can be useful for managing blood glucose levels and making changes to the treatment plan include all of the following except:

A Using premeal testing to determine regular insulin dose for multiple injections

B Testing at 3 AM at least once a week when fasting glucose levels are elevated

C Testing daily for people who have asymptomatic hypoglycemia

D Using premeal testing before administering a supplemental insulin bolus during acute illness

See next page for answer key.

Post-Test Answer Key

Pattern Management of Blood Glucose

6

1	D		**6**	C
2	B		**7**	B
3	D		**8**	D
4	C		**9**	C
5	A			

A Core Curriculum for Diabetes Education
Diabetes Management Therapies

Insulin Pump Therapy and Carbohydrate Counting for Pump Therapy: Insulin-to-Carbohydrate Ratios

7

Insulin Pump Therapy
Ann Marie Brooks, MSN, RN, BC-ADM, CDE
St. Marks Hospital Diabetes Center
Salt Lake City, Utah

Carbohydrate Counting for Pump Therapy: Insulin-to-Carbohydrate Ratios
Karmeen Kulkarni, MS, RD, BC-ADM, CDE
St. Marks Hospital Diabetes Center
Salt Lake City, Utah

Introduction

1 Insulin pump therapy, also known as continuous subcutaneous insulin infusion (CSII), is a valuable asset in attaining normoglycemia.

2 Studies such as the Diabetes Control and Complications Trial (DCCT)[1] and the United Kingdom Prospective Diabetes Study (UKPDS)[2] have shown conclusively that glycemic control is essential for preventing diabetes complications.

3 Both the American Diabetes Association[3] and the American Association of Diabetes Educators[4] have position statements supporting the use of insulin pump therapy.

4 The benefits and limitations of insulin pump therapy must be considered in determining the appropriateness of this type of therapy for a patient.

5 Proper patient selection is critical to the success of insulin pump therapy. Specific criteria and ethical considerations are part of the selection process.

6 Currently eight insulin pumps are approved for use in the US. Each pump offers unique features that can serve as a guide in determining the best model to meet a patient's needs.

7 A number of steps are involved in initiating successful pump therapy. The diabetes educator plays an important role in this process.

8 Follow-up and fine-tuning are essential elements of successful pump therapy and achieving patient goals.

9 Insulin therapy should be integrated into the usual eating and exercise habits of the person with diabetes.[5] Insulin pump therapy provides an excellent means of achieving this goal.

10 Carbohydrate counting involving insulin-to-carbohydrate ratios is used to implement medical nutrition therapy for insulin pump therapy.

Objectives

Upon completion of this chapter, the learner will be able to

1 State the indications for patient use of insulin pump therapy.
2 Explain the limitations of insulin pump therapy.
3 Identify selection criteria for pump candidates.
4 Identify insulin pumps that currently are available in the US.
5 Describe correction factors used in insulin pump therapy.
6 State the skills necessary for using carbohydrate counting for insulin pump therapy.
7 Describe how to evaluate a person's understanding of and ability to use carbohydrate counting.
8 Explain how to determine insulin-to-carbohydrate ratios

Insulin Pump Therapy

1 The number of insulin pump users, or "pumpers," is increasing rapidly each year. According to the manufacturers of insulin pumps, there currently are more than 162 000 insulin pump users in the US.[6] This number is relatively low considering that there are more than 1 000 000 patients with type 1 diabetes. The number of type 2 patients with pumps is smaller.

2 Insulin pump therapy can help patients achieve near-normal blood glucose levels. The Diabetes Control and Complications Trial Research Group (DCCT) conclusively demonstrated the beneficial effects and impact of optimal glycemic control, which changed the way that diabetes is treated.[7]

3 The earliest model of the insulin pump weighed several pounds and looked like a back-pack. Current models weigh as little as 2+ ounces and can be worn on a belt like a pager or hidden under clothing.

  A The insulin pump is a miniature computer that mimics the functioning of the human pancreas as it delivers rapid-acting insulin or short-acting insulin in 2 ways:
  - Basal or metabolic/background insulin is preprogrammed to match pancreatic insulin release patterns.
  - Bolus insulin doses are given to cover food intake or to correct a high blood glucose level. The bolus can be given all at once to cover a high-carbohydrate meal or over time to mimic the insulin release needed for a more slowly digested meal.

  B The insulin is delivered via an infusion set that is placed just under the skin into the subcutaneous tissue, usually into the abdomen. The infusion site is changed about every 72 hours, relieving the patient of frequent injections with a syringe.

Benefits of Pump Therapy

1 Insulin pump therapy provides one means of helping patients improve their glycemic control, which has been shown to reduce the long-term complications of diabetes.

2 Immediate improvement in blood glucose levels is possible with insulin pump therapy "due to better insulin pharmacokinetics."[6]

  A Insulin dosing with an insulin pump can be precise to within one twentieth of a unit.
  B Difference in absorption from various sites is reduced.
  C Incidence of absorption loss from the site depot is reduced.
  D Continuous delivery improves insulin absorption.
  E Dawn phenomenon effects are easier to manage with insulin pump therapy because the basal rate can be increased to accommodate the rise in insulin requirements that occurs during the early morning hours.

3 Insulin pump therapy provides an improved safety profile.

  A The fear of nocturnal hypoglycemia can be minimized when basal rates are reduced during the period of low physiological requirements.[8]
  B Users experience greater safety while operating machinery or an automobile due to an increased ability to modify insulin delivery patterns.

C Pump users are better able to make adjustments for sick days by using a temporary basal rate that matches their changed needs.

4 Insulin pump therapy can increase the user's lifestyle flexibility and satisfaction.
  A Food/meals can be customized to fit the user's schedules and preferences.[9]
  • The need for forced snacking is reduced.
  • Motivated individuals who desire weight loss may find it easier with insulin pump therapy. Initially, improved glycemia may promote some weight gain but less than with conventional intensive therapy.[6] This is likely because less total insulin is required with pump therapy.[10]
  • Pump users have a flexible schedule of variable food choices.
  • There are fewer problems with picky eaters, such as children, because the bolus can be given after the food consumption has been determined.
  B Pump users can exercise more safely because basal rates can be reduced during the activity, or the basal delivery can even be suspended.
  C The increased flexibility makes it easier for pump wearers to travel. Once the destination is reached, the clock on the pump can be changed and all of the former settings are retained.
  D Schedule changes can be accommodated. Many pump wearers find the insulin pump useful for shift work or other kinds of unpredictable life situations.

Limitations of Pump Therapy

1 There are also drawbacks to or limitations of insulin pump therapy for the user.
  A There is a high learning curve associated with pump therapy; some individuals are unable to master the learning curve.
  B Successful adaptation to pump therapy may take months; some individuals give up before realizing success.
  C Being connected to a pump is a visual reminder of having a chronic disease.
  D Technical failures do not occur with insulin and syringes but are possible with a pump.
  E There may be an increased risk of ketosis when only rapid-acting or short-acting insulin is available.
  F Some patients experience problems with skin irritation and infections. The special adhesive patches and occlusive dressings may irritate some types of skin.
  G Site changes require 3 to 10 minutes and may interrupt a busy schedule.
  H Some patient populations, such as children, may require assistance from a caregiver.

2 Many healthcare providers are unfamiliar with pump therapy and may be unable to provide needed patient support.

3 The cost of an insulin pump is usually over $5000 and supplies are about $1000 to $1500 per year. Insurance companies typically cover only about 80% of pump expenses. Because coverage varies from state to state and from plan to plan, this needs to be checked on an individual basis. Reimbursement for diabetes education to support the patient is also variable. (See Chapter 8, Payment for Diabetes Education, in Diabetes Education and Program Management.)

4 Many of these problems can be overcome, and motivated patients are usually successful.

Medical Indications for Pump Therapy

1 The need to improve overall glycemic control is a common indication for insulin pump therapy.

   A Tighter blood glucose control has been shown to reduce the incidence of diabetic complications. The DCCT[1] and the UKPDS[2], as well as the Kumamoto[11] studies, have demonstrated that well-controlled blood glucose levels reduce complications for patients with type 1 as well as for patients with type 2 diabetes.

   B Insulin pump therapy can improve outcomes and prevent deterioration of existing diabetes complications.

     • Bolus options may help the patient with gastroparesis avoid postprandial high and low blood glucose readings.

     • Patients who achieve normoglycemia may experience an improvement in neuropathy.

     • Patients with diabetic foot ulcers may have an improved chance of healing.

     • Patients may have an improved sense of energy and well-being.

2 Insulin pump therapy has been shown to reduce the incidence of hypoglycemia, even in patients with tighter control.[8]

   A Exercise-induced hypoglycemia is easier to prevent because the basal rate can be reduced, eliminated, or suspended. There is less risk that long-acting insulin will cause an unexpected dip in glucose levels.

   B Nocturnal hypoglycemia can be controlled and the naturally occurring reduction in the need for insulin (typically between midnight and 3 AM) can be anticipated.[8]

3 To control the dawn phenomenon, the basal rate can be increased to adjust for the hormone-mediated predawn increase in blood glucose.

4 Insulin sensitivity, which is typically seen in smaller adults and children, can be managed more easily with insulin pump therapy. Basal rates as low as 0.05 unit per hour are possible; with dilution, even more minute basal rates are possible.

5 Insulin pump therapy benefits appropriate women with type 1 diabetes during pregnancy.[12] Problems with hypoglycemia may occur during the first 20 weeks of pregnancy, such as nausea and vomiting of food after an insulin injection is given. With the pump, the patient can use a bolus dose on a bite-by-bite basis. In addition, tight control has been found to improve maternal and fetal outcomes.[13] Additional studies have shown women with type 2 and gestational diabetes requiring large insulin doses also benefit from insulin pump therapy.[14]

6 A variable lifestyle and changing work and activity schedules are handled more smoothly with insulin pump therapy.

   A People who must travel frequently may find they have better control with insulin pump therapy. They may change the clock on the pump once they arrive at the new destination. They may also make small corrections or adjustments more easily as they encounter changes in meal times and sleep times.

B People who perform shift work can find insulin pump therapy beneficial in adjusting to variable patterns of eating and sleeping.

C Pump patients may find they can have a more flexible lifestyle, including sleeping late, snacking, missing or delaying meals, or losing weight.

7 Insulin-requiring patients with type 2 diabetes may benefit from pump therapy, enjoying greater flexibility in their lifestyle and the benefits of tight control.[15]

Successful Pump Candidates

1 Motivation is the most important ingredient for success. In addition, the successful pump candidate must be able to handle a variety of tasks and responsibilities.

A Pump users must overcome the learning curve associated with new therapy, equipment, and problem-solving situations. They must be able to troubleshoot problems, keep records, and adjust insulin.

B Emotional maturity is essential for effective problem solving and acceptance of the disease. It is generally thought that the average child would be able to manage the basic operations of an insulin pump by the age of 10.[16] However, decisions regarding the use of an insulin pump by children should be made on a case-by-case basis as emotional maturity may not be related to age.[16] Some children may benefit from the addition of nighttime pump therapy. [17,18]

C Testing and record keeping are vital to success with insulin pump therapy.

D Users must master carbohydrate counting, which involves the use of insulin-to-carbohydrate ratios and is used to implement nutrition therapy for optimal pump therapy. They must know how to determine the correct amount of insulin for a bolus dose based on the foods they have chosen. The user must be able to weigh or estimate portions accurately and make adjustments for high-fat or high-fiber foods. Without carbohydrate counting, the benefits and flexibility of insulin pump therapy are greatly reduced and pump therapy is of little value over the traditional approach of using fixed meals and insulin doses.

E Insulin therapy should be integrated into the usual eating and exercise habits of the person with diabetes.

F The user needs sufficient dexterity to be able to operate the pump.

G Visually impaired persons can successfully use insulin pump therapy but will require increased education and motivation.

H If the pump wearer lacks the competence to handle this type of therapy (eg, a child or mentally challenged person), a motivated and continually accessible caregiver is necessary.

I Financial resources are necessary for using pump therapy. Most candidates rely on insurance, which generally covers about 80% of the cost. Highly motivated individuals tend to be more successful in securing financial support.

Contraindications to Pump Therapy

1 Unrealistic expectations, such as thinking that insulin pump therapy will cure diabetes, will lead to failure using pump therapy.

2 Severe depression or other serious psychological disorders are incompatible with successful insulin pump therapy. Patients have been known to use the device to harm themselves.

3 Inability or unwillingness to calculate bolus doses is a contraindication for insulin pump therapy, with the noted exception of when a caregiver performs all or most of the functions.

4 A history of poor compliance and healthcare practices, such as failure to perform self-monitoring of blood glucose, keep appointments, and weigh and estimate portions, will signal failure.

5 Intense needle phobia will make it difficult, if not impossible, to use and benefit from insulin pump therapy.

6 Denial of the disease and fear of diabetes exposure are contraindications because the pump is a visible reminder of the reality of having diabetes.[19]

7 Educators need to be cautious in referring patients for pump therapy because negative outcomes hurt other candidates. Insurance companies look at failure rates and may deny pumps to appropriate candidates. Many companies have tightened eligibility requirements for insulin pump therapy to include 4 to 6 months of meticulous blood glucose records. Insurance companies may also increase copayments, thus making it more difficult for responsible candidates. A screening protocol is useful in identifying successful candidates.[19,20]

Selecting an Insulin Pump

1 Once the candidate for insulin pump therapy and his/her support team have decided to proceed, the process of selecting a pump begins in earnest.

2 The physician or educator may have suggestions as to the best model to meet the patient's unique needs.

3 There currently are 8 insulin pumps approved for distribution in the US. Others are in clinical trials and pending FDA approval.
   A The Animas pump has 2 models, the R-1000 and R-1000A. Features include menu-driven programming, 3-minute basal delivery, backlighting, multiple languages, waterproofing, and fashion covers.
   B The Dahedi pump is waterproof for surface activities and has a keypad for people with visual impairment. It is lightweight and can be easily concealed in clothing.
   C The Disetronic D-Tron pump features waterproofing for surface activities, 5 bolus alternatives, variable profiles, menu-driven programming, 3-minute basal delivery, backlighting, and occlusion detection.
   D The Disentronic D-Tron Plus pump is water resistant for surface activities; it has tactile buttons and 3-minute basal pulses; and it includes 2 pumps for the price of 1.

E The Mini-Med 508 pump features 3 sets of basal rates, multiple bolus options, remote programming capability, multiple profiles, child blocking, a watertight design, and backlighting; it is menu driven.

F The Mini-Med Paradigm has 3 basal patterns, back lighting, and remote programming capability; it is waterproof to 8 feet and has a rapid insulin pulse and bolus options.

G The Cosmo (Deltec) pump features include light weight (2.7 oz), personalized bolus and correction features, and new tracking features.

H The Dana pump is lightweight, simple, and affordable. It is distributed as a durable medical device.

Obtaining the Chosen Model

1 An insulin pump requires a doctor's prescription.

2 Insurance companies require a letter of medical necessity from the physician.

3 Once the insurance company is notified of the patient's desire for insulin pump therapy, it assesses the letter of medical necessity as well as the pump user history. Blood glucose records and other records may be required.

4 After authorization has been granted, the patient, educator, or insurance company contacts a vendor who handles the chosen insulin pump.

5 The patient and the medical team—physician, educators, and other healthcare providers—schedule pump training and follow-up visits. The pump user may wear the pump and initially use normal saline to become familiar with the mechanics and elements of daily living with the pump.

6 Most pumps come with a training video that helps users become familiar with the mechanics of using the pump and demonstrates insertion techniques.

7 At one time, patients stayed in the hospital for a day or more when pump therapy was initiated. Currently, most pump starts are performed on an outpatient basis. Because the training sessions may last only a few hours, greater effort and preparation on the part of the patient is required.

Getting Started With Pump Therapy

1 Patient education is crucial to success with insulin pump therapy.

2 The pump user needs to master the mechanics of the selected model.

3 An insulin-to-carbohydrate ratio is calculated based on the individual's weight, current insulin dose, and usual meal carbohydrate content. The effectiveness of this ratio is reflected in a comparison of preprandial and postprandial blood glucose levels. Some practitioners prefer a flat result, or no increase in blood glucose after a meal, while others prefer a 30 to 40 mg/dL (1.7 to 2.2 mmol/L) increase after a meal to prevent the need for snacking before the next meal. A user may not have the same insulin-to-carbohydrate ratio for all meals because needs and insulin requirements may vary during the day.

4 The education team, including the pump candidate, determines a reasonable target blood glucose level. Insulin bolus adjustments are based to this target, which might be 100 mg/dL (5.6 mmol/L) for individuals in tight control. Those who have not experienced tight glucose control might need to start with a higher target. A pregnant woman might have a target of 80 mg/dL (4.4 mmol/L).

5 A correction factor, or insulin-sensitivity factor, is also an important consideration. The patient adds or subtracts insulin from the meal bolus based on how much 1 unit of insulin might be expected to decrease the blood glucose level. A formula can be used such as the one in the Insulin Pump Therapy Handbook,[21] or even more importantly, from patient input.

   A Two commonly used formulas are used as starting points to determine the insulin-sensitivity factor: the 1800 and the 1500 rule.

     • The 1800 rule is usually used for rapid-acting insulin; 1800 is divided by the total daily insulin dose. The answer is the mg/dL of glucose that is decreased by 1 unit of rapid-acting insulin. For example, the total daily insulin dose is 48 units; 1800 ÷ 48 = 37.5 (round up to 40). The insulin sensitivity factor is 40 mg/dL; 1 unit of rapid-acting insulin decreases glucose by 40 mg/dL.

     • The 1500 rule is usually used for short-acting insulin; 1500 is divided by the total insulin dose. The answer is the mg/dL of glucose that is decreased by 1 unit of short-acting insulin.

     • The following example shows how a correction factor is used. The patient's target is 100 mg/dL, correction factor is 40. If the premeal blood glucose level is 140 mg/dL, add 1 unit to the meal bolus. If the premeal blood glucose level is 60 mg/dL, subtract at least 1 unit and give the bolus with the meal.

6 The basal profile or rate is vital for insulin pump therapy. About 50% of the insulin requirement is reflected in the basal or background rate. Children may require less insulin in the basal rate, perhaps 40% to 45%.[22] Most patients require more than 1 rate. Insulin pumps currently offer 12 to 48 basal rates or profiles. These profiles begin at midnight and can be programmed to adjust for nocturnal hypoglycemia, dawn phenomenon, or any routine physiological change.

   A The user's weight and current insulin dose guide the clinician in establishing basal rates; clinicians often start by reducing current doses by 25% or even 30%.

   B Fasting blood glucose levels and readings between meals reflect the efficacy of the basal rates.

   C Some pump models offer up to 4 basal routines, such as for weekends, sick days, or exercise days.

   D Most pumps offer temporary basal rates for unusual circumstances, such as surgery, exercise, or illness.

   E Basal profiles can reflect unique patient needs. Some patients may require more insulin in the early morning hours and some at the dinner hour. Other patients require little or no insulin at night or a reduction during the late afternoon.

F Insulin lispro and insulin aspart are frequently used with insulin pump therapy.[3,23,24] Some patients may experience various clinical differences in the two fast-acting insulins and may select one over the other.

7 The healthcare team helps the pump candidate select an appropriate infusion site and an appropriate infusion set.

A Most pump wearers select a site on the abdomen. Absorption is usually best in this area and the sites are less obtrusive; sites in the arms, thighs, buttocks, and breasts are also used successfully. Scars, or scar tissue, such as seen with lipodystrophy, prevent even insulin absorption and should be avoided, as well as the area immediately around the umbilicus.

B The tip of the infusion cannula must be in subcutaneous or fatty tissue. In some very thin persons the subcutaneous is just a compartment or layer between the dermis and the muscle. These individuals must roll and pinch up the skin to locate the correct site area.

C The site is prepared by cleansing the skin thoroughly in a circular motion from the inside to the outside. Users may develop an allergy to cleansers that are too harsh. Many pump wearers cover the site with an occlusive dressing or tape and then insert the infusion set.

D Infusion sets are available in a wide variety of styles, features, and prices. Most are interchangeable between the various brands of pumps. Some sets can be disconnected at or near the site to facilitate bathing, swimming, or intimate moments. Others must remain in place at all times. The sets should be changed every 2 to 3 days. A plugged, infected, or misplaced site must be changed at once.

E Several pump manufacturers now make an insertion device that facilitates site changes. This works well for persons with needle phobia, vision, or dexterity problems.

8 The insulin pump therapy candidate must be able to troubleshoot pump problems. Without long-acting insulin, diabetic ketoacidosis can develop more rapidly. Pump users must be able to

A Adjust for and prevent hypoglycemia or hyperglycemia.

B Deal with alarms, batteries, and mechanical or site problems.

C Understand sick-day management.

D Understand exercise adjustments and precautions.

E Know when to test and how to interpret the results. When insulin pump therapy is initiated, patients may need to test at 2 to 3 AM for a while to be able to understand the correct nocturnal insulin requirements.

F Locate a dependable source for insulin pump supplies. They must still carry insulin and syringes for emergencies.

G Have reasonable expectations because success requires time and patience in mastering the learning curve.

H Select additional support references such as those listed in the suggested readings.

Follow-Up: The Key to Success

1 Insulin pump therapy is most successful when the patient has support from a multi-disciplinary team. The patient, physician, and educators (nurse and dietitian) can assess patient records and responses. This ongoing follow-up and reassessment help the patient achieve individualized goals. Life itself—needs, habits, and activities—changes and evolves constantly. This is reflected in changing insulin requirements and a need for continuous fine-tuning.[25]

Looking Ahead

1 Glucose sensors reflect a breakthrough in technology.[26] The sensor is placed under the skin just like an infusion set, and it checks blood glucose every 5 minutes for 3 days. The wearer returns the device to a healthcare provider at the end of 3 days and the blood glucose data are downloaded to a computer so the data are analyzed.

   A This device helps identify physiological glucose patterns that were previously unknown to the patient and healthcare providers. The information can be used to better determine basal rates, insulin ratios, and periods of hypoglycemia or hyperglycemia. Even those individuals in tight control may experience glucose excursions of which they are unaware.

   B Glucose sensors, which currently are available on a limited basis, may one day provide a closed-loop system in which glucose is sensed and insulin is released in response, mimicking the functioning of the human pancreas. This technology offers persons with diabetes the hope of tight control over their lifetime. Bode, Tamborlane, and Davidson[6] predict insulin pump therapy will "...eventually be used by more than 40% of people with type 1 diabetes" and by many more type 2 patients.

2 A Diaport system offers further hope of normoglycemia. In this system, which currently is undergoing safety trials in the US and Europe, a port that is placed in the peritoneal cavity automatically senses glucose levels. (Interested readers may want to read the EVADIAC experience noted in the suggested readings.)

Key Educational Considerations for Pump Therapy

1 Insulin pump therapy has been shown to be an effective tool for helping persons with diabetes achieve better glycemic control.

2 Insulin pump therapy has many advantages, including lifestyle flexibility, reduction of hypoglycemia, and prevention of dawn phenomenon (hyperglycemia).

3 Disadvantages include cost, risk of diabetic ketoacidosis, and a comprehensive learning curve.

4 Candidates must be selected carefully to ensure success with insulin pump therapy.

5 A number of different insulin pumps are currently available, and they offer a variety of features.

6 The pump candidate selects a pump and an infusion set to match personal needs.

7 Insurance companies usually cover 80% of the costs of insulin pump therapy, although some cover 100%.

8 Insulin-to-carbohydrate ratios, basal rates, and target/correction factors help pump users achieve tight control safely.

9 User success is facilitated by a team approach. Frequent follow-up is vital to maximize insulin pump use.

Self-Review Questions on Pump Therapy
1 State the indications for and limitations of insulin pump therapy.
2 What are the characteristics of successful insulin pump therapy users?
3 Identify contraindications to insulin pump therapy.
4 What insulin pumps are currently available in the US?
5 What steps are necessary to obtain an insulin pump?
6 State the key educational requirements for pump therapy users.
7 What are the most vital elements for continuing success with insulin pump therapy?

Learning Assessment: Pump Therapy Case Study 1
Jared, age 22, has asked his physician for an insulin pump to "fix" his diabetes. He has heard about the pump and is adamant about having one. Jared has had type 1 diabetes since he was 11 years old. He tests his blood glucose level occasionally and takes his insulin when he remembers. Jared's current A1C is 14.2%. He has microalbuminuria and complains of increasing numbness in his feet. His family is pressuring the diabetes team to "stop the complications." Jared's insurance company requires 4 months of glucose testing records before reimbursing for an insulin pump, but he has thus far not produced the records. Twice he failed to show up for his carbohydrate counting session. Either Jared or his mother calls the diabetes team almost daily, and they believe the team is letting Jared down.

Questions for Discussion
1 Is Jared an appropriate candidate for insulin pump therapy? Why or why not?
2 What are the obligations of the diabetes team in helping this patient obtain an insulin pump?
3 What could Jared do to change this situation?

Discussion
1 At the present time Jared is not an appropriate insulin pump therapy candidate. His glycemic control would not likely improve with an insulin pump, and he might be even more likely to experience an episode of diabetic ketoacidosis because he would no longer be using any long-acting insulin.

2 Jared has not learned carbohydrate counting so he would not be able to match his insulin dose with his carbohydrate intake.

3 Jared has been unwilling to submit the blood glucose records that the insurance company requires before approving reimbursement for an insulin pump. The insurance company's rules protect patients, the company, and healthcare providers.

4 The team has tried to help Jared achieve better control. He must make the effort to change his situation. He may need psychiatric help or counseling to accomplish this goal.

5 If Jared fails to use his insulin pump properly and requires additional hospitalization, his failure may influence the availability of the program and benefits for other candidates.

6 Jared can change this situation. He can start doing regular blood glucose testing, keep records, and attend a carbohydrate counting session. He also can begin taking multiple daily insulin injections. Performing these tasks in a responsible manner may then qualify Jared for insulin pump therapy and the chance to benefit from this type of therapy.

Learning Assessment: Pump Therapy Case Study 2

Denise, age 27, and her husband are planning a pregnancy. Denise has had type 1 diabetes since the age of 15. She has had laser surgery for background retinopathy but has not experienced any other known complications. She manages her diabetes with insulin injections 3 times daily: 20 units NPH insulin and 6 units regular insulin in the morning, 6 units regular insulin at dinner, and 12 units NPH insulin at bedtime. Denise tests her blood glucose 3 times a day. She weighs 130 lb and is 5 ft 5 in tall. Her current A1C is 7.6%. Her physician would like her to have tighter control before becoming pregnant,[27] and has recommended an insulin pump.

Questions for Discussion

1 What kind of preparation will Denise need before she begins insulin pump therapy?
2 What A1C level would be optimal for pregnancy?
3 How might Denise's insulin need change during pregnancy?

Discussion

1 Denise will need to master carbohydrate counting as part of her preparation for insulin pump therapy. She can see a dietitian and begin this process at once.

2 She will want to change her insulin regimen to multiple daily injections (MDI), possibly using insulin glargine or Ultralente and a rapid-acting insulin, to match her insulin and carbohydrate intake.

3 Denise will need an eye exam if she has not had one in the last 6 to 9 months to ensure the stability of her retinopathy. Some physicians may also require a 24-hour urine clearance test.

4 She will need to check her blood glucose level at least 4 times daily to facilitate the MDI and provide better glucose management data for her diabetes team.

5 The physician or educator may help Denise choose her insulin pump. She will require alternative infusion sites once she is pregnant and as her abdomen enlarges.

6 The A1C goal for Denise will be below 7.0%, preferably closer to 6.0%, during her pregnancy.

7 She will need close contact with her diabetes management team throughout her pregnancy because her basal insulin needs will change (increase) as her pregnancy progresses.[26]

Pump Therapy References

1 Diabetes Control and Complications Trial Research Group. The effect of intensive treatment of diabetes mellitus on the development and progression of long-term complications in insulin-dependent diabetes. N Eng J Med. 1993;329:977-986.

2 UK Prospective Diabetes Study (UKPDS) Group. Intensive blood-glucose control with sulphonylureas or insulin compared with conventional treatment and risk of complications in patients with type 2 diabetes (UKPDS 33). Lancet. 1998;352:837-853.

3 American Diabetes Association. Continuous subcutaneous insulin infusion (position statement). Diabetes Care. 2003;26(suppl 1):S125.

4 American Association of Diabetes Educators. Position statement: education for continuous subcutaneous insulin infusion pump users. Diabetes Educ. 2003;29:97-99.

5 American Diabetes Association. Nutrition recommendations and principles for people with diabetes mellitus (position statement). Diabetes Care. 2003;26(suppl 1):S51-S61.

6 Bode BW, Tamborlane WV, Davidson PC. Insulin pump therapy in the 21st century. Postgraduate Medicine. 2002;3:69-77.

7 Skylar J. Introduction. In: Fredrickson L, ed. Insulin Pump Therapy Book. Sylmar, Calif: MiniMed Technologies;1995:3-8.

8 Bode BW, Steed RD, Davidson PC. Reduction in severe hypoglycemia with long-term continuous subcutaneous infusion in type 1 diabetes. Diabetes Care. 1996; 19:324-327.

9 DAFNE Study Group. Training in flexible, intensive insulin management to enable dietary freedom in people with type 1 diabetes: dose adjustment for normal eating (DAFNE) randomised controlled trial. BMJ. 2002;325:746-752.

10 Hanaire-Broutin H, Melki V, Bessieres-Lacombe S, Tauber J. Comparison of continuous subcutaneous insulin infusion and multiple daily injection regimens using insulin lispro in type 1 diabetic patients on intensified treatment. Diabetes Care. 2000; 23:1232-1235.

11 Ohkubo Y, Kishikawa H, Araki E, et al. Intensive insulin therapy prevents the progression of diabetic microvascular complications in Japanese patients with non-insulin dependent diabetes mellitus: a randomized prospective 6-year study. Diabetes Resources Clin Pract. 1995;8:113-117.

12 Jovanovich-Peterson L, Peterson C, Coustan D, et al. A randomized clinical trial of the insulin pump vs. intensive conventional therapy in diabetic pregnancies. JAMA. 1986;255:631-636.

13 Jornsay D. Pregnancy and continuous insulin infusion therapy. Diabetes Spectrum. 1998;11:26-32.

14 Simmons D, Thompson CF, Conroy C, Scott D. Use of insulin pumps in pregnancies complicated by type 2 diabetes and gestational diabetes in a multiethnic community. Diabetes Care. 2001;24:2078-2082.

15 Jennings A, Lewis K, Murdoch S, Talbot J, Bradley C, Ward J. Randomized trial comparing continuous subcutaneous insulin infusion and conventional therapy in type 2 diabetic patients poorly controlled with sulfonylureas. Diabetes Care. 1991;14:738-744.

16 Slipper F, deBeaufort C, Bruining G, et al. Psychological impact of continuous subcutaneous insulin infusion therapy in nonselected newly diagnosed insulin dependent (type I) diabetic children: evaluation after 2 years of therapy. Diabetic Med. 1990;16:273-277.

17 Maniatis AK, Klingensmith GJ, Slover RH, Mowry, CJ, Chase, HP. Continuous subcutaneous insulin infusion therapy for children and adolescents: an option for routine diabetes care. Pediatrics. 2001;107:351-356.

18 Kaufman FR, Kim C, Halvorsor M, Pitukcheewanont P. Use of insulin pump therapy at nighttime only for children 7-10 years of age with type 1 diabetes. Diabetes Care. 2000;23:579-582.

19 Tannenberg R. Candidate selection. In: Fredrickson L, ed. Insulin Pump Therapy Book. Sylmar, Calif: MiniMed Technologies;1995:21-30.

20 Sanfield JA, Hegstad M, Hanna RS. Protocol for outpatient screening and initiation of continuous subcutaneous insulin infusion therapy: impact on cost and quality. The Diabetes Educator. 2002;28:599-607.

21 Fredrickson L, ed. Insulin Pump Therapy Book. Sylmar, Calif: MiniMed Technologies; 1995.

22 Conrad SC, McGrath MT, Gitelman, SE. Transition from multiple daily injections to continuous subcutaneous insulin infusions in type 1 diabetes mellitus. Pediatr. 2002; 140:235-240.

23 Zinman B, Tildesley H, Chiasson J-L, Tsui E, Strack T. Insulin lispro in CSII: results of a double-blind cross over study. Diabetes. 1997;46:440-443.

24 Bode B, Strange P. Efficacy, safety, and pump compatibility of insulin aspart used in continuous subcutaneous insulin infusion therapy in patients with type 1 diabetes. Diabetes Care. 2001;24:69-72.

25 Lenhard MF, Reeves GD. Continuous subcutaneous insulin infusion: a comprehensive review of insulin pump therapy. Arch Intern Med. 2001;161:2293-2300.

26 Bode BW, Sabbah H, Robertson DG, Tolbert LC, Fredrikson LP. Clinical decision making: new opportunities for therapeutic changes with continuous glucose sensing. Diabetes Spectrum. 2000;13:171-174.

27 Drexler A. Pump therapy in preconception and pregnancy. In: Fredrickson L, ed. Insulin Pump Therapy Book. Sylmar, Calif: MiniMed Technologies;1995:145-150.

Suggested Readings on Pump Therapy

American Association of Diabetes Educators. Position statement: education for continuous subcutaneous insulin infusion pump users. The Diabetes Educator. 2003;29:97-99.

American Diabetes Association. Preconception care of women with diabetes (position statement). Diabetes Care. 2003;24(suppl 1):S91-S93.

American Diabetes Association. Diabetes Forecast Resource Guide. 2003;34,35,40.

Davidson P. Bolus and supplemental insulin. In: Fredrickson L, ed. Insulin Pump Therapy Book. Sylmar, Calif: MiniMed Technologies;1995:59-70.

DeVries JH, Snoek FJ, Kostense PJ, Masurel N, Heine RJ. A randomized trial of continuous subcutaneous insulin infusion and intensive injection therapy in type 1 diabetes for patients with long-standing poor glycemic control. Diabetes Care. 2002;25:2074-2080.

Fredrickson L, Rubin R, Rubin S. Optimal Pumping: A Guide to Good Health With Diabetes. Sylmar, Calif: MiniMed Technologies; 2001.

Gin H, Melki V, Guerci B, Catargi B, EVADIAC Study Group. Clinical evaluation of a newly designed compliant side port catheter for an insulin implantable pump. Diabetes Care. 2001;24:175.

Glucose Sensor. Sylmar, Calif: MiniMed Technologies; 1999. Publication D9195869.

Griffin ME, Feder A, Tamborlane WV. Lipoatrophy assisted with lispro insulin in insulin pump therapy. Diabetes Care. 2001;24:174.

Grossman J. Successful management of type 2 diabetes: are the benefits worth the costs? Practical Diabetol. 1999;June:12-22.

Insulin Pump Therapy Series. Reprint 5. Minneapolis, Minn: Disetronic Medical Systems; 1998. (Readers will find the entire series of 15 pamphlets helpful.)

MiniMed Corporation. Selected abstracts from the 17th International Diabetes Federation Congress (Glucose Sensors), Mexico City, Mexico, 2000.

Pickup J, Keen H. Continuous subcutaneous insulin infusion 25 years: evidence base for the expanding use of insulin pump therapy in type 1 diabetes. Diabetes Care. 2000; 25:593-598.

Pickup J, Mattock M, Kerry S. Glycaemic control with continuous subcutaneous insulin infusion compared to intensive insulin injections in patients with type 1 diabetes: a meta-analysis of randomised controlled trials. BMJ. 2002;324:705-710.

Rowe R. Insulin pump therapy. Diabetic Medicine. 2001;18:5-6.

Weissberg-Benchell J, Antisdel-Lomaglio J, Seshadri R. Insulin pump therapy. A meta-analysis. Diabetes Care. 2003;26:1079-1087.

Notes
Insulin pumps and supplies vary in price, as do amounts of insurance reimbursement. Readers may check with local vendors, the manufacturers, and local insurance carriers.

Thank you to the insulin pump manufacturers for providing synopses of pump features.

Carbohydrate Counting for Pump Therapy: Insulin-to-Carbohydrate Ratios

Introduction

1 Early research on continuous subcutaneous insulin infusion (insulin pump therapy) demonstrated that premeal insulin boluses were related solely to carbohydrate intake while basal insulin could be adjusted according to fasting blood glucose levels.[1] Additional research documented the relationship of insulin doses to carbohydrate.[2,3] Mixed meals (carbohydrate plus protein and fat) were shown to have very little effect on carbohydrate-based bolus insulin doses.

2 Recent research confirmed that the amount of the carbohydrate in the meal determines the bolus (mealtime) doses of insulin and that insulin should be adjusted accordingly.[4-6] Algorithms based on grams of carbohydrate are effective.[4]

A The glycemic index, fiber, fat, and caloric content of the meal do not affect the bolus (mealtime) insulin doses.[4,5]

B This finding is further supported by the DCCT, which showed that individuals on intensive insulin therapy who adjusted their meal insulin doses based on food carbohydrate content or on food exchanges had a lower A1C of 0.5% ($P<.03$).[6,7]

C Dose adjustment for normal eating (DAFNE) is a method for teaching individuals how to match insulin doses to their food choices (carbohydrate content) while keeping their blood glucose levels close to normal.[8] A clinical trial tested this method and showed that skills training in insulin adjustment promoted dietary freedom and improved the quality of life and glycemic control in people with type 1 diabetes without worsening of hypoglycemia or cardiovascular risk factors. This method, they concluded, has the potential to encourage more individuals to use intensive treatment.

3 Thus, research has provided evidence that using insulin-to-carbohydrate ratios is effective.[9]

Carbohydrate Counting and Insulin Doses

1 Steps involved in using insulin-to-carbohydrate ratios include

A Identifying the anticipated carbohydrate intake at meals and snacks and accurately determining the number of carbohydrate servings or the grams of carbohydrate intake.

B Identifying the units of insulin needed to cover carbohydrate intake.

C Administering a rapid-acting insulin (or short-acting insulin) bolus based on a predetermined insulin-to-carbohydrate ratio.

2 Two levels of carbohydrate counting have been defined: basic and advanced.[10,11]

A Mastery of the basic understanding of carbohydrate counting includes understanding the relationship between food, physical activity, and blood glucose levels. Advanced level carbohydrate counting includes an understanding of pattern management and using insulin-to-carbohydrate ratios.

B Basic Carbohydrate Counting[10] and Advanced Carbohydrate Counting[11] are patient education booklets that provide step-by-step guidelines for carbohydrate counting and are available from the American Diabetes Association and the American Dietetic Association. (For additional information, see the section on carbohydrate counting in Chapter 1, Medical Nutrition Therapy for Diabetes, in Diabetes Management Therapies.)

3 Before insulin pump therapy is initiated, the patient must demonstrate proficiency in adjusting insulin doses to meet blood glucose goals. This requires consistent use of food, blood glucose data, and insulin records for at least 1 to 2 weeks to determine and confirm the insulin-to-carbohydrate ratios.

   A An insulin-to-carbohydrate ratio is based on matching the rapid-acting insulin (or short-acting insulin) to the carbohydrate content of food to be eaten.

   B Individuals will have different insulin-to-carbohydrate ratios. Therefore, the insulin-to carbohydrate ratio must always be individualized.

Determining Insulin-to-Carbohydrate Ratios

1 There are different approaches and methods for determining insulin-to-carbohydrate ratios. In general about half of the total daily dose of insulin required is for basal or background insulin and about half is for bolus or mealtime insulin. Bolus or mealtime insulin doses can be based on the total grams of carbohydrate to be eaten or on the total number of carbohydrate servings.

2 The following steps are used when determining the insulin-to-carbohydrate ratio based on the grams of carbohydrate eaten.[11]

   A Use food records to determine the total amount of carbohydrate at each meal and snack for at least 3 days. Determine both the average intake of carbohydrate and the average range for each meal and snack. If this cannot be determined look for factors that may have interfered with the patient eating consistent amounts of carbohydrate, such as eating out or not knowing how to count the carbohydrate in combination foods.

   B Ask the patient to eat consistent amounts of carbohydrate at meals. It is helpful if the patient practices using different foods and a variety of resources (food labels, books) to locate carbohydrate information.

   C With the patient, study glucose records. Identify some meals where both the before-meal and after-meal glucose levels are within the target range.

   D Determine the insulin-to-carbohydrate ratio. Using the meals identified in the previous step, divide the number of grams of meal carbohydrate by the units of bolus or mealtime insulin. For example, if the patient ate 65 g of carbohydrate and took 8 units of rapid-acting insulin, and the postmeal glucose was within target range, divide 65 by 8. This equals 1 unit of insulin per 8 g of carbohydrate, which is a 1:8 ratio.

   • Therefore, on days when the patient is planning to eat 65 g of carbohydrate, he or she will take 8 units of bolus insulin; however, on days when he or she will be eating more or less carbohydrate, the bolus dose will be adjusted by 1 unit for every 8 g of carbohydrate. If the patient is planning to eat an additional 15 g of carbohydrate, he or she will take an extra 2 units of insulin (10 units). If the patient is planning on eating 15 g less of carbohydrate, he or she will take 2 units less of insulin (6 units).

- Another way to make adjustments is to divide the total planned intake of carbohydrate by the number of grams of carbohydrate covered by 1 unit of insulin. In the example above, 80 would be divided by 8, which would be 10 units of needed insulin.

   E For best results, fine-tune insulin-to-carbohydrate ratios. Determine the ratio for several meals on 2 other days to be sure it is correct. Keep in mind that ratios can vary by meal, on active days versus sedentary days, or because of circumstances such as illness or stress. Finding the best ratios often takes time.

3 A second method uses the following steps to determine an insulin-to-carbohydrate ratio based on the number of carbohydrate servings or choices eaten at meals or snacks.[12] One carbohydrate serving is the amount of a food containing 15 g of carbohydrate.

   A Determine the total bolus amounts of insulin used per day. This will be approximately one half of the total daily insulin dose.

   B Determine the total number of carbohydrate servings from meals and snacks per day.

   C Divide the total daily insulin dose by the number of carbohydrate servings. This will be the insulin-to-carbohydrate ratio. For example, if a patient takes a total of 20 units of bolus insulin per day and eats a total of 13 carbohydrate servings (4 at breakfast, 3 at lunch, 4 at dinner, and 2 at bedtime), the insulin-to-carbohydrate ratio is 1.5 units per carbohydrate choice (20 divided by 13 = 1.5). Therefore, the breakfast bolus would be 6 units, the lunch bolus 4.5 units, the dinner bolus 6 units, and the bedtime snack bolus 3 units. After 3 to 5 days, doses may need to be recalculated based on glucose monitoring data.

4 A third method has been proposed for determining insulin-to-carbohydrate ratio and involves the following steps:[13]

   A Add units of insulin taken in all doses per day to determine the total daily insulin dose.

   B Divide 450 by the total daily insulin dose. This is the number of carbohydrate grams covered by 1 unit of insulin.

   C Divide the number of carbohydrate grams by 15.

   D Round up or down to the nearest unit as appropriate. This is the insulin-to-carbohydrate ratio, or the units of insulin needed to cover 15 g of carbohydrate (1 carbohydrate serving).

Other Considerations When Using Insulin-to-Carbohydrate Ratios

1 There are a number of factors that affect insulin doses.

   A Patients may have more than 1 insulin-to-carbohydrate ratio.[14,15] For example, a patient may have a ratio of 1 unit of insulin to 10 g of carbohydrate at breakfast and a ratio of 1 unit of insulin to 15 g of carbohydrate at dinner.

   B Insulin-to-carbohydrate ratios may change with changes in body weight or level of physical activity.

   C Portion control is important to assure precise matching of insulin doses with anticipated carbohydrate intake.[16]

D With the shorter duration of action of rapid-acting insulin, the dose taken with the preceding meal may not provide adequate coverage of between-meal snacks. Snacks may need to be omitted, a lower carbohydrate snack may be needed, or an insulin bolus may be necessary at the time of a larger snack.

E While the premeal glucose reading is often used to determine insulin-to-carbohydrate ratios, checking glucose after meals is the best way to determine how well the bolus (mealtime) dose covers the meal.

2 There are additional food-related factors to consider when using insulin-to-carbohydrate ratios.

A The increased flexibility of carbohydrate intake for meals and snacks being covered by appropriate doses of insulin improves glycemic control; however, it can also place patients at risk for weight gain. Focusing only on carbohydrate and ignoring the amount of meat and meat substitutes and fat eaten also contributes to risk of weight gain. Reducing fat and monitoring total energy intake and/or increasing physical activity can help maintain desired weight.

B Because fat slows gastric emptying time,[17] a delay in the timing of the mealtime rapid-acting insulin (or short-acting insulin) may be necessary to match the peak of the insulin with the peak postprandial blood glucose response with very high-fat meals. However, the addition of fat does not change the area under the glucose curve.[3]

• If the pump has a square, dual, or extended wave bolus feature, the pump can be programmed to deliver the bolus dose over a specific amount of time. This feature is helpful for high-fat meals; adjustments are based on clinical observations.

C Dietary fiber generally is not digested and absorbed like other carbohydrates. Therefore, paying attention to the fiber content in high-fiber foods (those containing 5 or more grams of dietary fiber) can help patients more accurately match the insulin dose with the available carbohydrate. (Subtracting the dietary nonsoluble fiber grams from the total carbohydrate grams equals the available carbohydrate grams.)

• Meals that are high in slowly absorbed carbohydrate (eg, cooked dried beans) may require delivery of premeal short-acting insulin closer to the consumption time or delivery of rapid-acting insulin after consumption to match the peak insulin activity with the postprandial blood glucose peak.

D Patients may identify specific carbohydrate foods or meals that produce blood glucose responses greater or less than anticipated.[18,19] Such responses require changes in the insulin-to-carbohydrate ratios or timing of premeal insulin delivery, based on clinical observation in some insulin pump therapy users. For example, eating pizza may require additional amounts of insulin.

Key Educational Considerations for Carbohydrate Counting for Pump Therapy

1 The individual needs to understand insulin adjustment and supplementation before introducing a new element that requires making a specific insulin dose adjustment such as insulin-to-carbohydrate ratios.

2 After determining individual insulin-to-carbohydrate ratios, provide ample opportunities for the patient to complete paper-and-pencil exercises that simulate situations in which insulin adjustments would be needed for meals or snacks that are larger or smaller than usual. Examples can include a weekend brunch, pizza party, or a light lunch.

3 Assess the individual's ongoing ability to accurately estimate carbohydrate amounts. If portion control or estimating skills are questionable, the patient may need to review the basics of carbohydrate counting and continue practicing skills from those levels.

4 Periodically review the individual's food, blood glucose, and physical activity records to ascertain appropriate use of insulin-to-carbohydrate ratios.

5 Monitor the individual's weight. If weight gain is a problem, emphasize portion control, limiting calories and meat and fat intake, and using weight-management behaviors.

Self-Review Questions on Carbohydrate Counting

1 What are 3 basic steps used to determine insulin-to-carbohydrate ratios?
2 List 3 prerequisites for determining insulin-to-carbohydrate ratios.
3 What are the differences between basic and advanced carbohydrate counting?
4 Explain how to calculate insulin-to-carbohydrate ratios using the carbohydrate gram method.
5 How much insulin would be needed to cover 90 g of carbohydrate for someone using an insulin-to-carbohydrate ratio of 1 unit of insulin to 15 g of carbohydrate?
6 Explain how to calculate insulin-to-carbohydrate ratios using carbohydrate servings or choices.
7 Why do patients using insulin-to-carbohydrate ratios also need to be concerned about intake of meat and meat substitutes and dietary fat?

Learning Assessment:
Carbohydrate Counting Case Study

RO is a 31-year-old female who has had type 1 diabetes for 5 years with no complications except for trace microalbuminuria. She and her husband are interested in starting a family within the next year. Her A1C was 8.6% and 9% on her last 2 tests (normal = 4.4% to 6.1%). Her preconception blood glucose goals are preprandial 70 to 100 mg/dL and postprandial at 1 h <140 mg/dL and at 2 h <120 mg/dL. RO's blood glucose levels have ranged between 50 and 250 mg/dL for the past month. Her insulin regimen is 8 units NPH insulin and 9 units lispro at breakfast, 8 units lispro at lunch, 10 units lispro at dinner, and 9 units NPH insulin at bedtime. She has been advised to test her blood glucose more than 7 times per day (before meals, after meals, at bedtime, plus before and after exercise and when hypoglycemic). She uses a meter with memory but does not keep blood glucose records.

RO is 5 ft 4 in (163 cm) tall and weighs 140 lb (63 kg). She eats 3 meals daily plus afternoon and bedtime snacks. Her lunches are fast food and her afternoon snacks are from a vending machine. The amount of food that she eats varies greatly depending on where she is eating. She uses candy bars to treat hypoglycemia, and she usually eats more balanced, low-fat meals at home than when eating out.

RO's estimated daily calorie intake is 1500 to 2400 calories. Based on the dietitian's assessment, the recommended distribution of carbohydrate is as follows: breakfast, 60 to 65 g; lunch, 50 to 55 g; afternoon snack, 15 g; dinner, 70 to 75 g; and bedtime snack, 25 to 30 g.

RO is a married college graduate and a sales representative for a large company. She travels frequently (about 1 out-of-town trip per week) to large metropolitan areas. Her finances are adequate.

She has been experiencing problems with midmorning and late-afternoon hypoglycemia. Safety factors are a concern since she spends 2 to 4 hours a day driving. She is also concerned about weight gain from treating frequent insulin reactions. She recently switched from a split-mixed insulin regimen (NPH and regular twice a day) to the current MDI regimen. She is still not able to reach her blood glucose goals and continues to experience hypoglycemic reactions.

RO has been working on carbohydrate counting with her dietitian and has agreed to following a food/meal plan with specific carbohydrate goals for meals and snacks. RO has not kept 2 weeks of careful blood glucose levels, food intake, and activity records as requested. However, she states that she is interested in learning how to adjust insulin for varying amounts of food. She is also interested in getting an insulin pump, having learned from her medical team that it would promote euglycemia and help reduce hypoglycemic episodes. All of her preparation with MDI will help in starting her on insulin pump therapy.

Questions for Discussion
1 What level of carbohydrate counting is appropriate for RO's current skills?
2 What carbohydrate counting skills or activities should RO work on prior to using insulin-to-carbohydrate ratios? Where should you start?
3 How could you determine that RO is ready to learn insulin-to-carbohydrate ratios?

Discussion
1 RO needs flexibility with carbohydrate consumption at meals and snacks because her job involves frequent eating out and unpredictable meal times and locations. To achieve optimal glycemic control under these circumstances, she needs to learn how to adjust her mealtime lispro insulin for varying amounts of carbohydrate. But first RO must establish a consistent carbohydrate intake around which insulin doses can be adjusted. She must proceed from basic carbohydrate counting to advanced carbohydrate counting before she can develop accurate insulin-to-carbohydrate ratios.

2 Nutrition and behavior change options that can be presented to RO include recording blood glucose levels before each meal, 2 hours after meals whenever possible, and at bedtime. In addition, for the first few days, she should test her blood glucose at 3 AM. She could test and record her blood glucose more frequently before driving and before and after exercise. Other options can include
   A Faxing her blood glucose records to her diabetes educators weekly so that they can discuss insulin adjustments and supplementation.

B Following her individualized food/meal plan, which consists of 3 meals and a bedtime snack with an optional additional snack for exercise. Her food/meal plan includes mutually agreed-upon carbohydrate goals for meals. She should focus on consistency of carbohydrate intake based on her planned carbohydrate goals.

- Practicing portion control at home by weighing and measuring food for at least 2 weeks. She can buy a carbohydrate reference book that includes nutrition information about fast food and chain restaurants to help with making estimates when traveling.
- Keeping a food intake, blood glucose, and physical activity record for 2 weeks prior to her visit to the dietitian to learn insulin-to-carbohydrate ratios.

C Developing an insulin-to-carbohydrate ratio to use for adjusting insulin to anticipated food intake.

3 RO is very quick to grasp the principles of carbohydrate counting, and with adequate motivation and cooperation she can probably proceed quickly through the basics of carbohydrate counting to the advanced carbohydrate level of insulin-to-carbohydrate ratios.

4 At the initial visit and assessment (60 to 90 minutes), the dietitian and RO can develop a food/meal plan that includes food choices when eating away from home. The dietitian can explain the rationale for being disciplined about consistency in meal timing and carbohydrate portion sizes to facilitate insulin adjustments, emphasizing how these skills can lead to greater freedom and flexibility later when using insulin-to-carbohydrate ratios. The dietitian can also assess RO's skills in weighing, measuring, and estimating portion sizes by using measuring tools, food labels, and carbohydrate resources and references. The dietitian can emphasize that the possibility of developing insulin-to-carbohydrate ratios at the next visit depends on meeting carbohydrate goals and completeness of records. RO can send food records to the dietitian for feedback between visits.

5 At a follow-up visit 2 to 3 weeks later, the dietitian and RO review food intake, physical activity, insulin, and blood glucose records. If insulin doses have been adjusted around consistent and accurate carbohydrate intake and target glucose levels are met, then they are ready to determine insulin-to-carbohydrate ratios. RO can practice with sample meals and snacks using insulin-to-carbohydrate ratios to make insulin dosage adjustments. Areas to discuss include glycemic effects of fat and fiber, any possible insulin adjustments needed for consuming large amounts of these nutrients, and continued need for portion control and control of fat intake to maintain weight control. The need for follow-up based on telephone contact to discuss records or additional visits for more practice will be determined based on the results of this visit.

6 RO feels very comfortable with her insulin-to-carbohydrate ratio. She has completed the paperwork for her medical insurance for receiving an insulin pump, it has been approved, and she has plans to receive it in 2 weeks. She is scheduled to start the pump initiation.

7 RO goes through the insulin pump start (refer to the section on insulin pumps for details). She does very well with the mechanics of pump use and is able to use her insulin-to-carbohydrate ratio and the carbohydrate counting training to manage her food, physical activity, and blood glucose levels.

Carbohydrate Counting References

1 Hamet P, Abarca G, Lopez D, et al. Patient self-management of continuous subcutaneous insulin infusion. Diabetes Care. 1982;5:489-491.

2 Slama G, Klein JC, Delage A, et al. Correlation between the nature and amount of carbohydrate in meal intake and insulin delivery by the artificial pancreas in 24 insulin-dependent diabetics. Diabetes. 1981; 30:101-105.

3 Peters AL, Davidson MB. Protein and fat effects on glucose response and insulin requirements in subjects with insulin-dependent diabetes mellitus. Am J Clin Nutr. 1993;58:555-600.

4 Rabasa-Lhoret R, Garon J, Langlier H, Poisson D, Chiasson J-L. Effects of meal carbohydrate on insulin requirements in type 1 diabetic patients treated intensively with the basal-bolus (Ultralente-regular) insulin regimen. Diabetes Care. 1999;22:667-673.

5 Lafrance L, Rabasa-Lhoret R, Poisson D, Ducros F, Chiasson J-L. The effects of different glycaemic index foods and dietary fibre on glycaemic control in type 1 diabetic patients on intensive insulin therapy. Diabetic Med. 1998;15:972-978.

6 Delahanty LM, Halford BN. The role of diet behaviors in achieving improved glycemic control in intensively treated patients in the Diabetes Control and Complications Trial. Diabetes Care. 1993;16:1453-1458.

7 Diabetes Control and Complications Trial Research Group. Nutrition interventions for intensive therapy in the Diabetes Control and Complications Trial. J Am Diet Assoc. 1993; 93:768-773.

8 DAFNE Study Group. Training in flexible, intensive insulin management to enable dietary freedom in people with type 1 diabetes: dose adjustment for normal eating (DAFNE) randomised controlled trial. BMJ. 2002;325:746-752.

9 Gillespie SJ, Kulkarni K, Daly AE. Using carbohydrate counting in diabetes clinical practice. J Am Diet Assoc. 1998;98:897-905.

10 Daly A, Bolderman K, Franz M, Kulkarni K. Basic Carbohydrate Counting. Alexandria, Va and Chicago, Il: American Diabetes Association and American Dietetic Association; 2003.

11 Daly A, Bolderman K, Franz M, Kulkarni K. Advanced Carbohydrate Counting. Alexandria, Va and Chicago, Il: American Diabetes Association and American Dietetic Association; 2003.

12 Reader D, Davidson J. Diabetes Therapies: Insulin (handout). Minneapolis, Mn: International Diabetes Center; 2002.

13 International Diabetes Center. Insulin Basics Clinical Guidelines. Minneapolis, Mn: International Diabetes Center; 2002.

14 Kulkarni K, Franz MJ. A dietitian's perspective on medical nutrition therapy for diabetes. In: Franz MJ, Bantle JP, eds. American Diabetes Association Guide to Medical Nutrition Therapy for Diabetes. Alexandria, Va: American Diabetes Association; 1999:3-17.

15 Kulkarni K, Tomky D. Influence of carbohydrate counting on blood glucose patterns in intensive insulin therapy. On the Cutting Edge [newsletter]. July 1996.

16 Daly A, Gillespie S, Kulkarni K. Carbohydrate counting: vignettes from the trenches. Diabetes Spectrum. 1996;9:114-117.

17 Strachan MWJ, Frier BM. Optimal time of administration of insulin lispro. Importance of meal composition. Diabetes Care. 1998;21:26-31.

18 Ahren JA, Garcomb PM, Held NA, Pettit WA, Tamborlane WV. Exaggerated hyperglycemia after a pizza meal in well-controlled diabetes. Diabetes Care. 1993; 16:578-580.

19 Vlachokosta FV, Piper CM, Gleason R, Kinzel L, Kahn CR. Dietary carbohydrate, a Big Mac, and insulin requirements in type I diabetes. Diabetes Care. 1988;11: 330-336.

Resources on Carbohydrate Counting

American Diabetes Association, American Dietetic Association. Exchange Lists for Meal Planning. Alexandria, Va and Chicago, Il: American Diabetes Association and American Dietetic Association; 2003.

Franz MJ. Exchanges for All Occasions. 4th ed. Minneapolis: IDC Publishing; 1997.

Franz MJ. Fast Food Facts. 5th ed. Minneapolis: IDC Publishing; 1998.

Holzmeister LA. The Diabetes Carbohydrate and Fat Gram Guide. 2nd ed. Alexandria, Va and Chicago: American Diabetes Association and American Dietetic Association; 2000.

Kulkarni K, Fredrickson L, Graff M. Carbohydrate Counting. A Primer for Insulin Pump Users to Zero in on Good Control. Sylmar, Calif: MiniMed Technologies; 1999.

Monk A, Cooper N. Convenience Food Facts. 4th ed. Minneapolis: IDC Publishing; 1997.

Pennington JA. Bowes & Church's Food Values of Portions Commonly Used. 17th ed. Philadelphia: Lippincott; 1998.

Ross T, Geil P. Carbohydrate Counting Cookbook. New York: John Wiley & Sons; 1998.

Warshaw H. The ADA Guide to Healthy Restaurant Eating. Alexandria, Va: American Diabetes Association; 2000.

Warshaw HS, Bolderman KM. Practical Carbohydrate Counting. A How-to-Teach Guide for Health Professionals. Alexandria, Va: American Diabetes Association; 2001.

Warshaw H, Kulkarni K. The American Diabetes Association Complete Guide to Carbohydrate Counting. Alexandria, Va: American Diabetes Association; 2001.

Learning Assessment: Post-Test Questions

Insulin Pump Therapy and Carbohydrate Counting for Pump Therapy: Insulin-to-Carbohydrate Ratios   **7**

1 Basal profiles usually are not adjusted to reflect:
  A Decreased nocturnal insulin needs
  B Increased early morning insulin resistance
  C Mealtime insulin needs
  D Exercise adjustments

2 Red flags for potential insulin pump therapy failure include:
  A Expectations that insulin pump therapy will "cure" diabetes
  B Problems with glycemic control
  C History of complications
  D Problems with hypoglycemia

3 Which of the following conditions may not be helped by insulin pump therapy?
  A Pregnancy
  B Hard-to-control diabetes in children
  C Gastroparesis
  D Severe depression

4 How many basal profiles do most patients require?
  A 10
  B 2 or 3
  C 1
  D 5

5 The infusion set may not be:
  A Disconnected frequently
  B Inserted with a device
  C Placed in fatty tissue
  D Changed every 2 to 3 days

6 Mr. Jones has a correction factor of 40 and a target of 110 mg/dL. He needs 7 units of insulin to cover his lunch. His blood glucose is 190 mg/dL. How much insulin should he take as a bolus dose?
  A 5 units
  B 10 units
  C 9 units
  D 7 units

7 The DCCT demonstrated that tighter control of diabetes with insulin pump therapy was associated with all of the following except:
  A Decreased weight
  B Decreased nephropathy
  C Decreased retinopathy
  D Increased patient satisfaction

8 Benefits of insulin pump therapy include all of the following except:
  A Improved insulin absorption
  B Decreased insulin consumption
  C Increased mealtime flexibility
  D Reduced need for blood glucose testing

9 Which of the following statements is true?
  A Pump therapy makes diabetes less noticeable
  B Pump therapy involves an accelerated learning curve
  C Pump wearers are discouraged from participating in active sports
  D Insulin pump therapy is appropriate for all type 1 patients

10 What is the most important requirement for insulin pump success?
A Family support
B Fitness
C Motivation
D Proficiency in mathematics

11 Carbohydrate counting does not involve (best answer):
A Weighing or measuring portions
B Insulin-to-carbohydrate ratios
C Making allowances for grams of fat and protein
D Reading food labels

12 Advanced carbohydrate counting includes all of the following except:
A Knowing target blood glucose and when to take action
B Understanding the action of the insulin dose over a 24-hour period
C Using pattern management is not necessary
D Calculating an individual insulin-to-carbohydrate ratio

See next page for answer key.

Post-Test Answer Key

Insulin Pump Therapy and Carbohydrate Counting for
Pump Therapy: Insulin-to-Carbohydrate Ratios   **7**

1 C   7 A

2 A   8 D

3 D   9 B

4 B   10 C

5 A   11 C

6 C   12 C

A Core Curriculum for Diabetes Education
Diabetes Management Therapies

Hypoglycemia 8

Linda A. Gonder-Frederick, PhD
University of Virginia
Behavioral Medicine Center
Charlottesville, Virginia

John Zrebiec, MSW
Harvard University
Joslin Diabetes Center
Boston, Massachusetts

Introduction

1 It is extremely difficult to duplicate normal blood glucose metabolism with insulin therapies. Therefore, blood glucose levels in patients taking insulin tend to fluctuate between abnormally high (hyperglycemia) and abnormally low (hypoglycemia) levels due to under- and over-insulinization relative to food intake, physical activity, and metabolic needs.

2 Almost every person using insulin therapy, especially those with type 1 diabetes, eventually experiences hypoglycemic episodes. Persons with type 2 diabetes using insulin or insulin secretagogues alone or in combinations are also at risk for hypoglycemia.

3 Hypoglycemia tends to occur suddenly, and almost always requires immediate treatment to prevent blood glucose levels from continuing to fall to a dangerously low range.

4 Hypoglycemia is associated with a number of negative consequences for the individual with diabetes:
A Unpleasant physical symptoms
B Impaired cognitive function
C Embarrassment
D Emotional trauma
E Family conflict
F Accidents
G Bodily injury, including death

5 The problem of hypoglycemia has become even more significant as individuals with diabetes strive to maintain their blood glucose levels in a near-normal range by using more intensive insulin therapies as recommended by the Diabetes Control and Complications Trial (DCCT).[1] As blood glucose levels are lowered toward normal, the frequency of hypoglycemic episodes increases. For this reason, hypoglycemia has been called the major barrier to optimal control of type 1 diabetes.[2]

Objectives

Upon completion of this chapter, the learner will be able to
1 Define and describe mild and severe hypoglycemic episodes, including the symptoms associated with varying levels of severity.
2 Explain the physiological changes that occur with hypoglycemia.
3 Describe hypoglycemic symptomatology, the effects of hypoglycemia on emotions and behavior, and factors underlying symptom idiosyncrasy.
4 Identify causes of hypoglycemia and possible risk factors for individual patients.
5 Explain the treatment for different levels of hypoglycemia, including guidelines for when the person with diabetes is unable to self-treat due to a severe hypoglycemic episode.
6 Identify psychosocial sequelae of hypoglycemia.
7 Develop general education plans for teaching patients about hypoglycemia as well as more specific assessment and intervention plans for patients experiencing frequent or severe hypoglycemic episodes.

Definition of Hypoglycemia

1 It is difficult to define hypoglycemia on the basis of a specific plasma glucose concentration in people with diabetes. However, because lower glucose levels impair defenses against subsequent hypoglycemia, plasma glucose levels lower then approximately 72 mg/dL (4.0 mmol/L) can be defined as hypoglycemia.[3] Because hypoglycemic episodes vary greatly in their severity, severity of hypoglycemia is not defined by any specific blood glucose level per se, but rather is defined symptomatically.

A Mild hypoglycemia is characterized by symptoms such as sweating, trembling, difficulty concentrating, lightheadedness, and a lack of coordination. These symptoms are usually alleviated quickly by drinking or eating foods containing carbohydrates.

B Severe hypoglycemia is characterized by an inability to self-treat due to mental confusion, lethargy, or unconsciousness. Because the individual is unable to self-treat, others must provide treatment to raise the blood glucose level out of a dangerously low range.

2 Absolute blood glucose levels cannot be used to describe the severity of hypoglycemic episodes because glycemic thresholds for the onset of symptoms, as well as symptom magnitude, differ greatly among individuals and from episode to episode, depending on various mediating variables.

A Some individuals remain alert with only a few symptoms at a plasma glucose level of 50 mg/dL (2.8 mmol/L), while others become stuporous at the same glucose concentration.

B An individual may tolerate a plasma glucose level of 50 mg/dL (2.8 mmol/L) with few symptoms on one occasion, but become completely incapacitated at the same glucose concentration on another occasion.

3 The classification of hypoglycemic episodes as previously stated is based exclusively on whether individuals can treat themselves. Thus, the term mild does not necessarily mean that the symptoms experienced by the individual are mild or easily tolerated. In fact, an individual can be quite symptomatic (eg, sweating profusely, nauseous, disoriented, and uncoordinated) and still manage to self-treat. Therefore, even mild hypoglycemic episodes can be aversive and distressing from the individual's perspective.

4 Hypoglycemic episodes caused by insulin secretagogues are just as potentially dangerous as episodes caused by insulin.

A Mild hypoglycemia is common in persons with type 2 diabetes undergoing aggressive diabetes management.[4] However, the frequency of severe hypoglycemia from the use of oral medications is lower than that from insulin, and it is difficult to predict which patients are at risk. An exaggerated fear of hypoglycemia should not be a limiting factor in achieving good glycemic control in persons with type 2 diabetes.

B Different rates of hypoglycemia appear to be associated with different oral medications.

- The risk is highest with sulfonylureas.
- Of the sulfonylureas, the highest rates are found with those with long half-lives (ie, glyburide and chlorpropamide).
- Meglitinides (nonsulfonylurea insulin secretagogues), such as repaglinide, have short half-lives and generally are associated with less problems with hypoglycemia.

- When insulin sensitizers (ie, metformin, rosiglitazone, pioglitazone) are monotherapy, hypoglycemia is generally not an issue.
- When alpha-glucosidase inhibitors (ie, acarbose and miglitol) are used alone, hypoglycemia should not occur.

C Factors that increase the risk for hypoglycemia in persons with type 2 diabetes include
- Advanced age
- Poor nutrition
- Hepatic or renal disease

Hypoglycemic Symptoms

1 Two biological mechanisms are responsible for most hypoglycemic symptoms.

A Hormonal counterregulation involves autonomic symptoms caused by hormonal reactions that increase the glucose level to counteract hypoglycemia.

B Neuroglycopenia involves disruptions in mental and motor function secondary to depletion of glucose that is available to the central nervous system.

2 The symptoms that result from these biological mechanisms are typically the first warning signs that blood glucose levels arc too low, and thus play a critical role in the treatment of hypoglycemia and the prevention of severe episodes.[5]

3 Some of the most common hypoglycemic symptoms are shown in Table 8.1.

A The autonomic symptoms are generally adrenergically based, although sweating appears to be cholinergic.

B Because hypoglycemia causes such widespread physiological changes in hormonal and central nervous system (CNS) function, many different symptoms can occur; the list presented in Table 8.1 is not intended to be exhaustive.

C Hypoglycemic symptoms appear to be similar for persons with type 1 and type 2 diabetes.

4 Autonomic symptoms provide early warning signs of hypoglycemia.

A In the nondiabetic person, the primary counterregulatory hormones are glucagon, which enhances the release of glucose that is stored in the liver, and epinephrine, which increases the liver's production of glucose and inhibits glucose utilization.[5]

B After only a few years of diabetes duration (2 to 5 years), glucagon secretion is impaired in most persons with type 1 diabetes and epinephrine secretion becomes the primary mechanism for raising low blood glucose levels.

C If the epinephrine response to hypoglycemia is adequate, blood glucose levels will either stop falling or increase slightly before they become dangerously low. With prolonged hypoglycemia, growth hormone and cortisol may also play a role, although these hormones do not appear to contribute to early warning symptoms or early recovery.

D Over the course of type 1 diabetes, defective hormonal counterregulation can cause the epinephrine response to hypoglycemia to be diminished or delayed.[6] The result is that epinephrine secretion may not occur until blood glucose levels are quite low or the amount of epinephrine released is inadequate to stop blood glucose levels from falling further.

Table 8.1. Hypoglycemic Symptoms

Type of Symptom	Symptom
Autonomic	• Trembling/shaking • Sweating • Pounding heart • Fast pulse • Changes in body temperature • Tingling in extremities • Heavy breathing
Neuroglycopenic	• Slow thinking • Blurred vision • Slurred speech • Uncoordination • Numbness • Trouble concentrating • Dizziness • Fatigue/sleepiness
Unknown Etiology	• Hunger • Nausea • Weakness • Headache • General feeling of something not right

E Defects in hormonal counterregulation also delay or diminish the onset of autonomic symptoms, resulting in reduced hypoglycemic symptom awareness. Because the blood glucose level drops further before the individual recognizes that treatment is needed, the risk of becoming severely hypoglycemic increases greatly.

F Hormonal counterregulation and autonomic symptoms can disappear almost completely, resulting in what is called hypoglycemia unawareness. This term is somewhat misleading because even persons with significantly reduced hypoglycemia awareness typically still have some symptoms such as those associated with neuroglycopenia.[7] However, the recognition of symptoms may occur too late to allow timely treatment before significant neuroglycopenia.

G Persons with reduced hypoglycemia awareness are at increased risk of severe hypoglycemia and should be encouraged to test their blood glucose more frequently, especially at times when blood glucose levels are likely to be low or when hypoglycemia may be especially dangerous, such as while driving a motor vehicle or operating machinery.

H Several clinical risk factors associated with defective hormonal counterregulation and reduced hypoglycemia awareness[8,9] are shown in Table 8.2; all appear to increase the frequency of hypoglycemia.

I The clinical risk factors listed in Table 8.2 result in what has been called hypoglycemia-associated autonomic failure.[10] Research suggests that this autonomic failure may be reversible. For example, when patients with defective counterregulation meticulously avoid low blood glucose fluctuations over a period of several weeks, epinephrine response improves and autonomic symptoms increase in magnitude.[11,12]

Table 8.2. Clinical Risk Factors That Increase the Frequency of Hypoglycemia

- Use of intensive insulin therapies
- Near-normal glycosylated hemoglobin level
- History of frequent/recurrent episodes of severe hypoglycemia
- Autonomic neuropathy

J Research has shown that the occurrence of only 1 mildly low blood glucose episode can cause temporary deficits in epinephrine response and a reduction in autonomic symptoms for the next 24 hours.[13]
  - If another low blood glucose episode occurs during the subsequent 24 hours, glucose levels will drop much lower before hormonal counterregulation and autonomic symptoms occur.
  - Consequently, persons with diabetes need to be taught the importance of testing their blood glucose levels more frequently and monitoring themselves for symptoms more carefully for the next day or so after a hypoglycemic episode.

5 Neuroglycopenic symptoms provide early warning signs of hypoglycemia.
  A Traditionally, autonomic symptoms were considered to be the most reliable early warning signs of hypoglycemia. Neuroglycopenic symptoms, in contrast, were believed to have little utility as early warning signs. These symptoms were assumed not to appear until blood glucose levels were quite low and the patient was too mentally compromised to recognize the low blood glucose level.
  B More recent research[4-6] has demonstrated that autonomic and neuroglycopenic symptoms occur at similar glycemic thresholds and that patients experience neuroglycopenic symptoms as frequently as other symptoms.
    - The earliest signs of neuroglycopenia include a slowing down in performance and difficulty concentrating and reading.
    - Subjectively, the person feels as if it takes more effort to perform routine tasks that are usually done easily.
  C As the blood glucose level drops further and neuroglycopenia progresses, the onset of the following symptoms occurs: frank mental confusion and disorientation, slurred or rambling speech, irrational or unusual behaviors, and extreme fatigue and lethargy.
    - If the blood glucose level continues to fall, unconsciousness and seizures can occur.
    - Neuroglycopenia is typically the cause of accidents and physical injuries that occur during hypoglycemic episodes.
  D Teach all patients that changes in their ability to do routine tasks can be a sign that blood glucose levels are too low. Being alert for such changes is especially important for those with reduced autonomic symptoms who are more likely to experience neuroglycopenic symptoms as the first sign of impending hypoglycemia.

E Instruct patients to treat themselves as soon as possible when neuroglycopenic symptoms occur. Failure to do so can cause individuals to become so neuroglycopenic that they do not recognize that their blood glucose level is low.

F Neuroglycopenia during hypoglycemia can severely compromise decision-making and self-treatment behavior; it is common for the individual experiencing hypoglycemia to resist attempts by others to give them carbohydrates or even to become belligerent when others try to persuade them to drink or eat.

G Neuroglycopenia can also cause a number of changes in an individual's emotional states and social behavior.[14]

• Some of the most common emotional changes, most of which are negative (eg, irritability and anxiety), are listed in Table 8.3. In children, these emotional changes may result in crying, argumentativeness, and misbehavior.[15]

• Some individuals may also display positive emotional changes, such as inappropriate giddiness or euphoria.

H The effects of hypoglycemia on emotions can be a source of significant distress to persons with diabetes, who often are not aware that such effects are common and who may be too embarrassed to talk to healthcare providers about their behavior. Emotional changes are also a source of distress for family members and significant others because they have to contend with sudden negative shifts in mood. Relationships at school and work and with caregivers can also be strained by these emotions.

Table 8.3. Changes in Emotions and Social Behavior Associated With Hypoglycemia

Negative Moods	• Anxiety	• Frustration
	• Nervousness	• Anger
	• Tension	• Sadness
	• Irritation	• Pessimism
Positive Moods	• Giddiness	
	• Euphoria	
	• Disinhibition	
Behaviors	• Arguing	
	• Crying	
	• Resisting treatment	
	• Aggressive acts	
	• Inappropriate social/sexual behaviors	

6 Symptoms of hypoglycemia can differ between individuals and individual hypoglycemic episodes.

A Hypoglycemic symptomatology tends to be idiosyncratic.[5] Although a given individual often has similar symptoms during different hypoglycemic episodes, the most reliable warning symptoms for one individual may not be representative symptoms for another individual.

B It is important for individuals to learn to identify their own most reliable symptoms.

- This identification process can be done systematically using a symptom diary like the one shown in Figure 8.1. Individuals record their symptoms whenever they measure their blood glucose and then review the data to identify symptoms that occur reliably with hypoglycemia.
- A symptom diary also can be used to help persons with reduced hypoglycemia awareness (eg, loss of personally familiar symptoms) identify current reliable symptoms of hypoglycemia that they may not be aware of, such as neuroglycopenic symptoms.

C Individuals also differ greatly in their ability to recognize and interpret symptoms accurately.[5] This variability among persons may be due to differences in physiological responses to hypoglycemia as well as differences in psychological factors such as a tendency to attend to somatic cues.

- Because persons who tend to become neuroglycopenic do not seem to manifest early warning autonomic symptoms, these individuals need to be instructed to monitor more carefully and frequently in order to detect mild levels of low blood glucose that, if untreated, may lead to severe hypoglycemia.

D The type and magnitude of symptoms also can differ for a given individual from one hypoglycemic episode to the next.

- One reason why hypoglycemia episodes may vary within the same individual is because of delayed or reduced autonomic symptoms following a recent low blood glucose event.[13]

E Foods and medications may influence autonomic symptoms.

- In some studies,[16] caffeine consumption has been found to increase autonomic symptoms.
- Alcohol consumption can diminish awareness of hypoglycemic symptoms and impede glycemic recovery by interfering with hepatic glucose production (gluconeogenesis).
- Some medications, such as propranolol, also can mask early warning autonomic symptoms. In certain persons, beta blockers in higher doses may also mask perception of recovery from hypoglycemia.

Causes of Hypoglycemia

1 Certain regimen factors and self-treatment behaviors can increase the risk of hypoglycemia.

A All hypoglycemic episodes are caused by an excess of the medications used to lower blood glucose (insulin or insulin secretagogues) relative to food intake and activity level.

- The first step in determining what is causing frequent hypoglycemia is a careful examination of the individual's insulin regimen. Insulin excess and hypoglycemia are more likely to occur at those times of the day when insulin action is peaking.
- Some of the newer insulin analogs, including rapid-acting insulins (eg, insulin lispro or aspart) and long-acting (glargine) insulins, appear to reduce some of the problems with hypoglycemia.[17,18] In general, insulins that have a more dramatic peak in action, such as NPH, are more often associated with problems with hypoglycemia.
- Insulin pump therapy, which also better mimics normal insulin secretion, also appears to be associated with fewer hypoglycemia episodes for some individuals.

Figure 8.1. Symptom Diary

Instructions

1 Fill in date and time.

2 Check your physical and mental state (mind and body) for symptoms. Also consider other blood glucose cues such as changes in your food, insulin, and exercise. Write down all of your symptoms and cues.

3 Based on your symptoms and cues, estimate your current blood glucose level. Record this number in the "Estimate" column.

4 Measure and record your actual blood glucose level.

5 If your actual blood glucose level is <70 mg/dL, but your estimated blood glucose level was >70 mg/dL, recheck your physical and mental state (mind and body) for symptoms you may have missed. List any symptoms you notice in the "Missed Cues" column.

6 Finally, if your glood glucose level is <70 mg/dL, think about what might have caused it. For example, have you eaten less food, exercised more, or taken more insulin in the recent past?

Date	Time	Symptoms/Cues	Blood Glucose		Missed Cues	Causes of Hypoglycemia
			Estimate	Actual		

Common symptoms of hypoglycemia:
Use these as "prompts" to help you see how your body may respond to hypoglycemia.

- Trembling/shaking
- Sweating
- Pounding heart
- Fast pulse
- Body temperature change
- Tingling in extremities
- Heavy breathing
- Slow thinking
- Blurred vision
- Slurred speech
- Uncoordinated
- Numb
- Trouble concentrating
- Dizzy
- Fatigued/sleepy
- Hunger
- Nausea
- Weakness
- Headache
- General feeling something is not right

B Hypoglycemia is also more likely when no food has been eaten for several hours or when physical activity increases significantly.

- Many diabetes self-management behaviors related to food intake and physical activity can increase risk of hypoglycemia especially if appropriate changes are not made in medication. Some of these behaviors are shown in Table 8.4.
- Alcohol consumption without food intake may result in hypoglycemia.

Table 8.4. Diabetes Self-Management Behaviors That Increase the Risk of Hypoglycemia

Insulin	• Frequent insulin adjustments • Irregular timing of insulin dosages • Failure to decrease insulin when eating less • Inaccurate preparation of insulin dose
Food	• Skipping meals/snacks • Delaying meals/snacks • Irregular timing of meals • Irregular carbohydrate content • Not carrying carbohydrate source
Physical Activity	• Failure to eat additional carbohydrates • High degree of variability in daily/weekly activity schedule • Failure to recognize significant increases in caloric demand

C More than 50% of all episodes of severe hypoglycemia occur during the night.

- Because individuals may not be awakened by early warning symptoms with nocturnal hypoglycemia, the risk of severe episodes is greatly increased, especially in persons with deficient counterregulation. For individuals with adequate counterregulation, it is not uncommon to sleep through episodes of nocturnal hypoglycemia.
- The most common symptom to awaken an individual is sweating, although this symptom is absent in persons with reduced hypoglycemic awareness. Partners may be awakened by the individual's moaning and thrashing if sweating is not present.
- Nocturnal hypoglycemia is encountered frequently when strenuous physical activity is performed during the previous day.[19] When strenuous activity is performed, individuals should test blood glucose levels more frequently over the next 12 to 24 hours. This information can help them determine insulin and/or carbohydrate adjustment strategies needed to prevent the occurrence of hypoglycemia following strenuous physical activity. Performing additional self-tests during the night (eg, 3 AM) after strenuous physical activity may be needed to avoid nocturnal hypoglycemia in persons at high risk.

D Several additional factors can contribute to nocturnal hypoglycemia:

- Predinner injections of intermediate-acting insulin, such as NPH, may peak in action during the night and cause relative hyperinsulinemia overnight.
- Insulin requirements also appear to decrease between midnight and 3 AM, compared with insulin requirements at dawn.

E Significant increases in physical exertion, combined with failure to increase carbohydrate consumption and/or reduce the insulin dose, are one of the most common causes of both daytime and nocturnal hypoglycemia.[2]

- Teach patients that any strenuous physical activity can cause low blood glucose levels, even if they are not formally exercising. Caloric expenditure from strenuous activity does not necessarily cause hypoglycemia. Inappropriate adjustments for physical activity/exercise, duration, timing, etc are more likely to be factors.
- Individuals may not understand that activities such as shoveling snow are just as demanding as jogging and require the same adjustments in diabetes self-management (eg, eating extra carbohydrate or decreasing insulin dose[s]).

F By increasing glucose requirements and utilization by muscle tissues, strenuous physical activity can have both an immediate and a prolonged effect of lowering blood glucose levels (see Chapter 2, Physical Activity/Exercise, in Diabetes Management Therapies).

- Because of the depletion and need to replenish muscle glycogen stores, more carbohydrate may be required to raise blood glucose levels after prolonged strenuous physical activity.

G Concomitant use of sulfa antibiotics (such as, Septia™ and Bactrim™) with a sulfonylurea can cause profound and refractory hypoglycemia. Persons with diabetes need to be instructed to tell their physician that they are also taking a sulfonylurea if a sulfa-type of antibiotic is prescribed.

2 Other factors can increase the risk of hypoglycemia.

A Reproductive hormonal changes in women can affect blood glucose levels.

- The incidence of hypoglycemia increases significantly during the first trimester of pregnancy due to fetal demand for glucose and increased sensitivity to insulin. Frequent vomiting can also increase the risk of hypoglycemia.
- The risk and incidence of hypoglycemia decreases as pregnancy progresses, as increased levels of placental hormones result in an increase in peripheral insulin resistance (see Chapter 4, Pregnancy With Preexisting Diabetes, in Diabetes in the Life Cycle and Research, for more information).
- The incidence of hypoglycemia increases significantly during the postpartum period due to increased insulin sensitivity and, if breastfeeding, increased glucose use.
- Women using intensive treatment programs frequently report higher blood glucose levels just prior to menses, followed by a lowering of blood glucose levels after the start of menstrual flow.

B The delayed absorption of carbohydrates and delayed gastric emptying caused by gastroparesis can cause hypoglycemia.

C Insulin sensitivity can affect blood glucose levels.

- Leaner individuals tend to be more sensitive to insulin and have reduced insulin requirements.
- Physically fit persons also are more sensitive to insulin than those who have a more sedentary lifestyle.

D Decreased renal function in the elderly or renal insufficiency in persons with type 2 diabetes can extend the duration of the effects of sulfonylureas or insulin and cause hypoglycemia.

E Decreases in caloric intake for weight loss that are not accompanied by decreases in insulin or oral medications can increase risk.

Prevention of Hypoglycemia

1 Avoidance of nearly all episodes of hypoglycemia is the ideal goal, but this is difficult to achieve in many persons. Avoidance of severe hypoglycemia, which is associated with significant risk for injury, is critical.

2 The most powerful tool for preventing hypoglycemia is diabetes self-management training.

A Because the majority of hypoglycemic episodes are caused by overinsulinization relative to food intake and physical activity, the person's knowledge about their diabetes treatment regimen and the causes of hypoglycemia should be carefully assessed.

B Even well-educated and experienced individuals may have misunderstandings or inadequate knowledge about hypoglycemia. For example, many individuals do not know that high-fat foods have a delayed and depressed glycemic effect. Thus, eating a high-fat, low-carbohydrate meal after insulin injections or boluses can lead to hypoglycemia.

C Because knowledge does not always influence behavior, the individual's self-management habits also need to be assessed.

3 Until recently, frequent hypoglycemia was often regarded as a sign of good glycemic control, and many patients continue to hold this belief.

A It is now known that frequent episodes of mild hypoglycemia greatly increase the risk of an episode of severe hypoglycemia.

B Hypoglycemic episodes also have little or no effect on metabolic control, which is determined by the frequency of hyperglycemia.

- A1C values of 7.0% or less may be the result of wide high-low blood glucose fluctuations, which further emphasizes the importance of blood glucose record review.

4 It is especially important to prevent nocturnal hypoglycemia because during sleep an individual cannot rely on being awakened by early warning symptoms. Guidelines for preventing nocturnal hypoglycemia are provided in Table 8.5.

Table 8.5. Guidelines for Preventing Nocturnal Hypoglycemia

- Do not skip presleep snacks.
- Measure presleep blood glucose levels regularly.
- If the bedtime plasma glucose level is 126 mg/dL (7.0 mmol/L) or lower, increase the carbohydrate content of the snack.[20]
- If daytime strenuous exertion occurred, eat additional carbohydrate at the night snack.
- Rather than decreasing the predinner dose of NPH, which can lead to fasting hyperglycemia, other options are to move the predinner NPH to presleep or change the basal insulin to glargine.
- Measure 3 AM blood glucose levels at least once a week or more frequently if recurrent nocturnal hypoglycemia is a problem.
- Measure 3 AM blood glucose levels when daytime physical activity or food consumption was atypical and when insulin doses are being adjusted.

Treatment of Hypoglycemia

1 Recommended thresholds for treatment of hypoglycemia vary across different health-care providers and individual patients. A conservative recommendation is to treat all plasma glucose levels less than 72 mg/dL (4 mmol/L), based on the evidence that even very mild hypoglycemia can reduce early warning symptoms and counterregulation.[12]

2 Treatment guidelines are relatively straightforward.

   A Eat or drink 10 to 15 g of glucose per se or any form of carbohydrate that contains glucose, which should raise the plasma glucose level 30 to 45 mg/dL (1.7 to 2.5 mmol/L). Ten grams of oral glucose raised plasma glucose levels from 60 mg/dL (3.3 mmol/L) to 97 mg/dL (5.4 mmol/L) over 30 minutes with levels starting to decline after 60 minutes. Twenty grams of oral glucose raised plasma glucose levels from 58 mg/dL (3.2 mmol/L) to 122 mg/dL (6.8 mmol/L) over 45 minutes, with the glucose level again starting to decline after 60 minutes.[21] Different foods and drinks that supply this amount of carbohydrate are listed in Table 8.6.

     • Glucose or carbohydrates containing glucose are used to treat hypoglycemia so that blood glucose levels rise quickly. Drinks/food that are high in fat content slow gastric emptying and absorption of carbohydrate and, therefore, take longer to raise blood glucose levels. Adding protein to the treatment of hypoglycemia does not raise blood glucose levels and does not prevent subsequent hypoglycemia.[22]

Table 8.6. Carbohydrate Sources (15 to 20 g) for Treating Hypoglycemia

Source	Quantity
Glucose tablets	3 to 4
Lifesavers® candies	8 to 10
Brach's® hard candies	8 to 10
Raisins	2 tablespoons
Nondiet soft drinks	4 to 6 oz
Fruit juice	4 to 6 oz
Milk (no fat or low fat)	8 oz

   B If plasma glucose levels are less than 50 mg/dL (2.8 mmol/L), 20 to 30 g of carbohydrate may be needed.

   C If possible, test blood glucose level before beginning treatment. If pretreatment testing is not possible and symptoms are present, proceed with the treatment.

   D Test blood glucose level 15 to 20 minutes after initiating treatment. If the blood glucose level is still low, repeat the treatment even if symptoms have disappeared.

   E If the person is not scheduled to eat a meal or snack within the next hour, he or she should be cautious about additional hypoglycemia. Patients should be instructed that their blood glucose level may fall again if food is not eaten within the next hour. Blood glucose level should be tested again and treated if low.

F Following very mild episodes of hypoglycemia, the indivdual usually can resume normal activity fairly soon after treatment. With more significant hypoglycemia, recovery of mental and motor function lags behind glycemic recovery. When plasma glucose levels fall to 45 mg/dL (2.5 mmol/dL), cognitive recovery may take as long as 45 to 75 minutes.[23,24] Advise patients that it may not be safe to engage in any potentially risky activities (eg, driving) during this period.

3 The following guidelines are recommended for self-treatment of hypoglycemia.

A Do not keep eating after the initial treatment; wait 15 to 20 minutes, then test blood glucose level to determine whether further treatment is needed.

B Do not keep eating until symptoms disappear.

C Avoid using high-fat foods for treatment (Table 8.7).

D Always carry some type of carbohydrate.
- Keep something at your bedside to treat nocturnal hypoglycemia.
- Keep something in the car at all times to treat episodes of hypoglycemia that might occur while driving.

E Always wear diabetes identification.

4 Overtreatment will cause posttreatment hyperglycemia.

A Overtreating hypoglycemia is relatively common and can be attributed to both physiological and psychological factors. The individual may eat until autonomic symptoms abate completely, rather than consuming the recommended amount of carbohydrate and waiting to see if symptoms subside or blood glucose increases.

B Other individuals overeat because of the fear of losing control due to neuroglycopenia. This fear is especially common in those who live alone, care for small children, or have experienced a traumatic episode of severe hypoglycemia in the past.

C Using commercially available, portion-controlled glucose products may help individuals avoid overtreatment.

Table 8.7. Foods With High Fat Content That are Poor Choices for Treating Hypoglycemia

• Ice cream	• Pies, cakes	• Pizza
• Doughnuts	• Cheese	• French fries
• Candy bars	• Nuts	• Milkshakes
• Meat	• Cookie dough	• Potato chips

---

5 Appropriate treatment of hypoglycemia is also determined by such complicated psychological processes as decision-making and judgment.[25]

A These processes can be compromised by diminished cognitive ability and inaccurate risk appraisal, either due to neuroglycopenia or inaccurate beliefs about hypoglycemia.

B Once individuals know that their blood glucose level is low, they make several decisions based on the following questions:
- Treat immediately or wait?

- What to eat and how much?
- Stop current activity or continue?

C Deciding to delay treatment is relatively common and often leads to severe hypoglycemia.

- Reasons for delaying treatment include the desire to finish a task and embarrassment about eating when others are not.
- Some individuals may even deny they are becoming hypoglycemic because it is a reminder of their diabetes or perceived as an indication that they have made some mistake in diabetes management.

D It is important to assess individuals' attitudes and beliefs about hypoglycemia. Some persons believe there is no reason to treat low blood glucose levels unless they are below 50 mg/dL (2.8 mmol/L) or until they feel symptoms.

- Many individuals believe that their ability to function is not affected until blood glucose levels fall very low, which often is not the case. Research shows that measurable deficits in mental and motor task performance occur at glucose levels of 65 mg/dL (3.5 mmol/L).[25-27]

6 Treatment of hypoglycemia often must be done by family members or significant others.

A A person with type 1 diabetes who is experiencing hypoglycemia often has to be treated by others because of the effect of neuroglycopenia on judgment and behavior.

- Teach family members and significant others how to cope with episodes of severe hypoglycemia and what to expect in terms of the patient's behavior (eg, stupor or possible resistance). Some family members report that it is helpful to use favorite foods to coax the hypoglycemic individual to eat.
- Coworkers, friends, and teachers also need to know how to respond to symptoms of hypoglycemia, which can be a problem if individuals do not want to reveal their diabetes to others.

B The following basic guidelines are recommended for treating severe hypoglycemia.

- Persons who are able to swallow without risk of aspiration may be coaxed into drinking juice or a soft drink. If this is not possible, place some glucose gel, honey, syrup, or jelly inside the individual's cheek.
- Persons who are unable to swallow without risk of aspiration can be given glucagon by subcutaneous or intramuscular injection. Glucagon is a hormone secreted by the pancreatic alpha cells that stimulates hepatic glucose production. It increases both glycogenolysis and gluconeogenesis and is less effective in persons with glycogen depletion.[23] It can produce substantial hyperglycemia, but as with oral glucose, the glycemic response is transient with glucose levels beginning to fall after approximately 1.5 hours.[28]
- Teach patients to keep glucagon in their homes at all times. Individuals who may be required to administer the injection need to know how to use the glucagon kit; this may include a teacher, coworker, roommate, friend or neighbor. Glucagon kits can be obtained by prescription. Patients also need to be aware of the expiration date on their glucagon.
- Glucagon can be injected subcutaneously or intramuscularly. Recommended doses are 1 mg for adults and older children, 0.5 mg for children <5 years old, and 0.25 mg for infants.[29]
- The glycemic effect of glucagon is quite short lived, so as soon as the individual is able to swallow, carbohydrate liquid (eg, juice, soft drink, low-fat milk) should

be administered to maintain normoglycemia (see Chapter 3, Pharmacologic Therapies for Glucose Management, in Diabetes Management Therapies, for more information on glucagon).

- Nausea and vomiting often follow treatment of hypoglycemia with glucagon.[30]
- In circumstances in which the individual expected to assist the person experiencing hypoglycemia is likely to be too anxious to administer the glucagon injection, that "assistant" should be instructed to call 911.
- Frequent blood glucose monitoring is needed over the next several hours to detect blood glucose levels that are falling again or to detect hyperglycemia due to overtreatment.
- Instruct patients to notify their healthcare provider following episodes of severe hypoglycemia.

C If episodes of severe hypoglycemia become frequent or recurrent, it is often helpful for the patient and team members to discuss how best to cope with these episodes. This discussion should only be attempted when the person is not hypoglycemic.

Psychosocial Impact

1 Individuals with diabetes may develop emotional distress and fear of hypoglycemia after experiencing mild or severe hypoglycemia episodes.

A Negative moods, social embarrassment, and potential danger associated with hypoglycemia can clearly cause emotional distress for persons with diabetes. Results from the DCCT[31] showed that the occurrence of severe hypoglycemia alone was not necessarily related to emotional distress, but recurrent episodes appeared to have a negative impact on quality of life.

B Persons with diabetes may also develop significant anxiety about hypoglycemia and go to extreme measures to avoid its occurrence. The Hypoglycemia Fear Survey[32] is an assessment tool used to measure the extent to which individuals worry about hypoglycemia and engage in behaviors to avoid hypoglycemia and its negative consequences. Characteristics of those at high risk for excessive fear of hypoglycemia are identified in Table 8.8.

Table 8.8. Characteristics of Those at High Risk for Excessive Fear of Hypoglycemia

Patient Characteristics

- Have just begun taking glucose-lowering medication
- Have little or no experience in coping effectively with episodes of hypoglycemia
- Have frequent and/or recurrent episodes of hypoglycemia
- Have experienced emotionally traumatic episodes of hypoglycemia
- Tend to be overly anxious
- Have ineffective coping skills
- Have visual impairment or other physical disabilities

C High levels of fear can contribute to inappropriate diabetes management, such as keeping blood glucose levels above the target range to avoid hypoglycemic episodes or phobic avoidance of certain situations such as being alone or driving. Individuals may also be reluctant to make necessary increases in medications or insulin because of fear of hypoglycemia.
  • Conversely, low levels of fear can also contribute to inappropriate or high-risk behaviors, such as delaying treatment in response to symptoms.
  • Assess the possible psychological sequelae of hypoglycemia on a routine basis, especially after an individual experiences an episode of severe hypoglycemia.

2 There are numerous aspects of hypoglycemia that contribute to conflicts between persons with diabetes and significant others and individuals with whom the person has frequent interaction (eg, roommates and caregivers).
  A The emotional changes associated with hypoglycemia (tension, irritation, and pessimistic thinking) can lead individuals to become argumentative with others.
  B When hypoglycemia is frequent or recurrent, the persons with diabetes may feel as if others blame them, so they become defensive and resentful; these behaviors can increase the likelihood of resisting treatment.
  • Similarly, family members and significant others can become angry and resentful if they believe their loved one is not exerting enough effort to prevent hypoglycemia or behaving in ways that increase the risk.
  • Spouses of persons with diabetes who experience frequent, severe hypoglycemia report increased rates of marital conflict about diabetes-related issues, including the prevention and treatment of hypoglycemia.[33]
  C In some families and households, power struggles occur over the management of hypoglycemia; these struggles may reflect other areas of unresolved conflict. The educator can offer to refer those in such relationships for counseling.

3 Family members and significant others may experience similar emotional distress and fear of hypoglycemia similar to that of persons with diabetes.
  A Family members and those living with the persons with diabetes also can develop significant fear of hypoglycemia, especially if they have experienced episodes associated with very frightening or traumatic consequences for their loved one.
  • Spouses of individuals who have experienced frequent, severe hypoglycemia show very high levels of fear compared with spouses of those who have experienced only mild episodes.[33]
  • Parents of children with type 1 diabetes report very high levels of fear in general, but especially if their child has been unconscious or had a seizure while hypoglycemic.[34]
  B If nocturnal hypoglycemia has been a problem, family members, roommates, and nighttime caregivers may even develop sleep disorders such as insomnia or restless sleep if they feel they must remain vigilant during the night to recognize symptoms.[33]

Assessment and Intervention

1 Assessment of knowledge about hypoglycemia and individual risk factors is essential for developing effective educational and intervention plans.
  A Hypoglycemia risk, treatment, and prevention are determined by many different factors, both general and specific for each individual, that may change over time.

Therefore, education and intervention must be ongoing, individually tailored, and reassessed regularly to reflect changing needs of the person with diabetes.

B The frequency and severity of hypoglycemic episodes can change over the course of diabetes due to a variety of factors:
- Changes in diabetes treatment
- Physiological changes (eg, insulin sensitivity, hormonal counterregulation)
- Changes in symptoms
- Lifestyle and schedule changes

C Objectively assess knowledge about hypoglycemia whenever possible. Patients often are reluctant to ask questions or admit that they do not understand the information they receive. Knowledge assessment can be done verbally, and written instruments also are available, such as the Hypoglycemia Knowledge Questionnaire.[35]

D In addition to basic knowledge, assess the patient's (or parents' if the patient is a child) personal habits and routine behaviors for treating and preventing hypoglycemia.
- It is important to identify beliefs about hypoglycemia and its treatment. Sample questions that can be used to identify personal risk factors and beliefs about hypoglycemia are listed in Figure 8.2.

Figure 8.2. Sample Questions to Determine Patient Risk Factors and Beliefs About Hypoglycemia

To What Extent Do You:	Not At All		Somewhat		A Great Deal
1 Always carry some type of food or drink with sugar?	1	2	3	4	5
2 Skip meals?	1	2	3	4	5
3 Skip snacks?	1	2	3	4	5
4 Worry about hypoglycemia?	1	2	3	4	5
5 Try to keep your BG levels below 100 mg/dL?	1	2	3	4	5
6 Delay eating when trying to finish a task?	1	2	3	4	5
7 Think having low BG is a sign of good control?	1	2	3	4	5
8 Eat extra food when you're going to be more active?	1	2	3	4	5
9 Recognize low BG symptoms?	1	2	3	4	5
10 Eat as little as possible to avoid gaining weight?	1	2	3	4	5
11 Increase your insulin whenever your blood glucose is too high?	1	2	3	4	5
12 Wait until you feel strong symptoms to treat a low BG?	1	2	3	4	5
13 Only treat very low BG levels (between 40 and 50 mg/dL)?	1	2	3	4	5
14 Believe you can function fine when your BG is below 50 mg/dL?	1	2	3	4	5

- Include possible emotional and social barriers to hypoglycemia management and treatment in the assessment. For example, adolescents often dislike having to eat a morning snack during school because it makes them feel different from their peers. Young women who are overly concerned about weight gain may be at increased risk of hypoglycemia due to low carbohydrate intake, even when blood glucose levels are low (see Chapter 6, Psychological Disorders, in Diabetes Education and Program Management, for more information).

E Some aspects of hypoglycemia management can be assessed directly. For example, patients can be asked to show the educator their diabetes identification and the emergency glucose they are carrying.

F Symptoms and the ability to recognize low blood glucose levels should be assessed on a regular basis. Changes in symptoms (eg, loss of autonomic symptoms) and decreased ability to tell when blood glucose is low require additional education and intervention. Symptoms of hypoglycemia can change as often as every 2 years.

G At each routine visit, ask patients if any hypoglycemic episodes have occurred since their last appointment. If so, a structured interview can be given to evaluate the following factors. This type of structured evaluation is especially important after episodes of severe hypoglycemia to help identify specific risk factors and problem areas for individual patients.
- Date, time, and location of the hypoglycemic episode
- Severity of the episode
- Possible causes of the episode (eg, events during preceding 24 hours)
- Degree of symptomatology and ability to recognize the need for treatment
- Ability to self-treat and/or respond to attempts by others to provide treatment
- Decisions made about when and how to treat
- Barriers to treatment (eg, no available food/drink)
- Type and amount of food eaten
- Negative consequences of the episode (eg, distress, accidents, or embarrassment)

H After severe, distressing, or traumatic episodes of hypoglycemia, patients need to be assessed for possible negative psychosocial sequelae. Objective measures of distress, such as the Hypoglycemia Fear Scale,[32] can be used. This assessment can also be accomplished by asking patients questions such as the following about the negative emotional and social effects of their hypoglycemic episode:
- How upsetting was the episode for you?
- How worried are you about another episode like that happening again?
- Have you changed your diabetes management to avoid another episode?
- Did the episode cause any problems between you and other people?

2 The core intervention for hypoglycemia management and treatment is effective education, although behavioral interventions may be needed when individuals have a solid knowledge and understanding of hypoglycemia, yet continue to have problems.

A Goal setting and contracting can be used by patients to make specific behavioral changes.

B Teaching problem-solving techniques to the person with diabetes also can be effective for dealing with barriers to hypoglycemia management.

C When reduced hypoglycemic awareness is a problem, individuals can use a diary to improve their ability to recognize and avoid hypoglycemia (Figure 8.1). Using a diary provides important benefits:

- Increased awareness of hypoglycemic symptoms and other predictors of low blood glucose levels
- Objective assessment of symptoms that are reliable signs of low blood glucose levels
- Objective assessment of how accurately low blood glucose is recognized
- Means of identifying patterns in hypoglycemic episodes (eg, causes, time of day)

D When frequent and/or severe hypoglycemic episodes continue in spite of medical, educational, and behavioral interventions, patients need referral to a mental health specialist who has experience working with diabetes-related psychosocial issues (see Chapter 6, Psychological Disorders, in Diabetes Education and Program Management, for more information).

- Individuals who remain rather unconcerned or refuse to change their behavior, even after potentially dangerous episodes, also need referral for a psychological assessment.
- Referrals for counseling or psychotherapy also are appropriate when patients are experiencing emotional problems due to hypoglycemia, such as anxiety, phobias, or conflicts in their marriage or relationships with significant others.

E Currently, one psychoeducational intervention, Blood Glucose Awareness Training (BGAT)[36,37] has been demonstrated empirically to improve ability to recognize low blood glucose levels, reduce the frequency of low blood glucose levels, and reduce the incidence of severe hypoglycemia without jeopardizing diabetes control.

- BGAT involves 8 weekly sessions using a manual with 8 chapters (1 per week) that provides training in recognizing hypoglycemic symptoms and predicting low blood glucose levels due to changes in insulin, food, and physical activity.
- Each chapter also provides activities (eg, symptom diary) to be done during the rest of the week to increase awareness of hypoglycemia.

Key Educational Considerations

1 Provide persons with type 1 diabetes basic information about hypoglycemia at diagnosis. This initial education includes

A An explanation of hypoglycemia and its primary causes

B A description of hypoglycemic symptoms

C Guidelines for treatment

D Measures to prevent hypoglycemia

2 At diagnosis, patients and their families or significant others are attempting to assimilate new information and are likely to process only a fraction of what they are taught.

A For this reason, give patients written materials such as handouts and articles about hypoglycemia for later review.

B Ask newly diagnosed patients and their families to call back soon after the first hypoglycemic episode occurs to determine how they managed the episode and to receive further education.

3 Teach patients and their families, those with whom the patient resides, and those who provide care that hypoglycemic symptoms are idiosyncratic and that patients need to learn to recognize how they feel when their blood glucose level is low.

A They need to know that hypoglycemic symptoms can sometimes be difficult to recognize and distinguish from other types of symptoms (eg, nervousness, sweating due to exertion).

B Describe the emotional and behavioral changes that can occur with hypoglycemia as biologically based and a normal manifestation of hypoglycemia.

4 In spite of the initial information overload, patients' families, those with whom the patient resides, and those who provide care need to be taught immediately how to administer glucagon when severe hypoglycemia occurs. This information must be repeated and reinforced on subsequent visits because those who have not had to use glucagon may forget how to use it, forget where they have placed it, or fail to check the expiration date.

5 Persons with type 2 diabetes who are taking oral glucose-lowering medication also need to be taught about hypoglycemia, even though they appear to be at less risk for severe hypoglycemia.

A Patients who are changing from oral medications to insulin may have considerable fears and concerns about hypoglycemia and need to be taught to monitor themselves for warning symptoms, especially at those times of the day when they are at most risk (eg, just before lunch). These patients may also need to increase the frequency of self-monitoring of blood glucose.

B Many type 2 patients are not adequately educated about hypoglycemia and are not aware of the risks that hypoglycemia can impose. Knowledge about hypoglycemia, including warning symptoms, needs to be assessed even in patients who have been taking medication for a long period of time.

C Hypoglycemia is treated by carbohydrate consumption, following the guidelines prescribed for patients with type 1 diabetes. However, glucagon is not appropriate for treatment of insulin secretagogue-induced hypoglycemia because glucagon also stimulates insulin secretion.

D Sulfonylurea-induced hypoglycemia can be quite prolonged and can recur. For this reason, hospitalization may be necessary.

E While more research is needed, persons with type 2 diabetes requiring insulin may have the same risk for hypoglycemia as persons with type 1 diabetes.

6 Education about hypoglycemia is an ongoing process.

A After diagnosis and initial education, the next important step in the learning process occurs when patients experience their first episode of hypoglycemia. Every hypoglycemic episode can be an opportunity for increasing knowledge.

B Use of the structured interview procedure can help teach patients about diabetes management behaviors that lead to lower blood glucose levels, their symptoms, and treatment decisions that increase the risk of severe episodes.

C Evaluation of specific episodes also provides an opportunity to give patients positive feedback when they have used their knowledge and judgment to avoid more severe problems with hypoglycemia.

7 Initial education about hypoglycemia provides an opportunity to instill treatment habits such as using commercially packaged glucose tablets and consuming carbohydrates immediately when blood glucose is low.

8 Ask patients and their families to describe their concerns about hypoglycemia; their input provides focus and direction for the educational efforts. Because areas of concern differ greatly across different patient groups and developmental stages, educational priorities are based on the personal needs of individual patients.

A Parents of infants with type 1 diabetes may justifiably worry about the negative long-term effects of hypoglycemia on their child's intellectual abilities; provide this group with more intensive diabetes education aimed at prevention.

B The lifestyle changes and attitudes of adolescent patients often place them at increased risk of hypoglycemia. For example, adolescents will try alcohol and periodically skip meals or eat inappropriate foods. Adolescents need to be reminded frequently about the effects of alcohol and drug use, increased exercise, dietary indiscretion, and other risky behaviors on blood glucose levels.

9 Patients and their families need to be instructed about the risks of hypoglycemia and driving.

A These risks include automobile accidents and injury as well as being mistakenly arrested for driving while intoxicated, which can happen when an individual is not wearing diabetes identification.

B At each visit, ask patients if they keep some kind of emergency carbohydrate in their car and, if so, what kind of food/drink they carry. They can also be asked to show their
  • Diabetes identification
  • Emergency carbohydrate they carry at all times in their purse or pocket.

C Assess patients' beliefs about driving and hypoglycemia.
  • Ask how low they believe their blood glucose needs to be before they will not drive.
  • Many individuals believe that they can continue to drive safely with blood glucose levels quite low.[38]
  • Patients should be instructed not to drive when their plasma glucose is <80 mg/dL (4.4 mmol/L) because they may have motor impairments they do not recognize and because their blood glucose can quickly become lower while they are driving.[39]

D Teach individuals about the importance of checking their blood glucose before driving. This is especially important for individuals who have previously experienced problems with hypoglycemia while driving or who have hypoglycemia unawareness.

E A surprisingly high number of patients report that they have never received any counseling from healthcare providers regarding driving and hypoglycemia.[40] All persons need to know the 4 basic guidelines listed below:
  • If possible, check BG before driving, especially if there is any reason to suspect that BG may be low or become low during the drive.
  • Always carry foods or beverages that contain carbohydrate where it is easy to reach in the car. Because the food or drink may not be used for a long period of time, check them from time to time to make sure that they are still edible.
  • If signs of hypoglycemia occur while driving, pull off the road as soon as possible. Do not attempt to drive to some destination before treatment.
  • Treat immediately and do not resume driving until cognitive and motor function are recovered. Recovery of function can lag behind glycemic recovery.

10 Patients also need to be educated about the risk of hypoglycemia in other potentially dangerous situations, such as when caring for young children or when using heavy tools (eg, electric saws, lawn mowers).

Self-Review Questions

1 What are the different levels of hypoglycemia?

2 List 10 symptoms associated with hypoglycemia and name the physiological basis for each of the symptoms.

3 What are 3 reasons why hypoglycemic symptoms can vary across individual patients and different episodes?

4 Explain what reduced hypoglycemic awareness is and what causes it.

5 What are emotional and behavioral changes that can occur with hypoglycemia?

6 List 3 of the most common causes of hypoglycemia.

7 Why can prolonged, vigorous exercises have a delayed effect on blood glucose levels?

8 Describe the guidelines for treating a patient with a plasma glucose between 50 and 72 mg/dL (2.8 to 4 mmol/L); with a plasma glucose lower than 50 mg/dL (2.8 mmol/L).

9 Name 3 foods that are not as effective for treating hypoglycemia and explain why these foods are inappropriate choices.

10 Describe 2 beliefs about hypoglycemia that can lead patients to risky treatment behaviors such as delaying treatment.

11 Describe fear of hypoglycemia and the types of patients who are most likely to exhibit it.

12 Name 3 possible effects that hypoglycemia can have on family members and significant others.

13 What are 4 basic rules that reduce risk of hypoglycemia while driving?

Learning Assessment: Case Study 1

LE is a 23-year-old female who has had type 1 diabetes for 12 years. Her metabolic control was fair during her adolescent and college years. LE currently is working full-time and living in an apartment with a roommate. For the last year, her glycemic control has been improving with regular insulin and NPH injections before breakfast and before dinner. She measures her BG before each insulin injection and sometimes before lunch. Because her fasting BG levels have been high, she has recently increased her predinner NPH. For weight control, LE jogs 3 miles after dinner several times each week and she only eats a bedtime snack if she feels hungry. At a routine office visit, LE reports that she is having 2 or 3 episodes of nocturnal hypoglycemia per week. In addition, she had many BG measurements during the day that were less than 50 mg/dL (2.8 mmol/L) and felt no symptoms at all. LE also reports that during a recent episode, her roommate had to force jelly into her mouth to treat her.

Questions for Discussion

1 What clinical and behavioral factors increase LE's risk of hypoglycemia?

2 What steps can be taken by LE and her diabetes care team to reduce the frequency of LE's nocturnal hypoglycemic episodes without jeopardizing her improved metabolic control?

Discussion

1 Several factors are contributing to LE's increased hypoglycemic risk:

  A Increase in predinner NPH dose

  B Failure to decrease predinner regular and/or NPH insulin dose before postdinner strenuous physical activity

  C Failure to eat regular bedtime snacks and larger snacks after evening jogging

  D Failure to test bedtime BG levels

  E Reduction in hypoglycemic symptoms due to deficient and/or delayed hormonal counterregulation secondary to LD's frequent low BG episodes.

2 Ask LE to identify her concerns regarding hypoglycemia. Problem-solve with her about strategies to reduce nocturnal hypoglycemia. She can also make these behavioral goals.

3 Strategies she might identify are

  A Consistently eat a bedtime snack. Check BG levels before eating the snack and make appropriate increases in the size of the snack depending on physical activity and BG level.

  B If nocturnal hypoglycemia continues despite these interventions, LE could move her predinner NPH to bedtime and her predinner regular insulin could be adjusted. She also could switch to a long-lasting basal insulin analog, such as insulin glargine, with mealtime rapid-acting insulin. The effect of insulin regimen changes should be assessed after a few days, with additional dose changes implemented, if necessary. Frequent contact with the healthcare provider is critical while insulin adjustments are being made.

  C Because of her reduced hypoglycemia awareness, LE could do more frequent blood glucose monitoring and keep a blood glucose awareness diary. She should be taught to measure her blood glucose before driving or engaging in any other potentially risky activities.

  D Provide LE with a prescription for glucagon. LE can teach her roommate how to use it and place it where her roommate can easily find it.

Learning Assessment: Case Study 2

MJ is a 66-year-old man who is overweight and was diagnosed with type 2 diabetes 4 years ago. His blood glucose has been poorly controlled using a meal plan and physical activity program, so glyburide each morning before breakfast was added. MJ was instructed that it was critical that he eat breakfast soon after taking his medication. He said that this would be no problem, describing himself as an old-fashioned, meat-and-potatoes man who always has a hearty breakfast. When MJ returned to the clinic for his 3-month checkup, his blood glucose records showed that most of his fasting and predinner levels were in a normal range. However, MJ reported that his medication was causing unpleasant side effects. He described feeling shaky, dizzy, and nauseous during the mid- to late-morning hours. While these symptoms seemed to eventually subside on their own, MJ found them to be quite aversive and disruptive to his work. He indicated that he wanted to stop taking the medication and attempt again to control his blood glucose levels with a meal plan and physical activity.

Questions for Discussion

1 What is the likely cause of MJ's unpleasant symptoms?

2 What can be done to help MJ continue to take his oral medications?

3 What food/meal factors would you want to assess as possible contributors to MJ's problem?

Discussion

1 Although it seems almost certain that MJ is experiencing midmorning hypoglycemia, this suspicion should be confirmed with daily midmorning BG measurements and additional measurements when symptoms occur.

2 Because MJ appears to be confused by his symptoms, additional education is needed about the following:

A Causes, warning symptoms, and treatment of hypoglycemia

B Importance of carrying carbohydrate at all times, including having food or drink at the office and in the car for quick treatment

3 MJ's meal pattern, especially breakfast foods, needs careful evaluation.

A He may eat a large breakfast that consists of high-fat, low-carbohydrate foods such as eggs, bacon, and milk. Consequently, his postmeal blood glucose levels may be lower than usual, causing him to become hypoglycemic.

B MJ should be given further nutrition education. Point out that by increasing his carbohydrate intake at breakfast he may prevent hypoglycemia.

C Another of his options is to eat a midmorning snack on a routine basis. This should be considered with caution given MJ's need to control his weight.

4 If MJ continues to have problems with hypoglycemia in spite of these interventions, his morning dose of glyburide may need to be decreased, or he may need to switch to an oral agent that does not increase the risk for low blood glucose levels.

Learning Assessment: Case Study 3

AG is a 44-year-old woman who has had diabetes for 25 years. Although AG has a long history of managing her diabetes quite well on multiple daily injections, and staying in relatively good control, she was recently diagnosed with retinopathy. In order to improve her diabetes control even further, AG began using an insulin pump about 6 months ago. During a clinic appointment, AG reports that in the past 2 months, she has experienced several episodes of severe hypoglycemia that have occurred approximately 2 hours after meals. One of these episodes occurred while she was driving, and she became so disoriented that she became lost and could not find her destination. She finally pulled off the road, and another driver stopped to see what was wrong. When AG could not answer any of his questions coherently, he called 911 for the rescue squad.

Questions for Discussion

1 What type of assessment is needed to identify the cause of AG's problem with severe hypoglycemia?

2 What types of education and intervention should be considered for AG?

Discussion

1 First, assess AG's self-management behaviors prior to these episodes (ie, insulin, food, and physical activity).
   A Determine whether AG's mealtime insulin bolus is appropriate for her meal carbohydrate.
   B Determine whether AG engaged in any recent strenuous physical activity before the episodes.
   C Review AG's recommended insulin regimen and correction factors for any problems.

2 Because AG has only been using her insulin pump for 6 months, it is also important to assess her understanding of the recommended regimen. If AG keeps a record of her daily insulin doses, review these. If she does not keep any record of her daily insulin, it might be helpful to ask her to begin doing so.

3 Psychological factors should also be considered.
   A Assess the degree to which AG is concerned about hyperglycemia and any impact this is having on her diabetes management.
   B Specifically, ask AG whether or not she is giving herself boluses after meals and the dose of these. It is not uncommon for individuals who are attempting to maintain normal BG levels to over-bolus after meals because they become very worried about postprandial increases in glucose. This type of "micromanagement" of postprandial glucose levels can lead individuals to deliver multiple boluses over relatively short periods of time.
   C Also assess the degree to which AG is now concerned about hypoglycemia and any impact this is having on her diabetes management. Given her traumatic episode of severe hypoglycemia while driving, AG could be experiencing extreme fear of hypoglycemia and engaging in self-management behaviors aimed at avoiding future episodes.

4 Depending on the results of the above assessment, several different types of education and/or intervention might be appropriate for AG.
   A AG's insulin regimen may need to be adjusted.
   B Any misunderstandings about insulin pump therapy and/or the recommended treatment regimen should be addressed through education.
   C If AG does appear to be over-bolusing after meals, she should receive education regarding this risk factor and be provided with treatment guidelines to manage postprandial rises in BG more appropriately.
   D If AG's concern about hyperglycemia and the development of long-term complications or her concern about future hypoglycemia appear to be a problem, she may need counseling to reduce her anxiety and identify more adaptive ways to cope with these risks.
   E Regardless of the cause of AG's episodes of severe hypoglycemia, she should receive education about the risk of driving when BG is low and the basic treatment guidelines for reducing this risk.

References

1 The Diabetes Control and Complications Trial Research Group. The effect of intensive treatment of diabetes on the development and progression of long-term complications in insulin-dependent diabetes mellitus. N Engl J Med. 1993;329:977-986.

2 Cryer PE. Hypoglycemia: the limiting factor in the glycemic management of type 1 and type 2 diabetes. Diabetologia. 2002;45:937-948.

3 Cryer PE, Davis SN, Shamoon H. Hypoglycemia in diabetes (technical review). Diabetes Care. 2003;26:1902-1912.

4 Miller CD, Phillips LS, Ziemer DC, Gallina DL, Cook CB, El-Kebbi IM. Hypoglycemia in patients with type 2 diabetes mellitus. Arch Intern Med. 2001;161:1653-1659.

5 Cox DJ, Gonder-Frederick L, Antoun B, Cryer PE, Clarke WL. Perceived symptoms in the recognition of hypoglycemia. Diabetes Care. 1993;6:519-527.

6 Clarke WL, Gonder-Frederick LA, Richards E, Cryer PE. Multifactorial origin of hypoglycemic symptom unawareness in IDDM: association with defective glucose counterregulation and better glycemic control. Diabetes. 1991;40:680-685.

7 Clarke WL, Cox DJ, Gonder-Frederick LA, Julian D, Schlundt D, Polonsky W. Reduced awareness of hypoglycemia in adults with IDDM. A prospective study of hypoglycemic frequency and associated symptoms. Diabetes Care. 1995;18:517-522.

8 Amiel SA, Sherwin RS, Simonson DC, Tamborlane WV. Effect of intensive insulin therapy on glycemic thresholds for counterregulatory hormone release. Diabetes. 1988;37:901-907.

9 Amiel SA, Tamborlane WV, Simonson DC, Sherwin RS. Defective glucose counterregulation after strict glycemic control of insulin-dependent diabetes mellitus. N Engl J Med. 1987;316:1376-1383.

10 Cryer PE. Iatrogenic hypoglycemia as a cause of hypoglycemia-associated autonomic failure in IDDM. A vicious cycle. Diabetes. 1992;41:255-260.

11 Cranston I, Lomas J, Maran A, MacDonald I, Amiel SA. Restoration of hypoglycaemia awareness in patients with long-duration insulin-dependent diabetes. Lancet. 1994; 344:283-287.

12 Fanelli CG, Epifano L, Rambotti AM, et al. Meticulous prevention of hypoglycemia normalizes the glycemia thresholds and magnitude of most neuroendocrine responses to, symptoms of, and cognitive function during hypoglycemia in intensively treated patients with short-term IDDM. Diabetes. 1993;42:1683-1689.

13 Heller SR, Cryer PE. Reduced neuroendocrine and symptomatic responses to subsequent hypoglycemia after 1 episode of hypoglycemia in nondiabetic humans. Diabetes. 1991;40:223-226.

14 Gonder-Frederick LA, Cox DJ, Bobbitt SA, Pennebaker JW. Mood changes associated with blood glucose fluctuations in insulin-dependent diabetes mellitus. Health Psychol. 1989;8:45-59.

15 McCrimmon RJ, Gold AE, Deary IJ, Kelnar CJ, Frier BM. Symptoms of hypoglycemia in children with IDDM. Diabetes Care. 1995;18:858-861.

16 Kerr D, Sherwin RS, Pavalkis F, et al. Effect of caffeine on the recognition of and responses to hypoglycemia in humans. Ann Intern Med. 1993;119:799-804.

17 DeWitt DE, Dugdale DC. Using new insulin strategies in the outpatient treatment of diabetes: clinical applications. JAMA. 2003;289:2265-2269.

18 Rosetti P, Pampanelli S, Fanelli C, et al. Intensive replacement of basal insulin in patients with type 1 diabetes given rapid-acting insulin analog at mealtime: a 3-month comparison between administration of NPH insulin four times daily and glargine insulin at dinner or bedtime. Diabetes Care. 2003;26;1490-1496.

19 Davis SN, Galassetti P, Wasserman DH, Tate D. Effects of antecedent hypoglycemia on subsequent counterregulatory responses to exercise. Diabetes. 2000;49:73-81.

20 Kalergis M, Schiffrin A, Gougeon R, Jones PJH, Yale JF. Impact of bedtime snack composition on prevention of hypoglycemia in adults with type 1 diabetes undergoing intensive insulin management using lispro insulin before meals. Diabetes Care. 2003;26:9-15.

21 Wiethop BV, Cryer PE. Alanine and terbutaline in the treatment of hypoglycemia in IDDM. Diabetes Care. 1993;16:1131-1136.

22 Gray RO, Butler PC, Beers TR, Kryshak EJ, Rizza RA. Comparison of the ability of bread versus bread plus meat to treat and prevent subsequent hypoglycemia in patients with insulin-dependent diabetes mellitus. J Clin Endocrinol Metab. 1996;81:1508-1511.

23 Blackman JD, Towle VL, Sturis J, Lewis GF, Spire JP, Polonsky KS. Hypoglycemic thresholds for cognitive dysfunction in IDDM. Diabetes. 1992;41:392-399.

24 Evans ML, Pernet A, Lomas J, Jones J, Amiel SA. Delay in onset of awareness of acute hypoglycemia and of restoration of cognitive performance during recovery. Diabetes Care. 2000;23:893-897.

25 Gonder-Frederick L, Cox D, Kovatchev B, Schlundt D, Clarke W. A biopsychobehavioral model of risk of severe hypoglycemia. Diabetes Care. 1997;20:661-669.

26 Gonder-Frederick LA, Cox DJ, Driesen NR, Ryan CM, Clarke WL. Individual differences in neurobehavioral disruption during mild and moderate hypoglycemia in adults with IDDM. Diabetes. 1994;43:1407-1412.

27 Driesen NR, Cox DJ, Gonder-Frederick LA, Clarke WL. Reaction time impairment in insulin-dependent diabetes: Task complexity, blood glucose levels, and individual differences. Neuropsychology. 1995;9:246-254.

28 Ryan CM, Atchison J, Puczynski S, Puczynski M, Arslanian S, Becker D. Mild hypoglycemia associated with deterioration of mental efficiency in children with insulin-dependent diabetes mellitus. J Pediatr. 1990;117:32-38.

29 Cryer PE, Fisher JN, Shamoon H. Hypoglycemia (technical review). Diabetes Care. 1994;17:734-755.

30 Collier A, Steedman DJ, Patrick AW, et al. Comparison of intravenous glucagon and dextrose in treatment of severe hypoglycemia in an accident and emergency department. Diabetes Care. 1987;10:712-715.

31 The Diabetes Control and Complications Trial Research Group. Influence of intensive diabetes treatment on quality-of-life outcomes in the diabetes control and complications trial. Diabetes Care. 1996;19:195-203.

32 Irvine A, Cox D, Gonder-Frederick L. The Fear of Hypoglycemia Scale. In: Bradley C, ed. Handbook of Psychology and Diabetes. Switzerland: Hardwood Academic Publishers; 1994:133-155.

33 Gonder-Frederick L, Cox D, Kovatchev B, Julian D, Clarke W. The psychosocial impact of severe hypoglycemic episodes on spouses of patients with IDDM. Diabetes Care. 1997;20:1543-1546.

34 Clarke WL, Gonder-Frederick LA, Miller S, Richardson T, Snyder A. Maternal fear of hypoglycemia in their children with insulin-dependent diabetes mellitus. J Pediatr Endocrinol Metab. 1998;11:189-194.

35 Drass JA, Feldman RH. Knowledge about hypoglycemia in young women with type I diabetes and their supportive others. Diabetes Educ. 1996;22:34-38.

36 Cox D, Gonder-Frederick L, Polonsky W, Schlundt D, Julian D, Clarke W. A multicenter evaluation of blood glucose awareness training—II. Diabetes Care. 1995;18:523-528.

37 Gonder-Frederick LA, Cox DJ, Clarke WL, Julian DM. Blood glucose awareness training. In: Snoek FJ, Skinner TC, eds. Psychology in Diabetes Care. Chichester, England: John Wiley & Sons; 2000:169-206.

38 Clarke WL, Cox DJ, Gonder-Frederick LA Kovatchev B. Hypoglycemia and the decision to drive a motor vehicle by persons with diabetes. JAMA. 1999;282:750-754.

39 Cox DJ, Gonder-Frederick LA, Kovatchev BP, Julian DM, Clarke WL. Progressive hypoglycemia's impact on driving simulation performance. Diabetes Care. 2000;23:163-170.

40 Cox DJ, Kovatchev BP, Gonder-Frederick LA, Clarke WL. Physiological and performance differences between drivers with type 1 diabetes with and without a recent history of driving mishaps: an exploratory study. Canadian Journal of Diabetes. 2003;27:23-28.

Suggested Readings

Clarke WL, Cox DJ, Gonder-Frederick L, Julian D, Kovatchev B, Young-Hyman D. Biopsychobehavioral model of risk of severe hypoglycemia. Diabetes Care. 1999;22:580-584.

Cryer PE. Hypoglycemia: Pathophysiology, Diagnosis and Treatment. New York: Oxford University Press; 1997.

Cryer PE, Davis SN, Shamoon H. Hypoglycemia in diabetes (technical review). Diabetes Care. 2003;26:1902-1912.

Gonder-Frederick L, Clarke WL, Cox DJ. The emotional, social, and behavioral implications of insulin-induced hypoglycemia. Semin Clin Neuropsychiatry. 1997;2:57-65.

Gonder-Frederick L, Cox DJ, Clarke WL. Helping patients understand and reduce hypoglycemia. In: Anderson BJ, Rubin RR, eds. Practical Psychology for Diabetes Clinicians, 2nd ed. Alexandria, Va: American Diabetes Association; 2002.

Ter Braak EWMT, Appelman AMMF, van de Laak MF, Stolk RP, van Haeften TW, Erkelens DW. Clinical characteristics of type 1 diabetic patients with and without severe hypoglycemia. Diabetes Care. 2000;23:1467-1471.

Other Resources

Blood Glucose Awareness Training was developed at the University of Virginia and is currently being used throughout the US, Canada, and Europe. Information about BGAT can be obtained by writing. The Behavioral Medicine Center, University of Virginia Health System, Box 800223, Charlottesville, VA 22908.

Learning Assessment: Post-Test Questions

Hypoglycemia

1   When a patient with type 1 diabetes of 10 years suddenly begins trembling, shaking, and experiencing other symptoms indicating a hypoglycemic reaction, the body responds by releasing:
    A   Acetylcholine
    B   Epinephrine
    C   Hydrocortisone
    D   Glucagon

2   Neuroglycopenic symptoms now have been shown to:
    A   Occur before autonomic symptoms
    B   Occur later than autonomic symptoms
    C   Be cholinergic in origin
    D   Occur at about the same time as autonomic symptoms

3   Which of the following is not a symptom of neuroglycopenia?
    A   Extremely high energy and excitation
    B   Slurred or rambling speech
    C   Mental confusion and disorientation
    D   Irrational or unusual behavior

4   When neuroglycopenic symptoms first occur, persons with diabetes should:
    A   Wait for help from a healthcare professional
    B   Not treat themselves because of the possibility of an accident
    C   Treat themselves immediately
    D   Wait before any treatment because their symptoms may eventually disappear

5   Consumption of coffee may:
    A   Be a first aid treatment for hypoglycemia
    B   Increase autonomic symptoms
    C   Enhance neuroglycopenia
    D   Interfere with gluconeogenesis

6   Hypoglycemia can be defined as any plasma glucose level of:
    A   85 mg/dL or lower
    B   80 mg/dL of lower
    C   75 mg/dL or lower
    D   70 mg/dL or lower

7   Physical activity by the person with diabetes:
    A   May require an increase in carbohydrate consumption and/or insulin reduction
    B   May be beneficial to prevent hypoglycemia
    C   Has no effect on hypoglycemia
    D   May require an increase in the insulin dose

8   Over the course of type 1 diabetes, defective hormonal counterregulation can cause:
    A   Neuroglycopenic symptoms to diminish
    B   Decreased epinephrine secretion leading to a diminished or delayed onset of symptoms
    C   Decreased glucagon secretion leading to a diminished or delayed onset of symptoms
    D   Fewer or delayed symptoms because of diminished cortisol secretion

9   Persons with type 1 diabetes and their families and/or significant others:
    A   Should not be given information concerning hypoglycemia on diagnosis because it increases their anxiety level
    B   Should be given written materials on hypoglycemia and instruction on administering glucagon
    C   Should be given written material, but no instruction on glucagon administration because it is dangerous for a nonprofessional to administer
    D   Should be given instructions in glucagon administration but not on hypoglycemia to avoid information overload

10 Persons with type 2 diabetes who are taking sulfonylureas and meglitinides:

  A Do not require instruction in hypoglycemia because they are less at risk due to a maintenance of integrity of hormonal counterregulation

  B Have an increased risk of hypoglycemia because of a lack of hormonal counterregulation

  C Need to be taught about hypoglycemia, although they appear to be at less risk for severe hypoglycemia

  D May experience occasional hypoglycemic attacks, but these are mild and never require corrective measures

11 Problems with hypoglycemia:

  A Are minimal for persons with type 2 diabetes receiving combination therapy

  B Are more significant because of current treatment approaches and blood glucose goals

  C Are less problematic as a result of the more intensive insulin therapies

  D Only occur with patients using insulin therapy

12 Symptoms associated with hypoglycemia:

  A May vary for a person from one hypoglycemic episode to the next

  B Are well documented and occur consistently in persons with diabetes

  C Are less likely to be affected by physiological or psychological factors

  D Are only slightly affected by food, alcohol, or medications

13 Most severe hypoglycemic episodes:

  A Occur within 2 hours after taking intermediate-acting insulin

  B Are likely to be nocturnal

  C Occur despite a consistent carbohydrate consumption and regularly scheduled meals

  D Are unrelated or unaffected by physical activity

14 Physical activity can have immediate and prolonged effects on blood glucose levels. One of these effects is:

  A Increased glucose utilization combined with decreased glucose production

  B Decreased glucose utilization by muscle tissue

  C Delayed insulin absorption

  D Accelerated glycogenolysis by the liver during exercise

15 Which of the following is not an appropriate recommendation for treating hypoglycemia?

  A Eat or drink 10 to 20 grams of carbohydrate, depending on how low the blood glucose level is

  B Avoid using beverages or foods that are high in fat content

  C Continue eating or drinking until symptoms subside in order to keep blood glucose levels from falling further

  D If a snack or meal is not planned for the next hour, eat some carbohydrate-containing food

16 Insulin regimens associated with a decreased risk for hypoglycemia include (check all that apply):

  A Long-lasting basal insulin analog such as glargine

  B Intermediate-acting insulins such as NPH

  C Rapid-acting insulins such as insulin lispro or aspart

  D Insulin pump therapy

17 Hypoglycemic unawareness:

  A May be reversed with meticulous avoidance of any blood glucose levels below 70 mg/dL (3.9 mmol/L)

  B Is almost always caused by autonomic neuropathy

  C Is typically psychological, not physiological in etiology

  D Only occurs in individuals who have had diabetes more than 10 years

See next page for answer key.

Post-Test Answer Key

Hypoglycemia
8

1	B	**10**	C
2	D	**11**	B
3	A	**12**	A
4	C	**13**	B
5	B	**14**	A
6	D	**15**	C
7	A	**16**	A,C,D
8	B	**17**	A
9	B		

A Core Curriculum for Diabetes Education
Diabetes Management Therapies

Illness and Surgery 9

Elaine Boswell King, MSN, RN, CS, CDE
Vanderbilt Diabetes Research and Training Center
Nashville, Tennessee

Janie Lipps, MSN, RN, CS, CDE
Vanderbilt Diabetes Research and Training Center
Nashville, Tennessee

Introduction

1 This chapter will address the knowledge and skills needed by healthcare providers and patients to manage diabetes during illness and surgery.

2 Illness can cause problems when managing diabetes. During times of illness, the body releases stress hormones that oppose the action of insulin and contribute to hyperglycemia and the formation and accumulation of ketones. If appropriate action is not taken, dehydration and ketosis or a hyperosmolar hyperglycemic state (HHS) can result, requiring hospitalization.

3 Surgical conditions can impact diabetes control. Persons with diabetes may require usual surgical interventions as well as surgery for associated complications of diabetes such as coronary artery disease, peripheral vascular disease, neuropathic ulcers, kidney disease, and proliferative retinopathy.

A Patients' usual treatment programs are affected when surgery is performed; typical adjustments involve nutrition therapy, medications, and mobility.

B Surgery can place persons with diabetes at risk for infections if their blood glucose remains above normal levels.

C The perioperative management of persons with type 1 and type 2 diabetes can differ.

4 An understanding of normal physiology is necessary to provide adequate support to the person with diabetes who is experiencing an illness or undergoing a surgical procedure. Special care is needed to achieve and maintain euglycemia, maintain fluid and electrolyte balance, provide adequate nutrition, and prevent further complications.

Objectives

Upon completion of this chapter, the learner will be able to

1 Describe the physiological effects of illness and surgery on blood glucose concentrations, ketone levels, and fluid and electrolyte balance.

2 Describe specific guidelines that healthcare providers can follow when managing the care of patients with intercurrent illnesses.

3 Identify sick-day situations that require evaluation and possible treatment in an office/clinic, emergency room, or hospital setting.

4 Identify assessment information needed preoperatively.

5 Describe methods of insulin/glucose management for the surgical patient.

6 Explain the importance of euglycemia during the perioperative period.

7 Explain postoperative concerns.

Physiologic and Clinical Effects of Illness and Surgery on Blood Glucose Concentrations, Ketone Levels, and Fluid/Electrolyte Balance

1 Metabolic homeostasis is maintained by the balance of the anabolic hormone insulin and the major catabolic hormones—glucagon, catecholamines, cortisol, and growth hormone. A major role of insulin is to lower glucose levels. Physiological stress caused by intercurrent illnesses, surgery, infection, injury, emotional trauma, or medications can disrupt homeostasis and cause hyperglycemia and ketosis.

2 During illness and surgery, there is an increase in the secretion of counterregulatory hormones, including cortisol, catecholamines (epinephrine and norepinephrine), growth hormone, and glucagon.[1,2]

A Catecholamines cause an increase in heart rate, increase blood pressure, and dilate the bronchi to maximize the amount of oxygen that is supplied to the body tissues. Blood is diverted from the vulnerable surface of the body to the core to supply the vital organs with essential oxygen. Since blood is diverted from the skin and subcutaneous fat, injected insulin may not be absorbed.

B Epinephrine decreases the uptake of glucose by the muscle tissue and inhibits the release of endogenous insulin.

3 In type 1 diabetes, counterregulatory hormones enhance the following metabolic changes: glycogenolysis, gluconeogenesis, lipolysis, and ketogenesis.[3,4]

A Counterregulatory hormones contribute to the release of glucose from the liver and oppose the action of insulin.

B Catecholamines and cortisol raise blood glucose levels by
- Causing glycogen that is stored in the liver to break down into glucose (glycogenolysis) and be released into the bloodstream.
- Causing the liver to create additional glucose (gluconeogenesis) from amino acids (alanine), glycerol, and lactate.
- Increasing peripheral insulin resistance.

C Catecholamines also suppress insulin release.

D Cortisol inhibits the uptake of glucose by the muscle tissue.

4 With hyperglycemia, urine volume is increased due to osmotic diuresis; fluid requirements also increase.

A Signs and symptoms related to increased fluid requirements include polydipsia, polyuria, thirst, and dry mouth.

B If hyperglycemia persists without fluid and electrolyte replacement, dehydration can occur. Adequate insulin replacement must be given to lower glucose, correct the osmotic diuresis, and prevent diabetic ketoacidosis (DKA).

C Signs and symptoms resulting from dehydration include muscle weakness and fatigue related to loss of sodium, potassium, phosphorus, and magnesium.

5 Ketogenesis and lipolysis are caused by an inadequate carbohydrate intake and/or insufficient insulin. Ketonuria and/or ketonemia are clinical manifestations of lipolysis and ketogenesis.

A Inadequate carbohydrate intake results in starvation ketosis. If glucose is not available, the body must switch to fat stores for energy.

B Symptoms of ketosis include nausea and anorexia. If ketosis caused by insufficient insulin goes untreated diabetic ketoacidosis can result.

C Warning signals of ketoacidosis include fruity acidic breath, abdominal pain, and/or rapid, labored breathing (Kussmaul respiration) (see Chapter 2, Hyperglycemia, in Diabetes and Complications, for more information on DKA).

D Hospitalization is appropriate for DKA when the plasma glucose is >250 mg/dL (>13.9 mmol/L) with arterial pH <7.30 and serum bicarbonate level is <15 mEq/L in the presence of moderate ketonuria and/or ketonemia.[5]

6 In type 2 diabetes, hyperosmolar hyperglycemic state (HHS) can occur as a manifestation of severe metabolic decompensation and dehydration. Although DKA and HHS are often discussed as distinct entities, they may overlap in a spectrum of decompensation.

A HHS is differentiated from DKA by the absence of significant ketosis. In HHS, volume depletion and dehydration result, but ketogenesis usually is suppressed because of levels of insulin high enough to prevent ketosis but not hyperglycemia.

B HHS is characterized by severe hyperglycemia (eg, plasma glucose >600 mg/dL) (>33.3 mmol/L) and hyperosmolarity (eg, >320 mOsm/kg) (>320 mmol/kg).[5,6]

C HHS is seen most often in the elderly, who have poor fluid intake or a diminished thirst mechanism.[7,8]

D If undetected or inadequately treated, lethargy, impaired mental status, or coma may result.[9]

E Recommendations for prevention and early treatment are similar to those for diabetic ketoacidosis. (See Chapter 2, Hyperglycemia, in Diabetes and Complications, for information on HHS.)

Guidelines for Sick-Day Management

1 Maintain adequate hydration because of the risk of dehydration from decreased fluid intake, polyuria, vomiting, diarrhea, and evaporative losses from fever.

A Instruct patients to drink at least 8 oz (240 mL) of calorie-free fluids every hour while they are awake. Examples of calorie-free liquids include diet soft drinks, water, broth, and sugar-free Kool-Aid® soft drink. Bouillon, consommé, and canned clear soups provide sodium and electrolytes as well as fluids and at least 8 oz should be consumed every third hour. A major cause of persistent ketoacidosis is inadequate sodium intake.

B If the patient is unable to tolerate fluids by mouth, antiemetic suppositories or intravenous fluids may be required. Vomiting that cannot be suppressed may require emergency room care.

2 Increase the frequency of blood glucose monitoring and initiate ketone monitoring during suspected or acute illness.

A The signs and symptoms of a developing acute illness can be preceded by elevated blood glucose levels and ketone levels.

B More frequent monitoring is indicated when the person experiences unusual physical symptoms such as malaise, fever, anorexia, and/or nausea or when blood glucose levels rise. These symptoms may disappear or may develop into an identifiable illness.

C The frequency of blood glucose monitoring may need to be increased to every 2 to 4 hours while glucose levels are elevated and/or until symptoms subside. Blood or urine ketone levels also need to be tested every 4 hours until negative results are obtained. Monitoring is performed at times when decisions regarding the insulin dose are needed.

D Instruct patients to record their monitoring results and response to treatment adjustments in order to more readily provide this information to the healthcare provider over the telephone, if needed.

3 Adjust medications during illness.

   A Insulin and/or most oral glucose-lowering agents are still needed during illness even when the patient is unable to eat. Omission of insulin is a common cause of ketosis.

      • Continue the routine dose of intermediate-insulin or long-acting insulin (NPH, Lente, Ultralente, glargine).

      • The full dose of daily insulin usually is required.

      • Individuals using insulin pump therapy should continue their basal insulin and may need to increase their basal rate. The pump should not be removed unless an adequate amount of insulin is administered via injections. Pump infusion site problems may result in hyperglycemia and ketoacidosis. Pump users should be instructed to change the infusion site in response to any unexpected metabolic decompensation. This is recommended even if the site has recently been changed, as the first sign of a site problem may be the development of hyperglycemia and ketosis.

      • Metformin should be stopped during a serious illness and insulin treatment may be initiated. Lactic acidosis is a rare but potential adverse effect in metformin-treated patients when an illness causes hypotension and decreases tissue perfusion.[10]

   B Supplemental doses of rapid-acting or short-acting insulins also may be required for continuously rising or persistently elevated blood glucose levels, large ketones, or persistent ketones.[11] Teach patients to call their healthcare providers for instructions on taking extra insulin if they have not previously been given an insulin algorithm for sick days.

      • Rapid-acting or short-acting insulins may be given every 1 to 4 hours.

      • The doses of rapid- and short-acting insulin depend on the severity of the illness. During most illnesses, 10% of the total daily dose can be given safely as a supplemental dose of rapid-acting or short-acting insulin. If the blood glucose level is higher than 300 mg/dL (16.7 mmol/L) with large ketones, 20% of the routine dose may be given as a supplement. There are a variety of alternative approaches to the acute treatment of hyperglycemia.

      • In the rare event that hypoglycemia exists, the rapid-acting or short-acting insulin doses can be decreased while maintaining the usual intermediate-acting or long-acting insulin doses. Hypoglycemia may occur with nausea and vomiting of short duration without systemic involvement such as fever.

   C Over-the-counter and prescription medications may contribute to hyperglycemia or hypoglycemia.

4 Substitute liquids or soft foods if patients are unable to tolerate usual foods at meal times because of nausea or anorexia.

   A In general, oral ingestion of approximately 150 to 200 g of carbohydrate per day in evenly divided doses (45 to 50 g, or 3 or 4 carbohydrate choices, every 3 to 4 hours) should be sufficient, along with medication adjustments, to prevent starvation ketosis. If regular foods are not tolerated, liquid or soft carbohydrate-containing foods, such as regular soft drinks, juices, soups, and ice cream, can be eaten.[12,13]

   B The foods and beverages shown in Table 9.1 contain approximately 15 g of carbohydrate and are appropriate for sick-day use.

5 Teach patients when to call their healthcare provider.

A Some patients hesitate to telephone their healthcare provider because they are concerned that their call might be a bother. Encourage patients to call anytime when questions and problems arise.

B Instruct patients to call a healthcare provider immediately if any of the conditions in Table 9.2 develop.

Table 9.1. Foods That Contain 15 g of Carbohydrate

- ½ cup apple juice
- ½ cup regular soft drink (not diet, caffeine-free)
- 1 Popsicle® stick
- 5 Lifesavers® candies
- 1 slice dry toast
- ½ cup cooked cereal
- 6 saltines
- ⅓ cup frozen yogurt
- 1 cup Gatorade® sports drink (replaces electrolytes)
- ½ cup regular ice cream
- ¼ cup sherbet
- ¼ cup regular pudding
- ½ cup regular gelatin/Jell-O®
- 6 oz. yogurt (not frozen) artificially sweetened or plain
- Milkshake (½ cup lowfat milk and ¼ cup ice cream)

Table 9.2. Conditions That Require Immediate Contact With a Healthcare Provider

- Vomiting more than once
- Diarrhea more than 5 times or for longer than 6 hours
- Difficulty breathing
- Blood glucose levels higher than 300 mg/dL (16.7 mmol/L) on 2 consecutive measurements that are unresponsive to increased insulin and fluids
- Moderate or large urine ketones or blood ketones above 0.6 mmol/L

Sick-Day Situations That Require Examination and Possible Treatment by a Healthcare Provider

1 The healthcare provider can determine whether telephone management is possible or if an assessment and evaluation in the clinic or emergency room is indicated.

2 Teach patients the signs and symptoms listed in Table 9.3 since they indicate a need for examination, treatment, and possible hospital care.

Table 9.3. Signs and Symptoms That Require Clinic or Hospital Treatment by a Healthcare Provider

- Persistent vomiting or an inability to tolerate fluids by mouth
- Persistent diarrhea and progressive weakness
- Orthostasis
- Chest pain
- Difficulty breathing; rapid and labored respirations
- Blood or urine ketones that do not improve
- Change in mental status

Perioperative Treatment for Patients With Diabetes

1 The goals of therapy during the perioperative period are prevention of hypoglycemia, excessive hyperglycemia, lipolysis, protein catabolism, and electrolyte disturbance.

   A Hyperglycemia has been associated with problems such as decreased effectiveness of leukocytes, increased risk of platelet aggregation, and increased rigidity of the red blood cell. This results in decreased circulation through the small vessels and deprivation of oxygen and nutrients.

   B Ketosis and ketoacidosis may ensue with persistent hyperglycemia, leading to a drop in pH. Patients with type 1 diabetes undergoing surgery are more prone to developing acidosis even with moderate hyperglycemia.[14]

   C All patients with glucose intolerance are susceptible to electrolyte abnormalities and volume depletion from osmotic diuresis.

   D Unrecognized and untreated hypoglycemia may endanger the life of the surgical patient. Because hypoglycemia in the anesthetized patient can be difficult to identify, frequent perioperative blood glucose monitoring is imperative.

2 Theoretically, enhanced healing depends on establishing and maintaining homeostasis. Normal glucose levels are essential for the normal protein synthesis that is required for wound healing without infection.[15] For maximum healing the blood glucose level should be less than 200 mg/dL (11.1 mmol/L).[16]

General Preoperative Assessment and Preparation for Surgery

1 Preoperative care includes a thorough history and physical examination.

2 Include the following information on the admission history:

   A Date of diabetes diagnosis

   B Any current signs and symptoms including those of uncontrolled diabetes

   C Medications, including type, dosage, and timing of insulin and/or oral agents

   D Over-the-counter medications

   E Assessment of metabolic control using A1C and records of self-monitoring of blood glucose if available

    F Current weight and maximum weight

    G Previous hospital admissions for surgery and other illnesses

    H For women, the last menstrual period and childbearing history

    I Allergies

    J Previous episodes of ketoacidosis, HHS, and severe hypoglycemia

3 Diagnostic laboratory data should be reviewed prior to admission for surgery with special consideration given to electrolyte balance and blood count.

    A An elevated A1C may indicate that the patient has been in poor control, is dehydrated, and may have a greater risk for ketoacidosis. A glycosylated albumin or fructosamine test may help determine the most recent level of glucose control.

    B Just prior to surgery, a complete blood count and electrolyte profile should be performed to assess for any metabolic derangements. Patients who have been hyperglycemic may be dehydrated. Patients with diabetic nephropathy may need monitoring to avoid fluid overload and hyperkalemia. An elevated white blood cell count (WBC) may indicate an underlying infection that would impede postoperative recovery.

4 Special considerations need to be given to the patient's cardiovascular, cerebrovascular, peripheral vascular, respiratory, neurological, and renal systems.

    A Certain cardiovascular assessments and considerations are necessary.

      • A thorough assessment is performed of any past cardiac problems and any cardiovascular symptoms. Cardiac problems are the leading cause of death in persons with diabetes. The presence of carotid bruits or transient ischemia attacks (TIAs) prior to surgery may indicate cerebrovascular disease. Metabolic and hemodynamic stresses may compromise the cardiovascular system and lead to myocardial infarction, congestive heart failure, cerebral vascular accidents, or acute renal failure. Anesthesia agents can depress heart muscle function and may induce rhythm disturbances. Several events during surgery can place additional stress on the myocardium: bleeding may result in hypovolemia, hypotension, tachycardia, or bradycardia; volume overload, fever, and shivering all may put additional stress on the myocardium. Patients with diabetes are also at risk for developing postoperative myocardial ischemia.[17]

      • If there is a history consistent with atherosclerotic cerebrovascular disease, the patient needs a vascular evaluation. All patients need, at minimum, auscultation of the carotids.

      • Preoperative and postoperative electrocardiograms should be obtained as well as measurements of cardiovascular enzyme activity, when indicated.

      • Blood pressure needs to be carefully monitored; antihypertensive medications should be reinstituted promptly after surgery.

      • It is important that a patient with a history of congestive heart failure (CHF) be assessed for fluid status. Caution is needed to prevent overhydration. The patient with CHF or hypertension may be at risk for hypokalemia due to previous diuretic therapy.

    B Certain neurological assessments and considerations are necessary.

      • If the patient has had recent TIAs, a neurological evaluation may be indicated.

      • The presence of some manifestations of neuropathy may affect recovery from the operation. Orthostatic hypotension, neurogenic bladder, hyperesthesia or hypoesthesia, and gastroparesis (including a history of early satiety) are some manifestations of diabetic neuropathies. Physical assessment needed to identify these problems includes lying and standing blood pressure readings, reflex and light touch assessment of the feet, and determination of residual urine, if there is any suggestion of autonomic neuropathy.

C Certain renal assessments and considerations are necessary.

- The presence of renal disease may alter the types and amounts of fluid infused and medication dosages. As part of the general assessment to guide diabetes management, measurement of urine protein and creatinine clearance may be indicated if the patient's diabetes has been diagnosed for more than 5 years and the tests have not been performed recently. Check a spot sample for the presence of microalbumin. If the result is positive and there is adequate time, perform a 24-hour urine collection for a quantitative evaluation. A serum creatinine should be included in the electrolyte screen.

- Arteriography procedures using radiocontrast material (nephrotoxic) need to be undertaken with caution in the patient with renal disease. The use of low osmolar dyes may be indicated; adequate hydration is essential and as small a dose as possible should be utilized.

Perioperative Concerns for Patients With Type 1 Diabetes

1 Several protocols for insulin management of the surgical patient with diabetes are available and effective. Ideally, a diabetologist or endocrinologist will be consulted for insulin and fluid management. In all insulin protocols, however, the usual insulin dosage is altered for the day of surgery and adequate glucose is supplied.[17,18]

A A glucose and insulin infusion regimen is the best option for providing optimal glucose control during surgery and the immediate postoperative period.

- Rapid-acting or short-acting insulin is mixed in a normal saline solution and infused intravenously using an infusion pump. An initial rate of 0.5 to 1.5 units per hour may be used. Beginning a dose at the low range is a safe way to start. Dose adjustments may be made frequently based on blood glucose monitoring. Different institutions use various formulas to calculate the additional insulin needed for elevated glucoses. One protocol uses a formula to calculate the patient's sensitivity factor. The sensitivity factor reflects the fall in blood glucose in mg/dl with 1 unit of regular insulin. The calculation is made by dividing the patient's total daily insulin dose into 1500 and so is known as the "1500 rule." Once the drop in blood glucose per mg/dL with 1 unit of regular insulin is determined, a correction scale for elevated glucoses can be ordered for the patient.[19]

- Also consider illness severity of the patient. Inflammatory responses in ill patients increase their insulin requirements. The basal insulin needs to be replaced either as intravenous regular insulin, as intermediate or long-acting insulin, or using an insulin pump. Insulin calculations should also cover the glucose in the intravenous solution. No one method for determining insulin doses has proven to be superior.

- Most protocols use a 5% or 10% glucose solution in a separate bag from the insulin solution. The glucose solution is administered in a piggyback fashion with the insulin solution. This method allows the insulin dose to be adjusted as needed while also allowing adjustment of the glucose infusion.

- Hourly capillary blood glucose measurements are used to determine the dose of insulin based on an algorithm.[17]

B Insulin is usually given subcutaneously with brief surgical procedures when the patient will be able to eat lunch.

- Subcutaneous rapid-acting insulin may be given with a 5% or 10% glucose intravenous solution to maintain the target glucose levels. Numerous methods have been used to calculate the dosage, from unit per kilogram body weight to percent total daily dose. The rate of insulin given usually varies from 0.5 to 5.0 units per hour.[11]

- Another approach is to withhold the morning rapid- or short-acting insulin and give one half to all of the morning intermediate-acting insulin. This method can lead to unpredictable glycemic excursions due to the variable absorption times of intermediate-acting insulin and the decreased peripheral perfusion during surgical procedures. However, if coverage is provided for basal insulin needs during a brief surgical procedure, rapid- or short-acting insulin can be given as needed based on bedside glucose monitoring.

C Persons wearing an insulin infusion pump may continue wearing the pump during surgery and be given additional intravenous insulin if needed.

2 Sufficient glucose to prevent hypoglycemia and to provide the basal energy requirement is administered during surgery in the insulinopenic patient. Administering 150 g of glucose over 24 hours (ie, 5 g per hour) will avoid ketosis.[18]

3 Electrolytes may be given as needed and added to the glucose solution.[18]

4 Persons who must be on fluid restrictions due to renal failure or heart failure may receive higher concentrations of glucose in smaller volumes of fluid using a central venous line.[18]

5 Surgery or tests that require the patient to have nothing by mouth (NPO) should be scheduled early in the morning whenever possible to prevent long periods of fasting. If the test or procedure is scheduled mid-to-late morning or in the afternoon, intravenous fluids and insulin should be initiated on the morning of the procedure to prevent hyperglycemia, hypoglycemia, and ketosis. For testing that requires an overnight fast in a person using an insulin pump or on an intensive insulin regimen, the basal insulin or intermediate insulin may be continued. Frequent blood glucose monitoring is needed to provide the information to make treatment decisions.

6 Frequent blood glucose and ketone monitoring are necessary to evaluate the adequacy of the insulin dose and calorie replacement.

A Urine or blood ketones should be monitored every 4 to 6 hours, or anytime the blood glucose level is greater than 240 mg/dL (13.3 mmol/L).

B The ease of obtaining and testing capillary samples using a blood glucose meter makes frequent blood glucose testing feasible with less expense. At minimum, blood glucose levels need to be checked preoperatively and postoperatively and before insulin administration. If the patient is receiving intravenous insulin, it is essential to monitor the blood glucose every hour if the patient is unstable or changes have been made in the insulin dose. Intraoperative blood glucose levels should be checked every 30 to 60 minutes.

Perioperative Concerns for Persons With Type 2 Diabetes

1 Type 2 patients who undergo surgery may be using insulin to manage their diabetes.

A These patients may respond metabolically like type 1 patients so the treatment approach may be the same.

B The main determinants for therapy in type 2 patients are the magnitude of the procedure and the metabolic state of the patient on the day of surgery.[16]

2 Patients whose diabetes is well controlled with medical nutrition therapy (MNT) or MNT plus oral glucose-lowering agents do not require specific therapy. Patients with fasting blood glucose levels lower than 140 mg/dL (7.8 mmol/L) treated with an oral agent can be given their medication and started on a glucose infusion the morning of surgery; however, it is sometimes suggested to stop the oral agent the evening before surgery. Discontinue the longer acting chlorpropamide 48 to 72 hours prior to the surgical procedure. Discontinue metformin the morning of the surgery. Metformin should not be resumed postoperatively until the patient has resumed a regular diet and has normal renal function.

3 Type 2 patients on oral agents whose diabetes is poorly controlled may need insulin during their perioperative period using the same regimens as type 1 patients.[17,18] Aggressive treatment of hyperglycemia and maintaining adequate hydration can prevent HHS and infection and improve wound healing.

Postoperative Care

1 Impaired wound healing can occur when the blood glucose level is greater than 200 mg/dL (11.1 mmol/L).[16]

A The wound needs to be observed carefully for any signs of inflammatory changes or drainage, and alterations in the patient's temperature noted. Meticulous wound care is essential to prevent infection.

B Maintaining and improving circulation to promote wound healing is particularly important for the person with diabetes who may have peripheral vascular disease.

2 Continue monitoring of blood glucose and electrolytes in the postoperative period. Hypoglycemia is a particular concern because the blood glucose level and insulin dose may decrease dramatically as the stress of surgery declines or as an infection is treated.

3 Postoperative nutritional management consists of 2 phases. Involvement of a registered dietitian will help to ensure a successful transition through these phases and the reinitiation of medications that are essential for successful outcomes.

A The first phase of nutritional management is the initial catabolic phase that extends from the period just before surgery into the period immediately following the operation. The second phase is the transition time during which the patient moves from NPO status to the usual meal plan.

B During the reintroduction of foods such as clear liquids, it is preferable to continue a low-maintenance dose of intravenous or subcutaneous rapid-acting or short-acting insulin along with fluids to maintain target blood glucose levels.

C Returning to the usual meal plan as soon as possible will promote healing and reestablish homeostasis. Adequate carbohydrate is needed daily to prevent starvation ketosis. Solid foods can be started as soon as tolerated.

4 Once food tolerance is established, the intravenous insulin infusion is stopped and a new treatment program is planned, considering such elements as infection, pain, steroids, or total parenteral nutrition (TPN). For patients treated with oral agents, the usual dose may be given with supplements of rapid-acting or short-acting insulin. For insulin-treated patients, a combination of intermediate-acting and rapid-acting or short-acting insulin may be given. When using only rapid-acting or short-acting insulin, care must be taken not to leave insulinopenic patients without basal insulin.

5 It is very important to note that subcutaneous insulin needs to be given at least 1 to 2 hours prior to the discontinuation of any intravenous insulin infusion to prevent hyperglycemia.

6 Capillary blood glucose monitoring is needed a minimum of 4 times per day, usually before meals and at bedtime to determine the effectiveness of the therapy.

7 Pain can cause the release of counterregulatory hormones that can increase the blood glucose level. Adequate pain management will help relieve this response. Because pain medication can make the patient drowsy, frequent assessment is necessary to recognize hypoglycemia. Hyperglycemia may heighten the perception of pain.

8 Peripheral neuropathy and peripheral vascular disease increase the risk of ulcerations. Careful monitoring of pressure areas and ambulation as soon as possible will help reduce the risk of these postoperative complications.

9 Written instructions are mandatory for postsurgical home care, with instructions for insulin, other medications, meal planning, physical activity, and wound care, if applicable.

Emergency Surgery

1 In situations that require emergency surgery, diabetes management will depend upon the metabolic condition of the patient. Surgical emergencies, particularly if there is underlying infection, can cause rapid metabolic decompensation, with dehydration and hyperglycemia, and ultimately ketoacidosis in the patient with type 1 diabetes. If the patient is in early or established DKA, the first priority is metabolic management.

2 If the patient is without severe metabolic disturbance, the initial diabetes management can involve intravenous insulin infusion. If the patient is dehydrated, normal saline is used for fluid replacement.[17]

Surgery in Children

1 Few published guidelines exist for the surgical management of diabetes in children. In general, adult regimens have been adapted for use.[17]

2 Caution needs to be taken in calculating fluid and insulin requirements. Consult a pediatric endocrinologist, if available.

Key Educational Considerations

1 Sick-day management is a survival skill and should be taught at an appropriate level to all patients with diabetes.

  A Sick-day instruction and reinforcement are a priority before a hospital discharge; before starting day care, school, or college; before the flu season and when administering the flu vaccine;[20] and before overnight travel away from home.

  B Learning is reinforced and retained when it is applied immediately. Because sick-day guidelines usually are taught when patients are healthy, evaluation needs to include assessing the patient's immediate and long-term recall of knowledge about sick-day management.

  C Give patients written instructions as reinforcement, keeping the guidelines as simple as possible.
  - If appropriate, ask the patient to copy the guidelines or highlight notes on a provided handout to enhance retention and personalize the written instructions.
  - Ask the patient where the guidelines will be posted or placed for easy access when needed.
  - Suggest that the patient pack a sick-day box with supplies and nonperishable items that can be stored for use during illness. Acknowledge that the patient may not be accustomed to keeping glucose-containing products such as Jell-O® gelatin, regular soft drinks, or regular sports drinks at home. Review the rationale for keeping these items on hand for sick days and determine if the patient is willing to prepare this kit. Ask about the site for storage or placement.

  D Evaluate patient's actual skills during and following an intercurrent illness.
  - During telephone contact and/or clinic visits on sick days, ask the patient to describe action taken during illness and assess results.
  - Ask the patient to describe how the sick-day plan worked and identify what changes are needed to make the plan work better.
  - During follow-up visits, props and simulations can be used for reinforcement and to assist the patient in recalling sick-day guidelines. For example, props such as rapid-acting or short-acting insulin vials, blood glucose and ketone testing materials, and an 8-oz plastic glass can be used to emphasize sick-day care. Simulations such as telephone call role-playing, review of blood glucose records, and actions to take may help to evaluate patient recall.

  E During an illness, many patients experience malaise, fatigue, and sleepiness, making self-care more difficult. Therefore, family members or significant others need to be familiar with sick-day guidelines and know where sick-day supplies and instructions are kept. Discuss a plan for their role and participation prior to an illness. They also need to know when to call a healthcare provider.

2 The preoperative assessment may provide insight into the educational needs of the patient and significant other(s). Assessing the patient's knowledge will help provide direction for preoperative and postoperative diabetes teaching. Include family members or significant others in the preoperative teaching, so they understand the postoperative recovery care needed.

A Explain to the patient how the insulin dose will be administered and adjusted during surgery. Many patients are fearful of giving others the decision-making responsibility for insulin adjustment.

B Explain the need for dextrose in the intravenous solution. Many patients know that dextrose raises the blood glucose level and they are concerned that an error may be made.

C Explain to patients with type 2 diabetes who are treated with oral agents that they may need insulin just for the time before, during, and immediately after surgery. Many patients are concerned that insulin therapy may permanently replace their previous treatment.

D Prepare the patient for frequent capillary blood glucose and ketone testing. Blood glucose levels may be checked every 1 to 2 hours.

3 Provide written discharge instructions for any medications, including insulin (if applicable), meal plan, physical activity, and surgical and medical follow-up. Work with the significant other(s) to plan menus for the first few days at home. Prior to discharge, provide updated information about nutrition therapy.

Self-Review Questions

1 What are the physiologic effects of illness and surgery on blood glucose concentrations, ketone levels, and fluid and electrolyte balance?

2 What are specific guidelines that healthcare providers may use when managing an intercurrent illness?

3 List situations that require examination and possible treatment in an office/clinic, emergency room, or hospital setting during an illness.

4 What effects can surgery have on the cardiovascular system?

5 Why is the prevention of hyperglycemia important to the surgical patient with diabetes?

6 What methods can be used to prevent hyperglycemia in the surgical patient?

7 What should be included in preoperative management?

8 List 2 alternatives for insulin therapy intraoperatively and immediately postoperatively. What are advantages and disadvantages of these alternatives?

9 List 4 potential postoperative problems that may be more common in the person with diabetes.

10 Which oral agent should be discontinued the morning of surgery?

Learning Assessment: Case Study 1

RS is a 32-year-old sales representative who was diagnosed with type 1 diabetes 1 year ago. He manages his diabetes with multiple daily injections of insulin consisting of long-acting and rapid-acting insulin before breakfast, rapid-acting insulin before lunch and dinner, and long-acting insulin before bedtime. He monitors his blood glucose 4 times per day, counts carbohydrates, and strives for consistency. RS has been instructed on the recognition and treatment of hypoglycemia, ketone testing, and sick-day management. He returns to the clinic for follow-up once every 2 to 3 months.

This morning RS calls you to report that he is feeling nauseated. He states that his blood glucose level before breakfast was 233 mg/dL (12.9 mmol/L), he administered his usual dose of insulin using his insulin algorithm, and then he was only able to drink 1 small glass of apple juice before becoming nauseated. It is now noon and he is still nauseated and does not feel like eating lunch or going to the office. RS reports that he vaguely recalls being instructed on sick-day management, but he is unsure what he should do because this is his first episode of being sick since his diagnosis.

Questions for Discussion

1 What additional assessment data would you obtain at this point?

2 What instruction and/or advice might be given?

Discussion

1 Gather information to determine if the patient's condition is stable.

   A Assess whether the patient has been vomiting or experiencing diarrhea, how often, and for how many hours.

   B Listen for symptoms of respiratory distress and ask whether the patient has had difficulty breathing.

   C RS reported no vomiting, diarrhea, or respiratory distress.

2 Once acute distress is ruled out, recent blood glucose and blood or urine ketone results are needed. Although diabetic ketoacidosis usually develops over hours, hyperglycemia and ketosis could be present yet unknown if self-monitoring of blood glucose and ketone testing is not performed or if testing is performed incorrectly.

   A RS had not tested his blood glucose since before breakfast and had not checked for ketones. He was asked to obtain blood glucose and blood or urine ketone measurements.

   B Depending on the circumstances, the healthcare provider may wait for the patient to report the testing results or ask the patient to call back immediately with the results.

   C RS reported a blood glucose value of 363 mg/dL (20.2 mmol/L) and a small amount of ketones.

3 Assess fluid and food intake.

   A Fluid intake was assessed and RS reported that he had been sipping on a diet soft drink during the morning because of thirst; because of nausea he had consumed only a total of approximately 8 oz.

   B He reported eating no solid foods.

   C The concept of avoiding dehydration by consuming adequate fluids was explained.

   D Because his blood glucose was 363 mg/dL, he agreed to have bouillon (a source of sodium and fluid) and a diet soft drink for lunch—both items were on hand and choices he likes. He also agreed to drink 8 oz of calorie-free fluids hourly during the afternoon and evening, drinking in sips if necessary.

4 Reinforce the rationale for not omitting insulin doses.

   A RS was given reassurance that administering his morning dose of insulin was appropriate.

B He then was instructed to use his insulin algorithm and administer his prelunch dose of rapid-acting insulin immediately after the telephone conversation.

5 Review plan of care and when to call.
  A RS was instructed to retest his blood glucose and blood or urine ketone levels in 3 hours, before supper (7 PM), and at bedtime.
  B He was reminded to call if his blood glucose values were higher than 300 mg/dL (16.7 mmol/L) and if he had moderate or large ketones.
  C RS was encouraged to telephone the clinic immediately if vomiting occurred more than once, if he experienced more than 5 episodes of diarrhea, or if he had difficulty breathing.

Learning Assessment: Case Study 2

CB is a 42-year-old female who was diagnosed with type 1 diabetes at age 17 years. She is being admitted for an elective cholecystectomy with general anesthesia. CB is hypertensive and being treated with ACE inhibitors. She also has background diabetic retinopathy and proteinuria. CB monitors her blood glucose 3 to 4 times per day and injects 15 units of Ultralente with 6 units of a lispro insulin before breakfast, 4 units of lispro before lunch, 8 units of lispro before dinner, and 15 units of Ultralente at bedtime.

In a team meeting the day before CB's admission for surgery, the resident suggests the following plan:
1 Based on CB's blood glucose level, make the following adjustments in insulin:
  • <150 mg/dL (8.3 mmol/L) = no insulin
  • 151 to 200 mg/dL (8.4 to 11.1 mmol/L) = 4 units
  • 201 to 250 mg/dL (11.2 to 13.9 mmol/L) = 6 units
  • 251 to 350 mg/dL (14.0 to 19.4 mmol/L) = 8 units

2 CB will be advised to take her usual Ultralente dose on the morning of surgery.

3 Capillary blood glucose readings are ordered every 4 hours and she will be given lispro insulin using a sliding scale.

Questions for Discussion
1 What problems do you see with the resident's plan?
2 What other options can be considered?
3 What pre- and post-operative teaching needs can you identify for CB and her family?

Discussion
1 Use of an insulin/glucose infusion would be optimal.
  A Use of an intermediate-acting or long-acting insulin prior to a lengthy surgical procedure could lead to difficulties with hypoglycemia or hyperglycemia.
  B Subcutaneous insulin is not given during surgery due to unpredictable absorption from changes in body temperature, varying blood volumes, and anesthesia. Subcutaneous insulin pump use is discontinued during surgery when the insulin/glu-

cose infusion method is used. The basal rate insulin of the pump or the intermediate- or long-acting insulin should be given 1 to 2 hours before discontinuing intravenous insulin. Rapid-acting or short-acting insulin given intravenously has a very short half-life.

C Intravenous fluids will be discontinued after CB is able to tolerate food.

D A patient with proteinuria may tolerate only small amounts of intravenous fluid. When necessary to meet the caloric needs of a patient with end-stage renal disease during surgery, a more concentrated dextrose solution may be used.

2 Blood glucose monitoring should be increased during the perioperative period.

A Blood glucose monitoring should be done every 30 to 60 minutes during surgery and until CB awakens from the anesthesia.

B Blood glucose monitoring should be done every 1 to 2 hours as long as CB receives intravenous insulin.

3 The ACE inhibitor could be given after surgery when CB fully awakens.

4 Both CB and her family have educational needs.

A Preoperative teaching should include information about the frequency of glucose monitoring, the surgical procedure, and postoperative care.

B CB will be discharged as soon as possible from the hospital with written instruction. Discharge instructions to CB and her family include wound care, assessment of her wound for infection, frequency of monitoring, safety issues related to the use of pain medication, when to call for assistance, and when to return for follow-up. When using narcotics, family members will need to ascertain that the patient has followed her diabetes self-care plan (eg, taken correct insulin dose, has eaten), and monitor her glucose for hypoglycemia.

References

1 Rosenbloom AL, Hanas R. Diabetic ketoacidosis (DKA): treatment guidelines. Clin Pediatr. 1996;35:261-266.

2 Schade DS, Eaton RP. Pathogenesis of diabetic ketoacidosis: a reappraisal. Diabetes Care. 1979;2:296-306.

3 Alberti KG. Role of glucagon and other hormones in development of diabetic ketoacidosis. Lancet. 1975;1:1307-1311.

4 Keller U, Schnell H, Girard J, Stauffacher W. Effect of physiological elevation of plasma growth hormone levels on ketone body kinetics and lipolysis in normal and acutely insulin-deficient men. Diabetologia. 1984; 26:103-108.

5 American Diabetes Association. Hospital admission guidelines for diabetes mellitus (position statement). Diabetes Care. 2003;26(suppl 1):S118.

6 Genuth S. Diabetic ketoacidosis and hyperosmolar hyperglycemic nonketotic syndrome in adults. In: Lebovitz HE, DeFronzo RA, Genuth S, Kreisberg RA, Pfeifer MA, Tamborlane WV, eds. Therapy for Diabetes Mellitus and Related Disorders. 3rd ed. Alexandria, Va: American Diabetes Association; 1998:83-96.

7 Ennis ED, Kreisberg RA. Diabetic ketoacidosis and the hyperglycemic hyperosmolar syndrome. In: LeRoith D, Taylor SI, Olesky JM, eds. Diabetes Mellitus: A Fundamental and Clinical Text. Philadelphia: Lippincott-Raven Publishers; 1996:276-286.

8 Matz R. Hyperosmolar nonacidotic diabetes (HNAD). In: Porte D Jr, Sherwin RS, eds. Ellenberg & Rifkin's Diabetes Mellitus. 5th ed. Stamford, Conn: Appleton & Lange; 1997:845-860.

9 Minaker KL. What diabetologists should know about elderly patients. Diabetes Care. 1990;13(suppl 2):34-46.

10 Bailey CJ, Turner RC. Drug therapy: metformin. N Engl J Med. 1996;334: 574-579.

11 Travaglini MT, Garg SK, Chase HP. Use of insulin lispro in the outpatient management of ketonuria. Arch Pediatr Adolesc Med. 1998;152:672-675.

12 American Diabetes Association. Translation of the diabetes nutrition recommendations for health care institutions (position statement). Diabetes Care. 2003;26(suppl 1):S70-S72.

13 Schafer RG, Bohannon B, Franz M, et al. Translation of the diabetes nutrition recommendations for health care institutions (technical review). Diabetes Care. 1997; 20:96-105.

14 Gaare-Porcari JM, O'Sullivan-Maillet JM. Care for persons with diabetes during surgery. In: Powers MA, ed. Handbook of Diabetes Medical Nutrition Therapy. Gaithersburg, Md. Aspen Publishers; 1996:601-615.

15 Palmisano J. Surgery and diabetes. In: Kahn R, Weir G, eds. Joslin's Diabetes Mellitus. 13th ed. Philadelphia: Lea & Febiger; 1994:955-961.

16 Golden SH, Kao WHL, Peart-Vigilance C, Brancati FL. Perioperative glycemic control and the risk of infectious complications in a cohort of adults with diabetes. Diabetes Care. 1999;22:1408-1414.

17 Alberti KGMM. Diabetes and surgery. In: Porte D Jr, Sherwin R, Eds. Ellenberg & Rifkin's Diabetes Mellitus: Theory and Practice. 5th ed. Stamford, CT, Appleton and Lange, 1997:875-885.

18 Hirsch, I, McGill, J. Role of insulin in management of surgical patients with diabetes mellitus. Diabetes Care. 1990:13:9:980-991.

19 Davidson PC. Bolus and supplemental insulin. In: Fredrickson L, ed. The Insulin Pump Therapy Book: Insights from the Experts., Sylmar, Calif: MiniMed Technologies;1995.

20 Stephenson I, Zambon, M. The epidemiology of influenza. Occupational Medicine. 2002;52:241-247.

Suggested Readings

American Diabetes Association. Hyperglycemic crises in patients with diabetes mellitus (position statement). Diabetes Care. 2003;26(suppl 1);S109-S118.

Avilés-Santa L, Raskin P. Surgery and anesthesia. In: Lebovitz H, ed. Therapy for Diabetes Mellitus and Related Disorders. 3rd ed. Alexandria, Va: American Diabetes Association; 1998;224-233.

Hieronymus L. The flu: More than just a nuisance. Available on the Internet at: http://www.diabetesselfmanagement.com/article.cfm?aid=427. Accessed March 2003.

Hirsch IB, Paauw DS. Diabetes management in special situations. Endocrinol Metab Clin North Am. 1997;3:631-645.

Kaufman FR, Dergan S, Roe TF, Costin G. Perioperative management with prolonged intravenous insulin infusion versus subcutaneous insulin in children with type 1 diabetes mellitus. J Diabetes Complications. 1996;10:6-11.

Lorber DM. Surgical management of the patient with diabetes. Pract Diabetology. 1996;15(2):2-4.

Malmberg K, Ryden L, Hamsten A, Herlitz J, Waldenstrom A, Wedel H. Mortality prediction in diabetic patients with myocardial infarction: experiences from the DIGAMI study. Cardiovascular Research. 1997; 34:248-253.

American Diabetes Association. When you're sick. Available on the Internet at: http://www.diabetes.org/main/application/commercewf. Accessed March 2003.

White NH, Henry DN. Special issues in diabetes mellitus. In: Haire-Joshu D, ed. Management of Diabetes Mellitus: Perspectives of Care Across the Life Span. 2nd ed. St. Louis. Mosby; 1996:378-384.

Learning Assessment: Post-Test Questions

Illness and Surgery   9

1 Which of the following is a sick-day management guideline?
  A Omit insulin dose when vomiting occurs
  B Increase frequency of blood glucose monitoring
  C Drink large amounts of carbohydrate-containing liquids
  D Only call healthcare providers if urine ketones are positive

2 Increased ketone levels in a postsurgical patient are most likely to be caused by:
  A Insufficient insulin and/or carbohydrate intake
  B Decreased lipolysis and/or carbohydrate intake
  C Decreased protein catabolism and/or carbohydrate intake
  D Increased protein anabolism and/or carbohydrate intake

3 In addition to completing an admission history, reviewing laboratory data, and performing a physical exam, what additional information would be most useful in a preoperative assessment of a 42-year-old patient with type 2 diabetes and no cardiovascular risk factors?
  A Medical records from previous hospital admission
  B Cardiovascular enzyme activity laboratory data
  C Information about the patient's cognitive and affective needs
  D Postoperative glucose and insulin protocol of hospital

4 Cardiac problems can be serious, even fatal, in a person with diabetes and should be assessed prior to surgery. During surgery, which of the following could occur?
  A Anesthesia agents could stimulate heart muscle function
  B Hyperglycemia could cause excessive bleeding
  C Patients risk hypotension, hypovolemia, and rhythm disturbances
  D Metabolic stresses cause carotid bruits to develop

5 A particular postoperative concern for a patient with diabetes whose blood glucose level is higher than 200 mg/dL is:
  A Fluid restrictions
  B Discontinuation of oral glucose-lowering agents
  C Peripheral vascular disease
  D Impaired wound healing

6 Surgical patients with type 2 diabetes who are taking oral glucose-lowering agents:
  A Will not need insulin before surgery
  B Will always need to take insulin after surgery as a permanent replacement of their previous treatment
  C Should be informed that they may need insulin before, during, and immediately after their surgery
  D All of the above

7 On discharge from a hospital, patients with diabetes need:
  A Oral instructions on sick-day management of their disease sufficient to avoid medical emergencies
  B To be told to contact healthcare providers only at certain times of the day so that proper attention can be given to their condition
  C Not be given any instructions on discharge since they will be too overwhelmed by all the procedures to grasp the meaning
  D Survival skills that include written instructions on sick-day management

8 When patients with diabetes are too sick to eat or tolerate large volumes of fluids, they are advised to consume something that contains 15 g of carbohydrate every 1 to 2 hours. An example of this would be:

A 1 cup Gatorade® sports drink

B 1 can diet Coca Cola® soft drink

C 1½ cup of sugar-free Jello-O® gelatin

D 2 Popsicle® sticks

9 Which guideline is important during postoperative care?

A Meticulous wound care

B Frequent monitoring of blood glucose

C Adequate pain management

D All of the above are important

See next page for answer key.

Post-Test Answer Key

Illness and Surgery   9

1	B		**6**	C
2	A		**7**	D
3	A		**8**	A
4	C		**9**	D
5	D			

A Core Curriculum for Diabetes Education
Diabetes Management Therapies

Index

A1C, 197, 220
  correlation with blood
    glucose levels, 199
Acarbose, 131, 136
ACE inhibitors, see Angiotensin-
  converting enzyme inhibitors
Acesulfame K, 15, 16
Actos, see Pioglitazone
ADA nutrition
  recommendations, 3
Albumin, 200
  excretion abnormalities, 201
Alcohol, 21–22
  and hypoglycemia, 22
Alitame, 15
Alpha-1 antagonists
  adverse effects, 137
Alpha-glucosidase inhibitors,
  131–33, 219, 232
    adverse effects, 131–32
    contraindications, 131
    pharmacology, 131
    therapy, 132
Amylin agonists, 133–34
Anabolic hormones, see
  Hormones, anabolic
Angiotensin II receptor blockers
  (ARBs), 17, 159, 165
    adverse effects, 165
    contraindications, 165
    monitoring, 165
    pharmacology, 165
Angiotensin-converting enzyme
  (ACE) inhibitors, 17, 159,
  163–64
    adverse effects, 164
    contraindications, 164
    monitoring, 163
    pharmacology, 163
Animas pump, 254
Antihistamines, anticholinergic
  adverse effects, 137
Antihypertensives
  adverse effects, 137
Antiinflammatory agents
  adverse effects, 137
Antioxidants, 21
ARBs, see Angiotensin II
  receptor blockers
Aspart, 100, 101
Aspartame, 15, 16
Avandia, see Rosiglitazone
BARs, see Bile acid resins
  (BARs)
Benzoic acid derivatives, 115
Beta-blockers, see Beta-receptor
  blockers

Beta-receptor blockers, 160,
  166–67
    adverse effects, 137
    contraindications, 166–67
    monitoring, 166
    pharmacology, 166
Biguanides, 115, 127–29; see
  also Metformin
    pharmacology, 127
Bile acid resins (BARs), 170,
  174–75
    adverse effects, 175
    interactions, 175
    pharmacology, 174
Blood glucose
  capillary, 323
  monitoring, 321
Blood Glucose Awareness
  Training (BGAT), 297
Blood glucose levels
  absolute, 280
Blood glucose meters
  accuracy, 192
  accuracy, considerations, 190
  accuracy, guidelines for
    determining, 192
  alternate sampling sites,
    192–93
  calibration, 191
  control solution, 191
  guidelines for patient
    education, 195
  quality assurance, 196
  sampling problems, 191
  strips, 191
Blood ketone concentrations, see
  Ketones, concentrations
Blood pressure
  classification, 159
Body mass index, 9
  determining, 10
Body weight, 7, 9, 14, 16
Caffeine, 160
Calcium channel blockers,
  167–68
    adverse effects, 137, 167
    monitoring, 167
    pharmacology, 167
Capillary blood glucose measurements, 321
Caprenin, 20
Carbohydrate, 9, 12, 36
  counting, 33–35
  counting and insulin pump
    therapy, 265–73
  in Diabetes Food/Meal Plan,
    14–16
  servings, 34

Carbohydrate-rich foods, 317
Case studies, see Learning
  assessments
Catabolic hormones, see
  Hormones, catabolic
CCBs, see Nondihydropyridine
  calcium channel blockers
Celiac disease, 37–38
Cellulose, 20
Chemotherapeutic agents
  adverse effects, 137
Children
  surgery, 323–24
Chlorthalidone, 160
Chocolate, 160
Cholesterol, 5, 6, 18, 53
Chromium, 21
Clonidine
  adverse effects, 137
Codeine
  adverse effects, 137
Comorbid conditions
  practice guidelines, 158
Continuous glucose monitoring,
  196
Continuous subcutaneous
  insulin infusion, see Insulin
  pump therapy
Continuous subcutaneous
  insulin infusion pump, 104;
  see also Insulin pump
Cortisol, 12, 98
Cosmo (Deltec) pump, 255
C-peptide, 96
Creatinine, 201
Cyclamates, 15
Cystic fibrosis–related diabetes,
  38–39
DAFNE, see Dose adjustment
  for normal eating
Dahedi pump, 254
Dana pump, 255
Dextrins, 20
Diabetes Control and
  Complications Trial (DCCT),
  279
Diabetes mellitus in pregnancy
  insulin therapy, 108
Diabetes mellitus type 1, 318
  insulin therapy, 108
Diabetes mellitus type 2
  as a progressive disorder, 8
  insulin therapy, 108
  oral medications, 115–133
Diabetic ketoacidosis,
  98, 314, 318
Diet, see Medical nutrition
  therapy

Diltiazem, see
Nondihydropyridine calcium
channel blockers (CCBs)
Disaccharides, 12
Disentronic D-Tron Plus pump,
254
Disetronic D-Tron pump, 254
Diuretics, 160–63
adverse effects, 137, 162
contraindications, 162
interactions, 162
monitoring, 162
pharmacology, 161
DKA, see Diabetic ketoacidosis
Dose adjustment for normal
eating (DAFNE), 7, 265
D-Phenylalanine derivatives,
115, 124
Drugs
adverse effects on body
systems, 139
effects on diabetes
complications, 138
interactions, concerns, 140
interactions, prevention, 141
Dyslipidemia, 157–82
lipid-lowering therapies and
their effect on lipid
profiles, 170
pharmacologic treatment,
168–75
suggested drug therapies, 169
Eating frequency, 11
Electrolyte balance, 313–15
Emergency surgery, 323
Energy requirements
adults, 29
youth, 30
Ephedra-based substances, 160
Ephedrine, 160
Epinephrine, 12, 98
Exchange list
macronutrient and caloric
values, 29
Exercise, 11, 61–86
aerobic, 72
anaerobic, 72
autonomic neuropathy
guidelines, 81
benefits, 61–63
carbohydrate adjustments,
68, 70
consequences of insufficient
insulin, 67
considerations, 67
considerations in the elderly,
76–77

considerations in the obese,
77–78
diabetic retinopathy
guidelines, 80
duration, 72
education, 40–42
frequency, 73
hormonal response and
metabolic effects, without
diabetes, 64
hypertension, 78
insulin adjustment, 68
intensity, 73
participation, 81–82
peripheral neuropathy
guidelines, 81
peripheral vascular disease,
79
physiology, with diabetes,
65–66
physiology, without diabetes,
63–64
program, 72–76
retinopathy, guidelines, 80
retinopathy, advanced, 79
safety precautions, 71–72
strengthening, 75–76
Fats, 13
diabetes food/meal plan, 20
insulin resistance, 11
monounsaturated, 18
omega-3 polyunsaturated, 18
polyunsaturated, 18
replacers, 20
saturated, 18
Fiber, 15
dietary, 12
Fibric acid derivatives (fibrates),
169, 172–73
adverse effects, 172
contraindications, 172
interactions, 173
monitoring, 172
pharmacology, 172
Fish oils, see Fats
Fluid balance, 313–15
Folate, 21
Food
diaries, 31
labels, 35
Fructosamine, see Glycosylated
serum albumin
Fructose, 12, 15
Galactose, 12
Gestational diabetes
insulin therapy, 108
Glargine, 100, 233

Glipizide, 219
Glitazones, 115
Glomerular filtration rate
(GFR), 160
Glucagon, 12, 98
adverse effects, 134
contraindications, 134
for severe hypoglycemia, 133
pharmacology, 133
therapy, 134
Glucophage, see Biguanides
Glucose recommendations
for adults with diabetes
mellitus, 5
Glucose sensors, 258
Glucose-lowering medications,
115–33
Glucotoxicity, 12
Glyburide, 127, 219
Glycemic index, 14–15
Glycosylated serum albumin,
198, 220
Glyset, see Miglitol
Growth
assessment, 202
hormone, 12, 98
Guarana, 160
HbA1c, see A1C
HDL cholesterol, 5, 168
Hemoglobin A1c, 197, 220
correlation with blood
glucose levels, 199
Herbal medicines, 21
HMG-CoA reductase inhibitors
(statins), 169, 170–72, 199
contraindications, 171
interactions, 172
monitoring, 171
pharmacology, 171
Hormones
anabolic, 313
catabolic, 313
counterregulatory, 314, 323
counterregulatory, diabetes
type 1, 314
Hydrochlorothiazide, 160
Hyperglycemia, 314, 318
activity-induced, 70–71
illness, 313
Hyperosmolar hyperglycemic
state (HHS), 98
diabetes type 2, 315
Hypertension, 157–82
major classes of drugs, 161
pharmacologic treatment,
158–68

Hypoglycemia, 96–98, 279–306, 318, 321, 322
  alcohol, 285
  assessment and intervention, 294–97
  autonomic symptoms, 281–83
  behaviors that increase risk, 287
  caffeine, 285
  carbohydrate sources for treatment, 290
  causes, 285–87
  clinical risk factors that increase frequency, 283
  common symptoms, 281
  decreased renal function, 288
  definition, 281
  emotional changes, 284
  excessive fear of, 293
  exercise, insulin pump therapy, 70
  family interactions, 294
  glucagon, 292
  guidelines for self-treatment, 291
  hormonal changes in women, 288
  in exercise, 65–66
  in exercise, prevention, 67–70
  in pregnancy and breastfeeding, 288
  incidence, 288
  insulin secretagogues, 280
  insulin sensitivity, 288
  mild, characteristics of, 280
  negative consequences of, 279
  neuroglycopenic symptoms, 283–84
  nocturnal, 17, 287
  prevention, 289
  overtreatment of, 7
  physical activity, 288
  postactivity late-onset (PAL), 66, 70
  posttreatment hyperglycemia, 291
  prevention, 289
  psychosocial factors, 291–92
  psychosocial impact, 293–94
  questions to determine patient risk factors, 295
  reduced symptom awareness, 282
  severe, characteristics of, 280
  sulfa antibiotics-sulfonylurea interactions, 288
  symptom diaries, 285, 286
  symptoms, 281–85
  symptoms, biological, 281
  treatment, 290–93
  treatment by others, 292–93
    psychosocial factors, 291-92
  treatment guidelines, 290
  weight loss, 288
Illness, see also Sick day management
  severity, 320
Illness and Surgery, 313–32
Insulin, 9, 12, 136; see also Pattern management
  1500 rule, 220, 256
  1800 rule, 220, 256
  algorithms, 220–21
  allergy, 105
  amino acid sequence difference between species, 100
  and medical nutrition therapy, 7
  and physical activity, 8
  available in US, 99
  biochemical formation, 97
  concentrations, 102
  determining bolus doses, 266
  endogenous, 98
  exogenous, 98
  fixed combinations, 99
  four-injection regimen, 113
  human, comparison, 101
  impurity, 105
  indications for use, 98
  intermediate-acting, 99
  long-acting, 99
  mixing, 106
  monotherapy, 109
  multiinjection regimen, 111–12
  physiology, 96–98
  premixed, 106
  pulmonary, 115
  pump therapy, 114
  purity, 102
  rapid-acting, 99, 320
  refrigeration, 103
  sensitivity, 62
  short-acting, 99
  sliding-scale approach, 221
  sources, 98–100
  storage, 103–4
  subcutaneous, 323
  subcutaneous rapid-acting, 321
  therapy, 107
  two-injection regimen, 109
Insulin administration
  equipment, 104
  syringes, 104
Insulin detemir (NN304), 102
Insulin glargine, 102
Insulin infusion regimen, 320
Insulin management
  surgical patient, 320
Insulin pump therapy, 249–64
  basal rate, 256
  benefits, 250–51
  carbohydrate counting, 265–73
  contraindications, 253–54
  definition, 250
  dosage, 256
  getting started, 255–57
  indications for use, 252–53
  infusion site, 257
  limitations, 251
  obtaining a pump, 255
  pump selection, 254–55
  requirements for patient success, 253
  troubleshooting, 257
Insulin therapy
  pregnancy, 108
  type 1 diabetes, 108
  type 2 diabetes, 108
Insulin-to-carbohydrate ratios, 35
  considerations, 267–68
  determining, 266–67
  for insulin pump therapy, 265
Interactions
  drug-disease and drug-drug, 120–23
  drug-food, 136
Interventions, pharmacologic, 95–142
Ketoacidosis, 314, 318
Ketogenesis, 314

Ketones
concentrations, 313–15
levels, 313–15
monitoring, 200
Ketosis, 318
illness, 313
Key educational considerations
carbohydrate counting,
268–69
hypoglycemia, 297–300
illness and surgery, 324–25
insulin pump therapy, 258–59
medical nutrition therapy,
40–42
monitoring, 203–4
pattern management, 237–38
pharmacologic therapies
for hypertension and
dyslipidemia, 175–76
physical activity and exercise,
83
Lactose, 12
Lantus, 100, see Insulin glargine
LDL cholesterol, 6, 168
Learning assessments
hypoglycemia, 300–303
counting carbohydrates,
269–71
illness & surgery, 325–28
insulin pump therapy, 259–61
medical nutrition therapy,
43–45
monitoring, 205–7
pattern management, 238–39
pharmacologic therapies,
143–47
pharmacologic therapies
for hypertension and
dyslipidemia, 176–80
physical activity and exercise,
84–86
Lente, 100
Lipodystrophies, 105
Lipolysis, 314
Lipoproteins
related to macrovascular
disease, 5
values for children and
adolescents, 6
Lispro, 100, 101
Low-carbohydrate/high-
protein diets, 17
Ma huang, 160
Magnesium, 21
Maltodextrins, 20
Mannitol, 15

Meal planning, 25
ethnic and cultural
appropriateness, 37
patient education, 33–36
resources, 35–36
Medical nutrition therapy, 3–55
basic and initial self-
management skills, 31
clinical practice, 33
education, 40–42
for use in healthcare facilities,
39–40
goals, 5, 6
medical nutrition therapy,
diabetes type 2, see
Nutrition
outcomes, 22–24
self-management, 33
strategies for type 1
diabetes, 7–8
strategies for type 2
diabetes, 8–12
Medications, see Interventions,
pharmacologic
Meglitinides, 124–27
Metabolic homeostasis, 313
Metformin, 115, 127, 136, 232,
233; see also Biguanides
adverse effects, 128
contraindications, 128
therapy, 128–29
Microalbumin screening, 201
Microalbuminuria, 201
Miglitol, 131, 136
Minerals, 13, 20–21
Mini-Med 508 pump, 255
Mini-Med Paradigm, 255
Modified food starches, 20
Monitoring, 189–210
for complication prevention,
199–202
long-term, 197–202
Monosaccharides, 12
Nateglinide, 126–27, 136, 219,
232
adverse effects, 126
pharmacology, 126
therapy, 127
Neotame, 15
Nephropathy
treatment, 17
Neutral protamine Hagedorn,
see NPH

Niacin, 173–74
adverse effects, 174
contraindications, 174
monitoring, 173
pharmacology, 173
Nocturnal hypoglycemia, 287
prevention, 289
Nondihydropyridine calcium
channel blockers (CCBs), 160
Norepinephrine, 12, 98
Nothing by mouth
surgical considerations, 321
NPH, 100, 101
NPO, see Nothing by mouth
Nutrition, see also Medical
nutrition therapy
medical nutrition therapy,
diabetes type 2, 322
postoperative care, 323
total parenteral, see Total
parenteral nutrition
Nutrition history, 25
example forms, 27
Obesity, 9
Oleic acid, 19
Olestra, 20
Oral glucose-lowering agents
in combination therapy, 116
type 1 diabetes, 116
PAL, see Hypoglycemia, postactivity late-onset
Pattern management, 215–46
concepts, 215
elements, 216
evaluating blood glucose
readings, 217
for high blood glucose
readings, 218
for insulin users, 221–27
for low blood glucose
readings, 218
in type 2 diabetes, 232–33
premeal and 2-hour postmeal
monitoring for 2 injections
per day, 225
premeal and 2-hour postmeal
monitoring for 3 injections
per day, 226
premeal and 2-hour postmeal
monitoring for 4 injections
per day, 227
premeal monitoring for 2-3
injections per day, 223
premeal monitoring for
4 injections per day, 224
problem-solving practice for
type 1 diabetes, 228–31

problem-solving practice for type 2 diabetes, 233–36
strategies, 218
Perioperative
assessment, 318–20
concerns—diabetes type 1, 320–21
concerns—diabetes type 2, 322
treatment, 318
Physical activity, see Exercise
Pioglitazone, 115, 129, 232
Polydextrose, 20
Polysaccharides, 12
Postoperative care, 322–23
hypoglycemia, 322
nutrition management, 323
Postsurgical home care, 323
Potassium, 21
Prazosin, see Alpha-1 antagonists
Precose, see Acarbose
Pregnancy
nonnutritive (low-calorie) sweeteners, 16
Proinsulin, 96
Protein, 13
in diabetes food/meal plan, 16–18
Rapid-acting insulin, see Insulin, rapid-acting
References
carbohydrate counting, 272
hypoglycemia, 304–6
illness and surgery, 328–29
insulin pump therapy, 261–63
medical nutrition therapy, 46–55
monitoring, 207–10
pattern management, 240
pharmacologic therapies, 147–51
pharmacologic therapies for hypertension and dyslipidemia, 180–82
Repaglinide, 124–26, 136, 219, 232
adverse effects, 125
contraindications, 125
pharmacology, 124
therapy, 125
Rosiglitazone, 115, 129, 232
Saccharin, 15, 16
Salatrim, 20
Salt, 20

Self-review questions
counting carbohydrates, 269
hypoglycemia, 300
illness and surgery, 325
insulin pump therapy, 259
medical nutrition therapy, 42–43
monitoring, 205
pattern management, 238
physical activity and exercise, 84
Self-monitoring of blood glucose, 189–96, 218–20
data for decision-making, 193
data management, 195
frequency and timing, 194–95, 218–19
psychosocial implications, 194
special needs, 196
Short-acting insulin, see Rapid-acting insulin
Sick day management, 315–16
blood glucose monitoring, 315
diet, 316
ketone monitoring, 315
medications, 316
severe conditions, 317
SMBG, see Self-monitoring of blood glucose
Sodium, 20
Sorbitol, 15
adverse effects, 137
Starch hydrolysates, 15
Statins, see HMG-CoA reductase inhibitors (statins)
Sucralose, 15, 16
Sucrose, 12, 14
Sugar alcohols, 15
Sugars, 14
Suggested readings
carbohydrate counting, 273
hypoglycemia, 306
illness and surgery, 330
insulin pump therapy, 263–64
monitoring, 209
pattern management, 241–42
pharmacologic therapies, 151
pharmacologic therapies for hypertension and dyslipidemia, 182
physical activity/exercise, 90
Sulfonylureas, 115, 116–24, 136
adverse effects, 119
contraindications, 119

pharmacology, 116
therapy, 124
Surgery
children, 323–24
emergency, 323
physiological effects, 315
Sweeteners, 15–16
Sympathomimetics
adverse effects, 137
Symptom diaries, 285, 286
Symptoms
hospital treatment, 318
severe, 317
Syringes, 104
prefilling, 106
Tea, 160
Terazosin, see Alpha-1 antagonists
Thiazolidinediones (TZDs), 115, 129–30, 136, 199, 219, 232
adverse effects, 130
contraindications, 129
pharmacology, 129
therapy, 130
Time action profiles
endogenous insulin, 107
four multiple-dose daily injections, 113
glargine vs. NPH insulin in type 1 diabetes, 103
insulin pump therapy, 114
one or two daily injections, 110
three multiple-dose daily injections, 112
two split-mixed daily injections, 111
Total Energy Expenditure (TEE), 29
Total parenteral nutrition, 323
TPN, see Total parenteral nutrition
Trans fatty acids, 18
Triglycerides, 5, 6, 168
Ultralente, 100
Urine glucose testing, 201
Verapamil, see Nondihydropyridine calcium channel blockers (CCBs)
Vitamins, 13, 20–21
Water, 14
Weight, 7, 9, 14, 16
assessment, 202
loss in diabetes mellitus type 2, 9
Xylitol, 15
Zinc, 21

Copyright Permission

a CORE Curriculum for Diabetes Education, 5th Edition
American Association of Diabetes Educators

Contact: AADE, 800/338-3633; fax 312/424-2427

TO WHOM IT MAY CONCERN:
Permission is hereby granted from the American Association of Diabetes Educators under the following terms:

ISSN/ISBN #1-881876-15-2

Book Title: _____

Chapter Title: _____

Page Numbers: _____

Permission Granted To: _____

Permission is granted for one-time use only and for educational purposes only.

Complete credit line should appear on all reproductions as follows:
"Reprinted with permission from A Core Curriculum for Diabetes Education, copyright _____, the American Association of Diabetes Educators."

_____   _____
AADE PUBLISHER   DATE